MW01672360

MOLECULAR and CELLULAR MECHANISMS of ANTIARRHYTHMIC AGENTS

edited by
Luc Hondeghem, M.D.
Professor of Medicine and Pharmacology
Director
Stahlman Cardiovascular Research Program
School of Medicine
Vanderbilt University

FUTURA

Futura Publishing Company, Inc.
Mount Kisco, NY
1989

Library of Congress Cataloging-in-Publication Data

Molecular and cellular mechanisms of antiarrhythmic agents / edited by
Luc M. Hondeghem.
p. cm.
Includes bibliographical references.
ISBN 0-87993-379-8
1. Myocardial depressants—Physiological effect. 2. Ion channels—Effect of drugs on. I. Hondeghem, Luc M.
RM347.M65 1989
615′.716—dc20 89-17112
CIP

Copyright © 1989
Futura Publishing Company, Inc.

Published by:
Futura Publishing Company, Inc.
2 Bedford Ridge Road, P.O. Box 330
Mount Kisco, New York 10549

L.C. No.: 89-17112
ISBN No.: 0-87993-379-8

All rights reserved.

No part of this book may be translated or reproduced in any form without written permission of the publisher.

Printed in the United States of America

Contributors

Jeffrey R. Balser
Department of Medicine and Pharmacology, Vanderbilt University, Nashville, Tennessee

Bruce Bean
Department of Neurobiology, Harvard Medical School, Boston, Massachusetts

Paul B. Bennett
Department of Pharmacology, Vanderbilt University, Nashville, Tennessee

Arthur M. Brown
Department of Molecular Physiology & Biophysics, Baylor College of Medicine, Houston, Texas

Daniel Chernoff
Anesthesia Research Labs, Brigham & Women's Hospital, Harvard Medical School, Boston, Massachusetts

David Chester
Department of Radiology and Biochemistry, Biomolecular Structure Analysis Center, University of Connecticut Health Center, Farmington, Connecticut

Robert DeHaan
Director, Program in Cardiac Cell Function, Department of Anatomy and Cell Biology, Emory University, Atlanta, Georgia

Harry Fozzard
Department of Medicine, Cardiology, The University of Chicago, Chicago, Illinois

H. Robert Guy
Department of Mathematical Biology, NCI, National Institutes of Health, Bethesda, Maryland

Leo Herbette
Departments of Radiology, Medicine and Biochemistry, Biomolecular Structure Analysis Center, University of Connecticut Health Center, Farmington, Connecticut

Luc Hondeghem
Department of Medicine and Pharmacology, Vanderbilt University, Nashville, Tennessee

Joseph Hume
Department of Physiology, University of Nevada, School of Medicine, Reno, Nevada

Glenn E. Kirsch
Research Assistant Professor, Department of Molecular Physiology and Biophysics, Baylor College of Medicine, Houston, Texas

Alexandros Makriyannis
Section of Medicinal Chemistry and Institute of Material Science, Storrs, Connecticut. F. Bitter National Magnet Laboratory, Massachusetts Institute of Technology, Cambridge, Massachusetts

Dan M. Roden
Department of Medicine and Pharmacology, Vanderbilt University, Nashville, Tennessee

Madison S. Spach
Duke University, Medical Center, Durham, North Carolina

Gary Strichartz
Anesthesia Research Labs, Brigham & Women's Hospital, Harvard Medical School, Boston, Massachusetts

Frank Starmer
Department of Medicine, Duke University Medical Center, Durham, North Carolina

David J. Triggle
Department of Biochemical Pharmacology, State University of New York at Buffalo, School of Pharmacy, Buffalo, New York

De-Ping Yang
Section of Medicinal Chemistry & Institute of Material Science, University of Connecticut, Storrs, Connecticut

Preface

Dr. Hondeghem's *Molecular and Cellular Mechanisms of Antiarrhythmic Agents* is important for two principal reasons. First, it gathers together the work of many of the best investigators and therefore many of the best theories and supporting data regarding mechanisms of antiarrhythmic drug action. Second, it provides a current compilation of basic research that has relevance to clinical application of antiarrhythmic drug therapy. Indeed, it is nearly unique in the extent to which it assembles current knowledge of the topic.

Clinicians frequently must use antiarrhythmic drugs in a pseudoscientific manner. The specific electrophysiologic phenomena that are responsible for arrhythmia are well delineated in only a few rhythm abnormalities. Also, the specific actions of an antiarrhythmic drug, which are responsible for its observed helpful or harmful effects upon an arrhythmia, are matters of speculation only. As a result, physicians have resorted to creating drug and arrhythmia classification schemes which, with the simplicity of a multiple choice paradigm, purport to bring just the right arrhythmia together with just the right drug.

This book has potential to improve the de facto trial and error method that the clinician uses to treat arrhythmia with drugs. It reviews the basic science and theories of antiarrhythmic drug action authoritatively and broadly. The electrophysiology, biophysics, biochemistry and pharmacology of sodium, calcium, potassium and gap junctional channels are examined. The potential importance to arrhythmias of the passive electrical properties of the myocardium, especially their anisotropic behavior, is discussed. Models of the drug-cell interaction are proposed. These models are especially important to the clinician, because they begin to reveal a scientific rationale for antiarrhythmic drug use.

Unfortunately, one only *sees* a potential for improvement in antiarrhythmic therapy through the knowledge offered in this book. It necessarily falls short of providing full-fledged recommendations for treatment because the basic molecular and cellular scientists have left the physiologists and clinicians in their dust, far behind. While the former have, almost literally, dissected apart the intricate molecular channels and ionic mechanisms responsible for the electrical activity of the cardiac cell and its modification by drugs, the latter have failed to comprehensively expose the critical abnormalities responsible for cardiac arrhythmias in man. When this latter step is achieved, one does see the basic sciences poised to solve many therapeutic problems.

This book provides an extraordinarily current and complete summary for molecular and cellular electrophysiologists interested in cardiac antiarrhythmic pharmacology. Perhaps its more important role, though, might be to stimulate the creativity of physiologists and clinicians to allow more extensive therapeutic application of this knowledge.

Jay W. Mason, M.D.
Professor of Medicine
Chief, Division of Cardiology
University of Utah School of Medicine
Salt Lake City, Utah

Introduction

During the past few decades our understanding of the basic mechanisms of ion channels, their involvement in arrhythmias and the mode of action of antiarrhythmic agents have greatly improved. In the present book, the highlights of this progress are reviewed. Emphasis is placed upon how this progress can have important clinical implications.

Most of our knowledge of the action of antiarrhythmic agents was first derived from $\dot{V}_{max}$ studies. Recently, it has become possible to study I_{Na} in isolated cardiac cells. In the first chapter, Drs. Fozzard, Hanck, and Sheets convincingly demonstrate that the availability between I_{Na} and $\dot{V}_{max}$ does not exhibit a linear relationship: $\dot{V}_{max}$ at times exceeds the value expected from I_{Na}. Thus, the use of $\dot{V}_{max}$ to evaluate drug action will at times tend to underestimate the drug effects. Although not yet demonstrated, it is very likely that similar discrepancies also will exist at 37°C. Since the action of antiarrhythmic drugs is so markedly dependent upon temperature,[1] it will be important to verify the relation between $\dot{V}_{max}$ and I_{Na} at body temperature, especially, now that this current can be clamped at 37°C.[2] Moreover, from single-channel results (Chapters 5 and 11) it is clear that availability of sodium channels may not linearly relate to macroscopic sodium currents either: at certain potentials available channels may yield multiple openings, while at others they may yield none. However, single-channel results, macroscopic sodium currents, and maximum upstroke velocity all have their strengths and weaknesses. Once we understand the behavior of the channels and their interactions with drugs more fully, it should be possible to fully reconcile the results of all three methods. Meanwhile, cautious use of all three techniques is essential.

In the second chapter, Drs. DeHaan, Chen, and Penrod discuss the importance of intercellular coupling via gap junction to conduction of the heartbeat. They point out that whereas adult junctions are relatively insensitive to membrane potential, those of neonatal hearts are strongly voltage-dependent. Moreover, under certain pathological conditions adult heart may appear to become sensitive again. In any event, gap junctions in both tissues appear to be very strongly modulated by intracellular Ca^{++}, pH, and by local hormones. Drugs that could selectively uncouple cells responsible for arrhythmias (e.g., ischemic cells) could form a potent tool for the treatment of arrhythmias. At this time no such drugs are available.

Electrical conduction in heartbeat is not only determined by the sodium current, the resulting $\dot{V}_{max}$ and the gap junctions. Indeed, as shown by Drs. Spach, Dolber, Heidlage, and Starmer, conduction may decline when $\dot{V}_{max}$ actually increases. This results from the fact that the electrical load sensed by the propagating waveform can markedly affect these parameters. Since the load and thus, conduction are anisotropic, the load is larger in the direction of fast conduction than in that of the slow conduction. As a result $\dot{V}_{max}$ is greater in the slow direction. Thus for $\dot{V}_{max}$ to be a reliable indicator of sodium channel availability it is important to verify that there was no microscopic change in direction of conduction. The authors also notice that poor transversal conduction becomes more marked with age. As a result older hearts are more prone to exhibit dissociated zig-zag conduction, before conduction failure. These new concepts are extremely important for understanding the action of antiarrhythmic agents.

Ionic channels, even sodium channels, are not only under control of membrane potential. In addition it is becoming increasingly clear that these channels are also under control of metabolic factors and G proteins. Drs. Brown, Yatani, Codina, and Birnbaumer review this important upcoming field in Chapter 4. Although no antiarrhythmic agents are known to act via these mechanisms, these sites could form an important target for future antiarrhythmic agents.

In Chapter 5, Dr. Kirsch compares the behavior of single sodium channels when incorporated in a whole cell, versus when a patch of membrane is excised from the cell. In view of the previous chapter, it is not surprising that the voltage-dependent kinetics of these channels are strongly modified when the channel is removed from its natural environment: individual channel openings become longer and multiple openings become more frequent. One would, therefore, expect that the actions of drugs might also be dramatically modified in an excised patch.

In Chapter 6, Dr. Bean reviews the channels that have calcium as their primary permeation. In the heart there appear to be two dominant calcium channels: L and T channels. These have different voltage dependences, kinetics of opening and inactivation, are modified differently by various inorganic blockers, and perhaps most importantly for the scope of the present book, are also interacting differently with drugs. Nevertheless, as for the sodium channels, the interactions of drugs with calcium channels are voltage- and time-dependent and can be characterized in terms of the modulated receptor theory. Agents that block T channels selectively do not yet exist, but such agents could be very useful in the treatment of disturbances in automaticity.

Dr. Hume gives an excellent overview of the important potassium channels in heart, in Chapter 7. He points out that of the many potassium currents, those that are primarily involved with action potential duration are I_{K1}, I_K and I_{TO}. Again, the channels that mediate these currents may provide important sites for the action of antiarrhythmic agents, especially those that act by class III mechanisms. It should be pointed out, however, that class III mechanisms are not limited to K^+ channel blockers.[3] The varied distribution of these channel types between cardiac tissues could form an important basis for drugs that have tissue-specific actions.

In Chapter 8, Drs. Roden, Balser, and Bennett point out that the interaction of drugs with potassium channels is also strongly modulated by voltage and time. Thus, whereas quinidine blocks the delayed potassium current primarily during diastole, when the channels are closed, amiodarone blocks these channels primarily when the channels are open during the plateau. The importance of these differences toward arrhythmogenicity and antiarrhythmic actions are discussed.

The sequence of many ion channels is becoming availble. Moreover, it is increasingly clear how these channels fold and cross cell membranes. This important information is reviewed in Chapter 9 by Dr. Guy. A three-dimensional model of the sodium channel is proposed, which accounts for activation, inactivation, and ion selectivity. Activation is proposed to result from a helical screw mechanism: when all 4 *screws* have rotated out of the channel, then the channel can permeate sodium until the inactivation particle closes the channel again. The model also proposes potential sites for the various types of sodium channel blockers and activators. Further development in this area will ultimately provide the tools to develop much better pharmacological agents.

In Chapter 10, Drs. Starmer, Nesterenko, Undrovinas, Packer, Gilliam, Grant, Rosenshtraukh, and Strauss characterize ion channel block using the guarded receptor. According to this view the receptor on the sodium channel has a constant affinity for drug interaction, but accessibility changes by trap and guard functions. Binding of the drug to its receptor blocks the channel, but it does not modify the voltage-dependent behavior of the channel. This simple model has the advantage of computing very quickly. In addition, by proposing an alternate view of drug-channel interactions, Dr. Starmer and his colleagues have stimulated a useful and probing debate into drug-channel interactions.

In Chapter 11, Drs. Hondeghem and Bennett demonstrate that the affinity for the receptor is modulated by voltage and time. Moreover, channels occupied by drug have a voltage-dependence that is shifted to more negative potentials. An analytical version of the modulated receptor hypothesis that can compute one action potential per msec is presented. In addition, a model of the sodium channel that can simulate single-channel results as well as macroscopic sodium currents is presented. The model incorporates many of the structural concepts presented in Chapter 9, and makes some novel predictions about drug effects at the single-channel level. Thus at the single-channel levels, antiarrhythmic drugs act primarily by reducing the probability of channel opening (sequestering them in a pool [ID] from which channel cannot open) and by shortening the channel open time. Fewer shorter openings result in less sodium current, reduced upstroke velocity, slower conduction, and widening of QRS. Since these effects are more marked at fast heart rates and in depolarized tissues, these drugs selectively interfere with arrhythmias while leaving the normal heartbeat less disturbed.

Drs. Chester and Herbette demonstrate (Chapter 12) that small molecules like ion channel blockers have a different structure in aqueous solution and in the membrane lipid; both are in turn different from the crystalline structure. Importantly, the authors show that drugs have a characteristic optimal depth of distribution in the membrane. It is proposed that this lipid bilayer distribution may be an important determinant for the interaction of the drug with its receptor on the ion channel protein: less drug at the correct depth in the membrane may provide a better interaction with the receptor than more drug at the less optimal depth. Based on this information I can only speculate that the charged and neutral forms of the antiarrhythmic agents may distribute at different depths. Could it be that the receptor *screws* into different positions in the membrane (see Chapter 9) and thus preferentially interacts with the neutral or charged form? The next decade will provide opportunities to answer such interesting molecular questions.

Although the structure-activity for sodium channel blockers is still in its infancy, that for agents interacting with calcium channels is much better understood. In Chapter 13, Dr. Triggle gives a detailed review of agonistic and antagonistic features. He discusses how agonist versus antagonist can be modulated by membrane potential and that only very minute molecular changes can account for these differences. Even stereoisomers can have different profiles. He discusses in great detail the importance of selectivity toward the therapeutic benefits.

Solid state nuclear magnetic resonance can determine minute changes in molecular structure of drugs in membranes. In Chapter 14, Drs. Makriyannis and De-Ping Yang demonstrate that very small changes in structure can dramatically alter the orientation of a molecule in a membrane. From Chapter 12, it would then not be surprising that such small changes could markedly alter the probability of interaction with the receptor on the ion channel. These powerful techniques may help us to design drugs that are oriented for optimal interaction in arrhythmogenic conditions (e.g., depolarized tissue), but under normal circumstances have an orientation for poor interaction, thus resulting in little or no effect.

In Chapter 15, Drs. Chernoff and Strichartz (the "father of use-dependent block") point out that *open* channel block may actually develop with a closed state prior to opening. Because of this possibility in our formulation of the modulated receptor hypothesis,[4] Bert Katzung and myself preferred the term *activation* block over open block. Block to a preopen state also follows directly from the new sodium channel model proposed in Chapter 11. Indeed, with 4 activation units there exist 16 activation unit combinations, only one of which is open; for 8 of these the unit containing the modulated receptor is activated, and only one of these is the open state. Hence there are 7 chances out of 8 that block during activation will occur *prior* to opening. The experimental results in Chapter 15 support this prediction. Conversely, since only one-eighth of the block may occur during opening, unless the drug under the experimental condition causes a large amount of activation block, one might not observe shortening of open time. If this hypothesis is correct, then it should also be possible to elicit activation unblock, without opening of the channels. Dr. Takafumi Anno has recently demonstrated this phenomenon in my laboratory.

Thus, as Chernoff and Strichartz elegantly point out, we should remember that the sodium channel has three primary states, but that each primary state may have numerous substates. All of the latter can be important to drug action.

I believe that over the past decade we have learned more about channel behavior than we have in the previous thousand years. More importantly, in the next decade we will surely progress even further. Point mutations in the ionic channels will unravel their functionality to the molecular level. The receptor(s) location(s) will be determined and the molecular basis for state-dependent binding will be unravelled in its smallest detail. This will soon be followed by predictable designs of new and better drugs. I am confident that during the next decade this great progress at the basic level will translate into better therapeutic agents for patients suffering from arrhythmias.

Luc Hondeghem, M.D.

1. Johns JA, Anno T, Bennett PB, Snyders DJ, Hondeghem LM. Temperature and voltage dependence of sodium channel blocking and unblocking by O-demethyl encainide in isolated guinea pigs myocytes. *J Cardiovasc Pharmacol* 13:826–835, 1989.
2. Murray KT, Anno T, Bennett PB, Hondeghem LM. Voltage clamp of cardiac sodium current in 145 mM sodium at 37°C. *J Mol Cell Cardiol* 1989. Abstract.
3. Hondeghem LM, Snyders DJ. Class III antiarrhythmic agents have a lot of potential, but a long way to go: reduced effectiveness and dangers of reverse use-dependence. *Circulation* 1989. In press.
4. Hondeghem LM, Katzung, BG. Time and voltage dependent interaction of antiarrhythmic drugs with cardiac sodium channels. *Biochim Biophys Acta* 472:373–398, 1977.

Contents

Chapter 1

The Relationship between $\dot{V}_{max}$ and I_{Na} in Cardiac Purkinje Cells and their Interpretation from Single Na^+ Channel Analysis

Harry A. Fozzard
Dorothy A. Hanck
Michael F. Sheets

INTRODUCTION

The sodium current (I_{Na}) is the principal current responsible for normal excitation and conduction in atrial muscle, ventricular muscle, and in the His-Purkinje conducting system. I_{Na} is also thought to play a major role in a large number of lethal arrhythmias (Fozzard and Makielski, 1985), and the Na^+ channel is a target for many of our more effective antiarrhythmic drugs (Grant et al., 1984). For these reasons, the normal and abnormal behavior of cardiac I_{Na} and the effects of antiarrhythmic drugs on the current have been major topics of study for many years. However, the study of I_{Na} has also been a source of controversy for the last 20 years (Johnson and Lieberman, 1971; Cohen et al., 1984), because the experimental methods have been less quantitative than those in nerve.

Hondeghem, Luc (ed): Molecular and Cellular Mechanisms of Antiarrhythmic Agents, Futura Publishing Company, Inc., Mount Kisco, NY, © 1989.

Consequently, much of our understanding of cardiac I_{Na} and the action of antiarrhythmic drugs has been derived from two sources: voltage clamp studies on nerve, and indirect measures of I_{Na} in heart muscle.

Quantitative study of cardiac I_{Na} by high quality voltage clamp similar to that of squid axon (Hodgkin and Huxley, 1952) has been either difficult or impossible. In place of the quantitative voltage clamp, most cardiac investigators have used the maximal depolarization rate of the action potential ($\dot{V}_{max}$) as a semiquantitative index of cardiac I_{Na}. Recently the technical barriers to quantitative voltage clamp studies in cardiac muscle have been overcome through the use of single cells and special low-resistance pipettes (Brown et al., 1981; Bustamonte and McDonald, 1983; Makielski et al., 1987; Follmer et al., 1987; Clark and Giles, 1987; Mitsiuye and Noma, 1987). These methods now permit both quantitative study of drug effects on cardiac I_{Na} and direct examination of the relationship between I_{Na} and $\dot{V}_{max}$.

The long-awaited technique of quantitative voltage clamp of cardiac muscle was achieved coincident with a revolution in the experimental study of ion channels. This revolution is occurring because of the discovery of a method to record openings of single channels in intact cells, in excised patches of membrane (Hamill et al., 1981), or in artificial bilayers containing reconstituted natural channels (Krueger et al., 1983). Whole cell voltage studies and patch clamp single channel studies combined with molecular biological techniques promise to permit dramatic advances in our understanding of the molecular structure–function relationships of the sodium channel. Simultaneous with the opportunity to study the effects of drugs on cardiac I_{Na} comes the necessity to reconcile I_{Na} with single Na^+ channel events and the opportunity to study drug effects directly on single Na^+ channels.

This chapter will address the question of the accuracy of $\dot{V}_{max}$ as a measure of I_{Na} and will attempt to interpret I_{Na} and $\dot{V}_{max}$ in terms of the possible single Na^+ channel events responsible for the rapid depolarization of the action potential.

I_{Na} AND $\dot{V}_{max}$: STATEMENT OF THE PROBLEMS

The action potential (AP) in atrial, ventricular, and Purkinje cells results from an increase in membrane permeability to Na^+, resulting in I_{Na}. This I_{Na} brings positive charge into the cell to offset charge stored by the membrane capacity of the cell membrane participating in the AP, and to provide current that helps to depolarize the next cell segment. The effect of I_{Na} is regenerative, in that I_{Na} depolarizes part of the cell membrane, which causes an increase in Na^+ permeability and I_{Na}, which depolarizes more membrane, etc. The process is self-limited, because sufficient depolarization brings the membrane potential near Na^+ equilibrium potential (E_{Na}) reducing I_{Na} because of the loss of driving force for Na^+ entry. During steady state with constant conduction velocity of an AP along a cable-like cell with negligible leak current, the following relationship holds:

$$I_{Na} = C_m\dot{V} \quad [1]$$

where C_m is the membrane capacitance.

This relationship implies that peak I_{Na} and $\dot{V}_{max}$ are related by the constant membrane capacity, C_m. However, two major problems arise in the application of this equation to estimate peak I_{Na} in heart muscle by $\dot{V}_{max}$. First, "C_m" is not a constant for the conducted AP (Fozzard, 1966). The complex geometry resulting from the organization of many cells into a muscle (even a muscle strand without t-tubules such as a Purkinje fiber), added to the presence of t-tubules in cells creates resistance in series with some of the membrane. This series resistance causes the effective "C_m" to be frequency-dependent, i.e., dependent upon $\dot{V}_{max}$. Adjustment for the effective C_m does make the relationship of equation 1 more predictive of experimental results (Walton and Fozzard, 1983a), but such an adjustment is experimentally difficult to make.

Second, the I_{Na} achieved by the AP is physiologically different from peak I_{Na} measured under voltage clamp (Cohen et al., 1985). The voltage clamp holds the membrane potential fixed and allows time for full activation of Na^+ channels at that potential. However, regenerative I_{Na} during the AP induces its own potential change. This change is usually so rapid that insufficient time is available to allow full activation of Na^+ channels before inactivation and reduction in driving force intervene. Therefore, I_{Na} during an AP results from only a portion of the Na^+ channels that open at peak I_{Na} under voltage clamp.

Computations of the fraction of peak I_{Na} achieved during simulated APs by Cohen et al., (1984) yielded values of 0.2–0.5. Measurements of the fraction achieved experimentally by Sheets et al.,

(1988) showed values of 0.25–0.6. The fraction achieved depended upon the maximal Na^+ conductance (i.e., Na^+ channel availability) and on channel kinetics. If the number of channels was reduced, then the rate of depolarization during the AP was slowed, and more time was available to open those channels that were available. This behavior helps the cell to maintain its excitability when it is depressed by pathological processes or drugs by allowing it to call on a reserve of channels not used during the normal AP. This ability to call upon a reserve of Na^+ channels may constitute part of the *safety factor* of conduction (Walton and Fozzard, 1983b).

Efforts to control the experimental conditions of AP stimulation to allow for compensation of the inevitable and well-documented differences between $\dot{V}_{max}$ and peak I_{Na} (Cohen et al., 1984; Sheets et al., 1988) include 1) stimulus adjustment to achieve a *constant latency* between stimulus and time of $\dot{V}_{max}$; and 2) compensation for the different membrane voltages at which $\dot{V}_{max}$ occurs, with the consequent changes in driving force. *Constant latency* was used in the experiments of Gettes and Reuter (1974) and the simulations of Walton and Fozzard (1979). In the simulations, the Hodgkin-Huxley model of I_{Na} was used, and constant latency was needed because inactivation proceeded rapidly. Constant latency kept inactivation similar between rapid upstrokes and slow upstrokes. Our recent experimental results indicate that inactivation occurs after a delay, contrary to the Hodgkin-Huxley model and that therefore, our previous ideas regarding the role of latency are wrong. The delay in onset of inactivation, which is also seen in nerve, can be explained by the Markov chain model of the Na^+ channel, where the channel activates through a series of steps before it can begin to inactivate. While the need for constant latency may exist under some conditions, we need to explore more carefully the underlying mechanisms before further defining its use. The membrane voltage at which $\dot{V}_{max}$ occurs also varies with rate of depolarization (Walton and Fozzard, 1979; Sheets et al., 1988). The following experiments were performed to address the questions of latency, voltage at $\dot{V}_{max}$, and the effect of these two variables on the relationship between I_{Na} and $\dot{V}_{max}$.

METHODS

The methods used in these experiments have been reported in detail elsewhere (Makielski et al., 1987; Sheets et al., 1988). In summary, single adult canine Purkinje cells were prepared enzymatically by the methods of Sheets et al., (1983). One end of a cell was drawn into the aperture of a glass double barreled pipette. After the cell sealed to the walls of the aperture, the end within the pipette was ruptured with a micromanipulator controlled wire, providing free access of the flowing pipette solution to the cell cytoplasm. The potential across the cell membrane external to the pipette could be clamped by a feedback amplifier. An electronic relay (Magnecraft 112) allowed the voltage clamp amplifier to be disconnected under computer control so that action potentials (spontaneous depolarizations) could be obtained.

The perfusate solutions were designed to allow only Na^+ currents. The external solution contained 45 mM NaCl, 104 mM CsCl, 1.8 mM $CaCl_2$, 1.O mM $MgCl_2$, and 10 mM HEPES (pH 7.2). The internal solution contained 15 mM NaF, 134 mM CsF, 10 mM EGTA, 5Oμ M MgATP and 10 mM HEPES (pH 7.2). Temperature was 18–2O°C and controlled by a thermoelectric device (TS4, Sensortek).

Command voltages were controlled by a 16 bit D/A converter and I_{Na} or AP were recorded by a 12 bit A/D converter (Masscomp 5500 System microcomputer). The response of the voltage clamp circuitry was 99% complete in 10 μsec. Capacity transients after series resistance compensation showed typical time constants of 5–10 μsec. Current signals were analog filtered with an 8-pole Bessel filter (Frequency Devices 848) at 50kHz and digitized at 100kHz. Subsequently they were digitally filtered at 5 kHz. Leak current, measured at the end of a 25 msec step was subtracted from peak current to determine I_{Na}. The relay required 80–110 μsec to open after command. Action potentials were measured by a high impedence ($10^{13}\Omega$) electrometer (Analog Devices, Model 515) filtered at 50 kHz with an 8-pole Bessel filter and digitized at 100 kHz. The digital signal was Gaussian filtered at 3–20 kHz (depending on the magnitude of $\dot{V}_{max}$) and then digitally differentiated to obtain dV/dt. For futher details see Sheets et al., (1988).

RESULTS

The experiments examined the effects of latency to $\dot{V}_{max}$ and membrane potential at $\dot{V}_{max}$ on the relationship between $\dot{V}_{max}$ and I_{Na}. The availability of Na^+ current from different conditioning voltages was first determined by measurement of I_{Na} during voltage

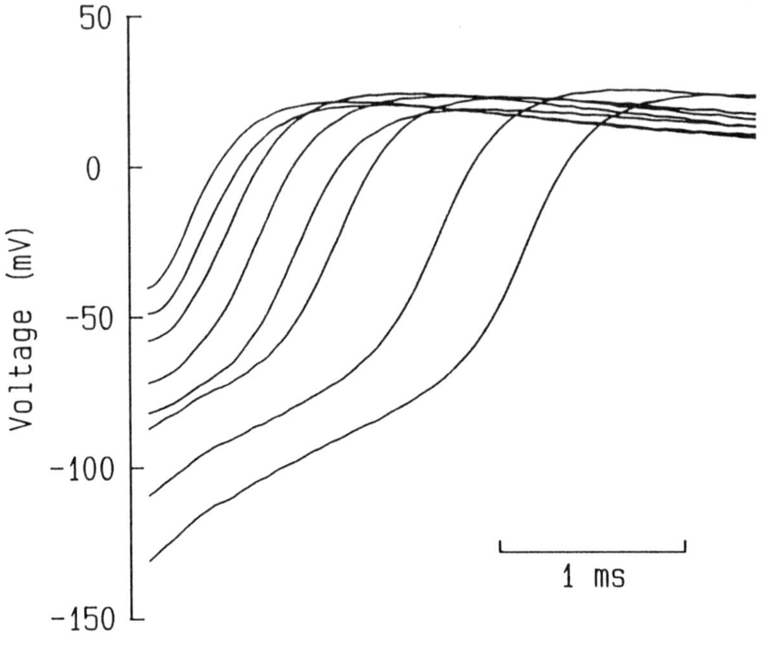

Figure 1. Recordings of action potential upstrokes after release from voltage-clamp when V_H was -120 mV. The membrane potential was changed to various pre-release potentials from -130 to -40 mV for 50 μsec before the cell was released from voltage clamp. Latency to $\dot{V}_{max}$ varied from 0.25–2.13 ms. Na_o/Na_i = 45/15 mM. Cell 33.03.28

clamp. Conditioning steps of 500 msec duration were made to various potentials prior to a test step to 0 mV. Normalized peak I_{Na} was plotted as a function of the conditioning potential (see Makielski et al., 1987). We chose two holding potentials, one that represented full availability of channels and one that inactivated approximately one half of the Na^+ channels. We then compared action potentials elicited from these two voltages when latency to $\dot{V}_{max}$ was varied by altering the potential from which cells were released from voltage clamp. This altered the latency because each release potential was further from or closer to I_{Na} threshold and the cell passively depolarized to threshold for I_{Na} activation before an AP upstroke was initiated.

Action potential upstrokes from a typical cell are shown in Fig. 1. In this case the cell was released from voltage clamp after pre-

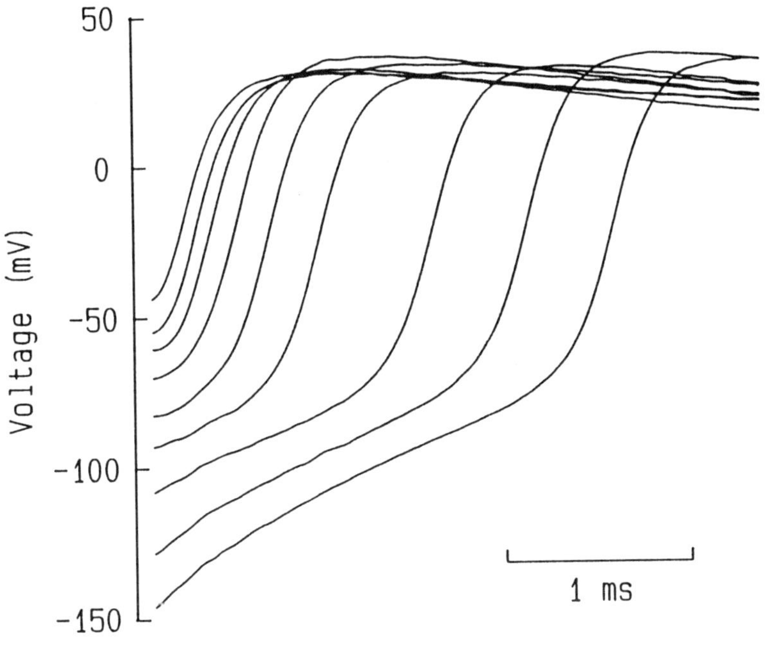

Figure 2. Recordings of action potential upstrokes upon release from voltage clamp when V_H was −150 mV. Protocol was similar to that in Figure 1. Note the large variation in latency to $\dot{V}_{max}$. Na_o/Na_i = 45/15 mM. Cell 33.03.27.

release conditioning steps of 50 μsec at release potentials from −130 mV to 40 mV. The holding potential (V_H) was −120 mV which by voltage clamp determination represented 57% availability. When the cell was released from more positive release potentials, latency to $\dot{V}_{max}$ became as short as 250 μsec; while when the cell was released from more negative potentials latencies became as long as 2130 μsec. Figure 2 illustrates the action potential upstrokes in the same cell with a similar protocol but when V_H was −150 mV where Na channel availability was 1.0. Again note the marked variation in latencies to $\dot{V}_{max}$.

The measurements of the latencies from voltage clamp release to the time of $\dot{V}_{max}$ are shown in Fig. 3A. Note that the latencies to $\dot{V}_{max}$ are slightly longer for the cell at a V_H of −120 mV compared

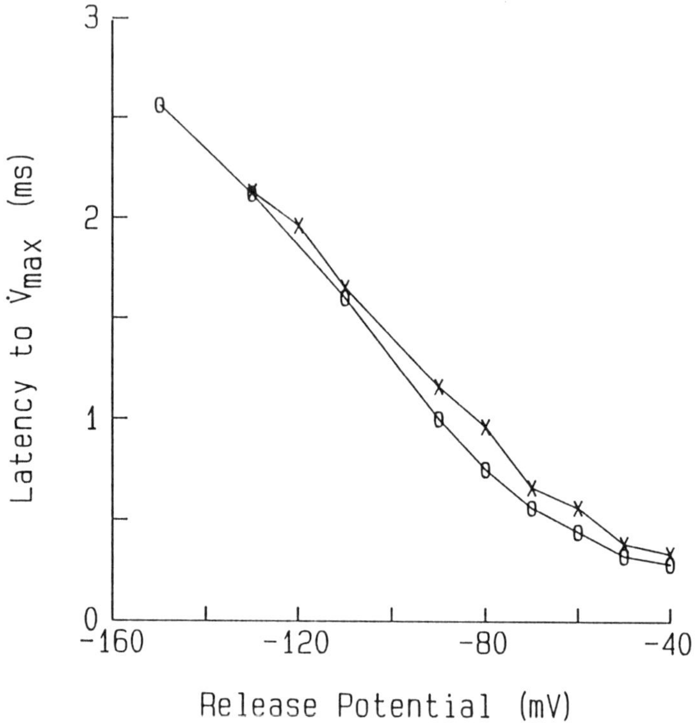

Figure 3. A. Latency from release from voltage clamp to $\dot{V}_{max}$ for different release potentials in the experiments shown in Figures 1 and 2. V_H was −150 mV (0) and −120 mV (X). B. $\dot{V}_{max}$ for the experiments shown in Figures 1 and 2. $\dot{V}_{max}$ averaged 144 ± 0.7 V/s (S.E., n = 9) for triggering potentials between −130 and −40 mV from a V_H of −120 mV (X). $\dot{V}_{max}$ averaged 243 ± 0.6 V/s (S.E., n = 9) for triggering potentials between −150 mV and −40 mV from a V_H of −150 mV (0).

to that of −150 mV consistent with the slower rise times, which results from the lower Na^+ channel availablity at the more positive conditioning potential. Figure 3B shows the magnitudes of $\dot{V}_{max}$ for each of the release potentials. As expected, $\dot{V}_{max}$ was greater (243 V/s ± 0.6, S.E., n = 9) when V_H was −150 mV than when V_H was −120 mV (144 V/s ± 0.7, S.E, n = 9). However, the values of $\dot{V}_{max}$ from each V_H were constant and did not vary as a result of the changing latency to $\dot{V}_{max}$. These experiments show that the value of $\dot{V}_{max}$ was related to the availability of Na^+ current just prior to the time of the triggering step, and that inactivation or desynchron-

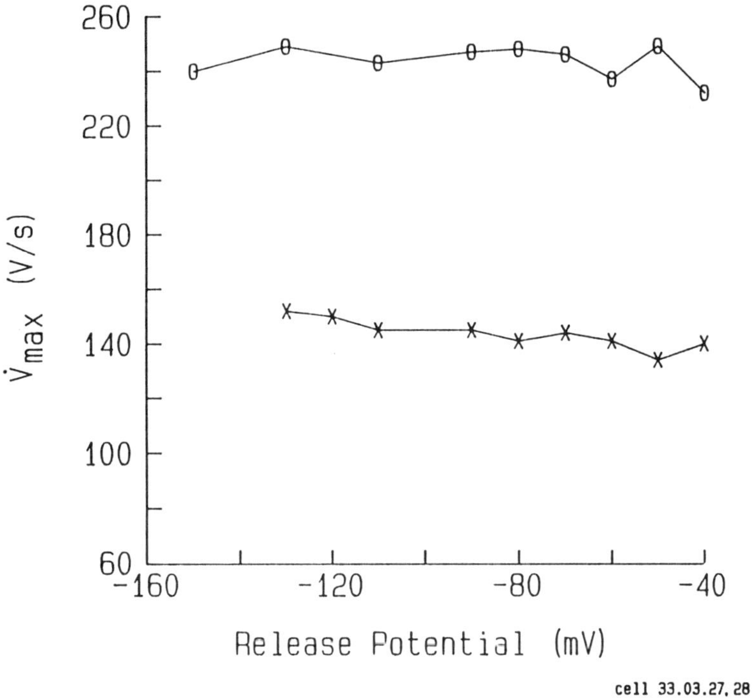

Figure 3B.

ization of channels did not occur during the slow approach to threshold by APs with long latencies regardless of prior partial inactivation of I_{Na}.

The membrane potentials at $\dot{V}_{max}$ for a V_H of −150 mV or for −120 mV are shown in Fig. 4. The membrane potentials at $\dot{V}_{max}$ for a V_H of −150 mV were constant and averaged −21.4 ± 0.4 mV (S.E.; n = 9) over a large triggering voltage range of −150 to −40 mV. From a V_H of −120 mV the membrane potential at $\dot{V}_{max}$ was also constant at −23.1 ± 0.4 mV (S.E.; n = 9). It is important to note that the membrane potentials at $\dot{V}_{max}$ did not change even though the availability of Na^+ channels (as assessed by I_{Na}) was decreased to 57% causing $\dot{V}_{max}$ to decrease to 144 V/s from 243 V/s.

The relationship between fractional I_{Na} and fractional $\dot{V}_{max}$ is shown in Fig. 5. The straight line is the expected relationship if fractional $\dot{V}_{max}$ is a linear estimate of fractional I_{Na}. The data show that $\dot{V}_{max}$ consistently overestimated the availability of Na^+ cur-

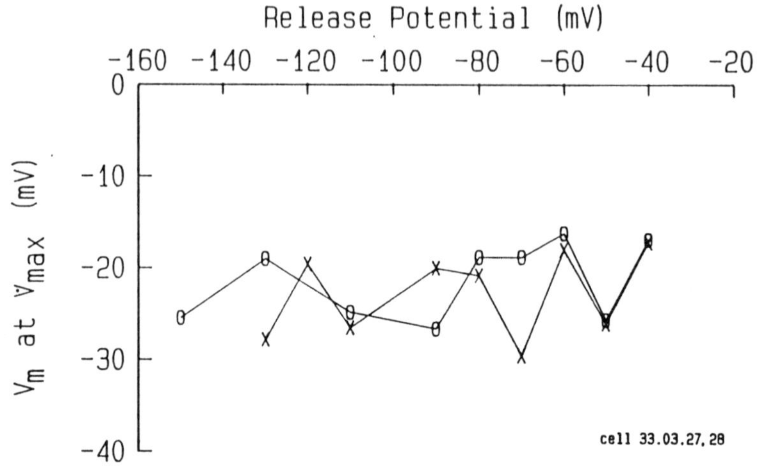

Figure 4. Membrane potentials at $\dot{V}_{max}$ when release potentials were varied. From a V_H of −150 mV (0), potentials at $\dot{V}_{max}$ averaged −21.4 ± .4 mV (S.E., n=9). From a V_H of −120 mV (X), potentials at $\dot{V}_{max}$ averaged −23.1 ± 0.4 V/s (S.E., n=8). Note that the membrane potential at $\dot{V}_{max}$ was nearly identical even though $\dot{V}_{max}$ decreased from 243 to 144 V/s.

rent as measured by peak I_{Na} during voltage clamp. Note that at a fractional current of 0.57, $\dot{V}_{max}$ overestimated I_{Na} by nearly 20% even though it has already been shown that the membrane potential at $\dot{V}_{max}$ did not change and that latencies to $\dot{V}_{max}$ did not affect $\dot{V}_{max}$ measurements under our experimental conditions.

These results agree with our previous studies of the relationship of $\dot{V}_{max}$ to I_{Na} where availability of Na^+ channels was modified by change in V_H, or by tetrodotoxin (Sheets et al., 1988). Over a twofold range of Na^+ channel availability, $\dot{V}_{max}$ failed to correlate with I_{Na}, in spite of a constant voltage at $\dot{V}_{max}$ and the absence of an effect of latency. We conclude that under our experimental conditions the physiological processes underlying peak I_{Na} and $\dot{V}_{max}$ are different.

DISCUSSION

The behavior of I_{Na} in squid giant axon was originally described by Hodgkin and Huxley (1952). Their scheme assumed that channels in the membrane selective for Na^+ are voltage-gated and that the channels are opened and closed by separate voltage-dependent pro-

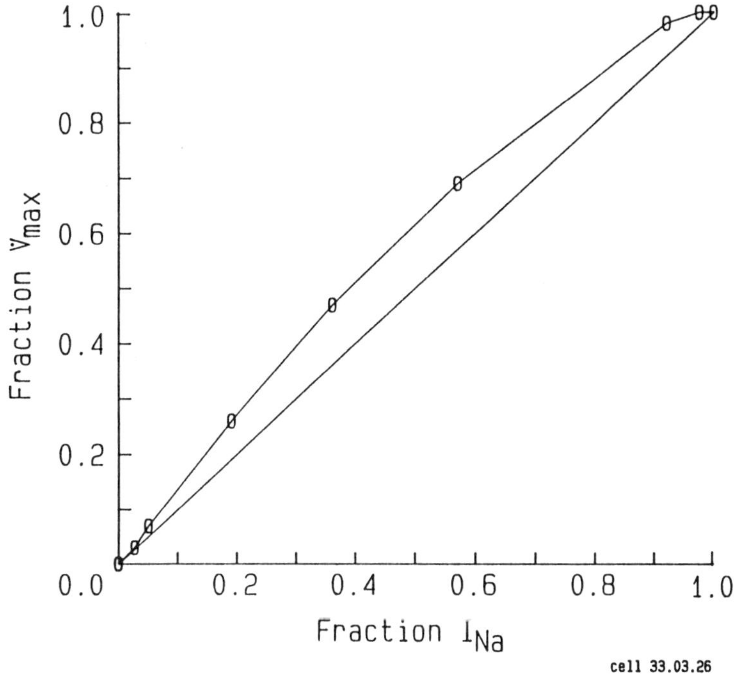

Figure 5. Fractional $\dot{V}_{max}$ compared to fractional peak I_{Na} obtained from Na channel availability plots as described in text. Also plotted is the line of identity. The experimental points deviate from a line of identity showing that fractional $\dot{V}_{max}$ overestimates I_{Na}. Even though fractional $\dot{V}_{max}$ decreased to 0.60, the membrane potential at $\dot{V}_{max}$ was not signifcantly changed. Cell 33.03.26

cesses. Cardiac I_{Na}, as well as that in most other cells containing voltage-dependent Na^+ channels, is generally described by the Hodgkin-Huxley models (McAllister et al., 1975; Beeler and Reuter, 1977), even though cardiac I_{Na} has some important kinetic differences from squid nerve. The effects of toxins, divalent ions, and drugs on cardiac I_{Na} and squid nerve are quite different, with the cardiac current particularly sensitive to *antiarrhythmic* drugs.

The failure of changes in latency to affect $\dot{V}_{max}$ is contrary to what would be predicted by the Hodgkin-Huxley model and implies that the model does not accurately reproduce the events occurring in the subthreshold and near threshold voltage regions. We will discuss our understanding of the excitatory I_{Na} and their underlying single channel events, to help us gain insight into the processes responsible for cardiac excitation and to guide us in modifying the Hodgkin-Huxley model.

I_{Na} Studied by the Voltage Clamp

I_{Na} is a large inward (depolarizing) current that is activated by depolarization to a threshold voltage. Its activation is accelerated by depolarization, so that depolarization causes the current to develop faster and to increase to a higher level. The current is transient, with its decay also being accelerated by depolarization. Peak current during voltage clamp is maximal at about −30 mV, with lower peak current as the voltage approaches the E_{Na}. Important characteristics are: 1) the steepness of the voltage-dependence of the current at threshold, so that inward current is activated fast enough to exceed any repolarizing currents; and 2) the peak current represents an index of the current available to produce conduction.

I_{Na} Studied by Single Channel Recording

Single channel recording requires isolating a small patch of membrane on the tip of a glass pipette about 1 micron in diameter and clamping the voltage across the membrane patch through the pipette. This permits recording of Na^+ current during channel opening when the patch is depolarized into the voltage range for activation of I_{Na}.

The behavior of a single channel is stochastic rather than deterministic. The voltage sets a probability that the channel will open; sometimes it will open early and sometimes it will open after a delay. The channel then closes in a probabilistic way with the greatest probability shortly after opening and with an exponential decline in the probability. A typical mean open time is 1 msec under similar experimental conditions. A summary of the characteristics of single Na^+ channels is as follows:

1. The Na^+ channel appears always to open to the same level of conductance. If there are subconductance states, they are not apparent under normal conditions (Cachelin et al., 1983; Patlak and Ortiz, 1985).

2. The mean open time is much shorter than the decay of I_{Na}. The channel may close to a state that allows reopening, or it may close to the inactivated (absorbing) state. The decay of I_{Na}, which we usually call inactivation, is produced by the declining probability that a channel will open, rather than inactivation as described by the Hodgkin-Huxley model (Aldrich and Stevens, 1987; Grant and Starmer, 1987; Kunze et al., 1985).
3. The channel may inactivate without ever opening. This occurs about half of the time at a temperature of 12°C (Scanley et al., unpublished observations).
4. Occasionally the channel does not inactivate for many msec, as if there is a failure of the normal inactivating process (Patlak and Ortiz, 1985).
5. I_{Na} in response to a voltage step results from the total population behavior of a large number of channels, all opening once or more, or not at all. However, if the behavior of one channel in response to a voltage step is summed for many depolarizing steps, it has the same time course as whole cell I_{Na}. This is to say, many channels opening during a single depolarization gives the same current as one channel opening many times (Fozzard et al., 1987).
6. There may be two populations of Na^+ channels in heart muscle. The second population is less than 20% as common, and it has a much lower single channel conductance, so its contribution to peak current should be small (Scanley and Fozzard, 1988).
7. The density of Na^+ channels appears to be very different in different parts of the heart. The Purkinje cells have a density near that of the squid nerve, but atrial and ventricular muscle cells may have a lower density (Hanck et al., unpublished observations).

Single Channel Events Underlying I_{Na} (peak) and $\dot{V}_{max}$

In order to understand why peak I_{Na} and $\dot{V}_{max}$ are different, it is important to consider the single channel physiological processes underlying these two events. I_{Na} (peak) is determined by six factors: 1) the density of Na^+ channels in the cell; 2) the fraction in the available (ready) configuration at onset of the voltage step (usually called h, after the Hodgkin-Huxley model terminology); 3) the fraction of available channels that open during the voltage step (as opposed to inactivating without ever opening); 4) the tendency of the opening channels to reopen; 5) the synchrony of opening within the channel population; and 6) the single channel current.

Because factor 1 is constant for both I_{Na} and $\dot{V}_{max}$ measurements, it can be discarded as a basis for differences between the two measurements. Factor 2, the fraction of available channels, is determined by the holding potential or the resting potential. In our experiments there was no difference in the fraction available for I_{Na} or $\dot{V}_{max}$. The fraction that opens (factor 3) varies between a few percent near I_{Na} threshold to 50%–60% near 0 mV (Scanley et al., in press). Although it is constant for a given voltage test step during voltage clamp, it would be expected to vary during a free-running action potential. The tendency of channels to reopen (factor 4) is greatest near threshold, where reopening may generate as much as 40% of the current (Scanley et al., unpublished observations). However, in the voltage range of $\dot{V}_{max}$ reopening is infrequent and this factor probably does not account for much of a role in the experimental differences between $\dot{V}_{max}$ and I_{Na}.

Factor 5, synchrony of opening, should be important, because it is very sensitive to voltage and time. Mobilization of channels requires time durations as long as a msec, with the delay shortening with more positive depolarizations. Peak I_{Na} is not reached for 0.5–2 msec, reflecting the time to generate channel openings. Free-running action potential depolarizations, on the other hand, are much quicker. As already discussed, $\dot{V}_{max}$ is usually achieved long before many channels can open. Therefore, the fraction of channels open at $\dot{V}_{max}$ is much less than those open at peak I_{Na}. Furthermore, this fraction at $\dot{V}_{max}$ varies as a function of the speed of depolarization of the action potential. This difference probably explains why $\dot{V}_{max}$ cannot be a reliable linear function of peak I_{Na}. The time dependency of synchrony of channel opening should make $\dot{V}_{max}$ a function of latency from the action potential stimulus. The most likely reason for the independence of $\dot{V}_{max}$ from latency in our experiments is found in the sharp voltage dependence of channel opening and inactivation, so that gradual depolarization in the subthreshold region fails to affect channel kinetics significantly and results in almost the same mobilization pattern for Na^+ channels.

Factor 6, single channel current, is determined by single channel conductance (obviously a constant), and the Na^+ electromechanical driving force. The latter is a sensitive voltage function, so variation in voltage during the upstroke is associated with large changes in single channel current. In our experiments, voltage at $\dot{V}_{max}$ was constant over a large range of Na^+ channel availability. The reason for this is not obvious. Membrane potential at $\dot{V}_{max}$ showed no change while $\dot{V}_{max}$ showed significant decreases. Only when $\dot{V}_{max}$ was severely reduced was the expected change in voltage at $\dot{V}_{max}$ seen.

What is the role of $\dot{V}_{max}$ in the study of Na^+ current and antiarrhythmic drug actions? Firstly, it should be recognized that $\dot{V}_{max}$ does reflect net maximal inward current during the action potential, which itself is a reflection of a wide variety of factors already discussed. Therefore, changes in $\dot{V}_{max}$ do reflect changes in Na^+ current, by a combination of factors related to Na^+ channel voltage dependence and kinetics. Proper study of antiarrhythmic drug action and mechanism requires both action potential-derived information and voltage clamp studies.

SUMMARY

1. Careful comparison of $\dot{V}_{max}$ and I_{Na} (from peak current measurements) shows that $\dot{V}_{max}$ is a monotonic but not a linear index of I_{Na}.
2. Na^+ channel kinetics and mechanism of channel block should be investigated by voltage clamp studies of I_{Na} and by single channel recordings, because $\dot{V}_{max}$ measurements may give misleading results.
3. $\dot{V}_{max}$ contributes to our understanding of Na^+ current and single Na^+ channel behavior during action potentials, and to antiarrhythmic mechanisms when studied in conjuction with voltage clamp studies.
4. Our previous interpretation of the role of latency from stimulus to $\dot{V}_{max}$ and voltage at $\dot{V}_{max}$ based on

the Hodgkin-Huxley model, is probably wrong, and requires reinterpretation by single channel studies.

Acknowledgements: Supported by USPHS grants POl HL 20592 and KJl HL 01971 (MFS).

BIBLIOGRAPHY

Aldrich RW, Stevens CF. Voltage-dependent gating of single sodium channels from mammalian neuroblastoma cells. *J Neuroscience* 7:418–431, 1987.

Beeler GW, Reuter H. Reconstruction of the action potential of ventricular myocardial fibres. *J Physiol* 268:177–210, 1977.

Brown AM, Lee KS, Powell T. Sodium currents in single rat heart muscle cells. *J Physiol* 318:479–500, 1981.

Bustamante JO, McDonald TF. Sodium current in segments of human heart cells. *Science* 220:320–321, 1983.

Cachelin AB, dePeyer JE, Kokubon S, Reuter H. Sodium channels in cultured cardiac cells. *J Physiol* 340:389–402, 1983.

Clark RB, Giles W. Sodium current in single cells from bullfrog atrium: voltage dependence and ion transfer properties. *J Physiol* 391:235–266, 1987.

Cohen CJ, Bean BP, Tsien RW. Maximal upstroke velocity as an index of available sodium conductances. *Circ Res* 54:636–651, 1984.

Cohen IS, Daytner NB, Gintant GA, Mulrine NK, Pennefather P. A note on the relation of maximum upstroke velocity to peak inward current recorded by the voltage clamp. *Circ Res* 57:482–484, 1985.

Follmer CH, Ten Eick RE, Yeh JZ. Sodium current kinetics in cat atrial myocytes. *J Physiol* 384:169–197, 1987.

Fozzard HA. Membrane capacity of the cardiac Purkinje fibre. *J Physiol* 182:255–267, 1966.

Fozzard HA, Hanck DA, Makielski JC, Scanley RE, Sheets MF. Sodium channels in cardiac Purkinje cells. *Experientia* 43:1162–1168, 1987.

Fozzard HA, Makielski JC. The electrophysiology of acute myocardial ischemia. *Ann Rev Med* 36:275–284, 1985.

Gettes LS, Reuter H. Slow recovery from inactivation of inward currents in mammalian myocardial fibres. *J Physiol* 240:703–724, 1974.

Grant AD, Starmer CF. Mechanisms of closure of cardiac sodium channels in rabbit ventricular myocytes: single channel analysis. *Circ Res* 60:897–913, 1987.

Grant AD, Starmer CF, Strauss HC. Antiarrhythmic drug action: blockade of inward current. *Circ Res* 55:427–439, 1984.

Hamill OP, Marty A, Neher E, Sakmann B, Sigworth FJ. Improved patch clamp techniques for high-resolution current recordings from cells and cell-free membrane patches. *Pfluegers Arch* 391:85–100, 1981.

Hodgkin, Huxley AF. A quantitative description of membrane current and its application to conduction and excitation in nerve. *J Physiol* 117:500–544, 1952.

Johnson EA, Lieberman M. Heart excitation and contraction. *Ann Rev Physiol* 33:479–532, 1971.
Krueger BK, Worley JF, French RJ. Single sodium channels from rat brain incorporated intro planar lipid bilayer membranes. *Nature* 303:172–175, 1983.
Kunze DL, Lacerda AE, Wilson DL, Brown AM. Cardiac Na currents and inactivating, reopening and waiting properties of single cardiac Na channels. *J Gen Physiol* 86:671–719, 1985.
Makielski JC, Sheets MF, Hanck DA, January CT, Fozzard HA. Sodium current in voltage clamped internally perfused canine cardiac Purkinje cells. *Biophys J* 52:1–11, 1987.
McAllister RE, Noble D, Tsien RW. Reconstruction of the electrical activity of cardiac Purkinje fibres. *J Physiol* 251:1–59, 1975.
Mitsuiye T, Noma A. A new oil-gap method for internal perfusion and voltage clamp of single cardiac cells. *Pfluger Arch* 410:7–14, 1987.
Patlak J, Ortiz M. Slow currents through single sodium channels of the adult rat heart. *J Gen Physiol* 86:89–104, 1985.
Scanley BE, Fozzard HA. Low conductance sodium channels in canine cardiac Purkinje cells. *Biophys J* 52:489–495, 1987.
Scanley BE, Hanck DA, Chay T, Fozzard HA. Kinetic analysis of single sodium channels from canine cardiac purkinje cells. *J Gen Physiol* 1989. In press.
Sheets MF, Hanck DA, Fozzard HA. Nonlinear relationship between $\dot{V}_{max}$ and I_{Na} in canine cardiac Purkinje cells. *Circ Res* 63:386–398, 1988.
Sheets MF, January CT, Fozzard HA. Isolation and characterization of single canine cardiac Purkinje cells. *Circ Res* 53:544–548, 1983.
Walton M, Fozzard HA. Experimental study of the conducted action potential in cardiac Purkinje strands. *Biophys J* 441–8, 1983a.
Walton M, Fozzard HA. The conducted action potential: models and comparison to experiments. *Biophys J* 44:9–26, 1983b.
Walton M, Fozzard HA. The relation of $\dot{V}_{max}$ to I_{Na}, G_{Na}, and $h\infty$ in a model of the cardiac Purkinje fiber. *Biophys J* 25:407–420, 1979.

Chapter 2

Voltage Dependence of Junctional Conductance in the Embryonic Heart

Robert L. DeHaan
Yan-hua Chen
Russel L. Penrod

INTRODUCTION

The cells of the heart are joined by gap junctions into an electrical syncytium that accounts for action potential propagation throughout the organ. Ischemia or fiber damage dramatically slows action potential (AP) conduction velocity in heart tissue and decouples cells, that is, it reduces junctional conductance (Hofmann, 1985; Kleber et al., 1986, 1987). Early studies of electrical coupling and intercellular dye diffusion, with a variety of more or less intact cardiac tissue preparations (reviewed in Page and Manjunath, 1986), indicated that the degree of coupling varied with changing conditions. But it was not possible to distinguish junctions from other resistive paths in multicellular tissues. Techniques for isolating healthy single cells from heart tissue (Powell et al., 1980; Wittenberg et al., 1986) and for recording the current passing from one member of a cell pair to the other, separately with independent voltage clamp circuits (Spray et al., 1981), have permitted more precise investigations of the regulation of junctional conductance

Hondeghem, Luc (ed): Molecular and Cellular Mechanisms of Antiarrhythmic Agents, Futura Publishing Company, Inc., Mount Kisco, NY, © 1989.

(Metzger and Weingart, 1985; Imanaga et al., 1987; Noma and Tsuboi, 1987). It is now well documented that the resistance of the junctions between cardiac cells is increased by many of the same agents that act in other tissues: elevated levels of Ca_i (Noma and Tsuboi, 1987), lowered cytosolic pH (Spray et al., 1985b), or perturbations in cell phosphorylating mechanisms (DeMello and van Loon, 1987). However, cell-to-cell conductance in adult heart tissue has been shown repeatedly to be independent of the potential across the junction (Kameyama, 1983; White et al., 1985; Weingart, 1986; Noma and Tsuboi, 1987). Recently, we have measured junctional conductance with patch electrodes applied to pairs of 7d chick embryo ventricle cells (Veenstra and DeHaan, 1986a; 1988a). Because the high input resistance of these small cells required holding currents only in the picoamp range, we were also able to record the currents through single cardiac gap junction channels. Current through cell-to-cell channels was readily distinguished from that through peripheral membrane channels since nonjunctional channel currents in either cell were recorded only in the electrode attached to that cell. In contrast, junctional channel current was measured as symmetrical signals of equal size and opposite polarity in the two electrodes, i.e., as inward current in one cell and outward from its neighbor. In recent experiments with this system, we have found that junctional conductance is dramatically affected by both the magnitude and polarity of the transjunctional potential (Chen, Penrod and DeHaan, 1988; Chen and DeHaan, 1989). In this chapter we will review the evidence that junctional conductance in embryonic heart cells is regulated by potential, and explore some possible mechanisms for that voltage dependence.

REGULATORS OF GAP JUNCTION CONDUCTANCE

Transjunctional Potential (V_j)

Voltage-regulated junctional channels are present in embryonic cells, but are uncommon in adult tissues (reviewed in Spray and Bennett, 1985a; Giaume et al., 1987; Brink et al., 1988). Spray et al. (1981) showed that the steady-state conductance of junctions between pairs of amphibian embryo blastomeres decreased as a steep function of transjunctional potential (V_j). Moreover, after a step change in V_j in these blastomeres, time-dependent activation and inactivation changes of junctional conductance were apparent (Harris et al., 1981). In contrast, Spray et al. (1986a,c) and Reverdin and Weingart (1988) found that gap junctions were voltage insensitive in intact pairs of adult rat liver cells. Even when junction protein was reconstituted in lipid membranes, Spray et al. (1986b) reported no voltage dependence for conductance. On the other hand, Young et al. (1987) found that the currents through channels formed by the liver 27kDa protein in lipid vesicles were not linear with voltage. As noted above, adult cardiac gap junctions have been shown to be voltage insensitive by several workers (Kameyama, 1983; White et al., 1985; Weingart, 1986). But DeMello (1986b) reported changes in the space constant in canine Purkinje fibers during the diastolic depolarization. He attributed the effect, in part, to a depolarization-induced increase in junctional conductance. Our initial results with embryonic chick heart cells (Veenstra and DeHaan, 1986a, 1988a) indicated that junctional conductance (g_j) behaved like that of adult cardiac cells, and was independent of membrane potential and V_j over the physiological range of potentials. But in our more recent experiments, described below, we have found that g_j has a pronounced time- and voltage-sensitivity (Chen et al., 1988b), comparable to that in fundulus blastomeres (Spray et al., 1984b). A major goal in understanding the relationship between g_j and V_j is to determine whether this voltage dependence results from a direct effect of a transjunctional electric field on junctional channels, or is secondary to voltage-induced changes in Ca_i, pH_i, or other molecular regulators. It will also be important to learn if this property is limited to embryonic cells, i.e., if the voltage sensitivity of early embryonic gap junctions diminishes with development.

Calcium Dependence

There is substantial evidence (Loewenstein, 1981; Obaid et al., 1983; Spray et al., 1985b) that cells of many tissues are uncoupled by conditions that increase intracellular free calcium concentration (Ca_i). With molecular markers of defined size, Simpson et al. (1977) found that elevation of Ca_i produced graded changes in permeability of junctions. In lacrimal gland cells, junctional channels were only slightly affected by $1x10^{-6}$ M free Ca_i, but closed within a few seconds with $1x10^{-5}$ M (Neyton and Trautmann, 1986b). In heart tissue,

Dahl and Isenberg (1980) reported that treatments that raised Ca_i into the micromolar range caused decoupling. Moreover, recent observations by Noma and Tsuboi (1987) with pairs of isolated cardiac myocytes suggest that relatively small increases in the intracellular concentration of divalent cations may have a regulatory effect on g_j, and raise the question whether g_j might fluctuate on a beat-to-beat time scale, as recently suggested by DeMello (1986b). With each beat in spontaneously active heart cells, Ca^i rises from an end-diastolic value of 100–200 nM (Blinks, 1986; Wier et al., 1987) to a peak-systolic level 5–6 times higher (Lee and Clusin, 1987). Junctional conductance in embryonic heart cells is clearly influenced by Ca_i, but appreciable changes in g_j on the time scale of the beat-to-beat fluctuations in Ca_i seem unlikely. When both members of a pair of embryonic chick ventricular cells were infused with solutions buffered with EGTA to a calculated free Ca_i of $1x10^{-6}$ M, g_j fell dramatically from an initial mean value of 14.6 nS to about 3 nS, but with a mean half-time for the decrease of about 5 min (Veenstra and DeHaan, 1988a). Some cell pairs registered as much as a 30-fold decline in g_j during 15–20 min after the beginning of high-Ca infusion. This decoupling resulted from a decrease in the open-state probability of the channels, not from a change in single-channel conductance or number of channels in the junction (Veenstra and DeHaan, 1988b). Ca-induced decoupling in pairs of adult rat lacrimal gland (Neyton and Trautmann, 1986a) and liver (Reverdin and Weingart, 1988) cells also took place on a time-scale of several minutes. When embryonic heart cell pairs were infused with a low-Ca solution ($<10^{-8}$ M), g_j rose (Veenstra and DeHaan, 1988a), again with a half-time of about 5 min. If prolonged depolarization can lead to Ca release from the sarcoplasmic reticulum and increased steady-state Ca_i levels (Cannell et al., 1987), this ion could act as an intermediary for voltage-dependent regulation of g_j.

pH Dependence

In many tissues, treatments that raise Ca_i also decrease pH_i (for review see Aickin, 1986). Several studies have compared the effects of Ca_i and pH_i on g_j. In pairs of squid or amphibian blastomeres, a decrease in pH_i of as little as 0.3 units, which is within the range of physiological fluctuation (Moolenaar, 1986), caused a dramatic reduction in junctional communication (Spray et al., 1984a). This effect was independent of the voltage-sensitive gate (Spray et al., 1986b), and was much more potent than Ca^{2+}-induced uncoupling (Spray et al., 1985b). In heart, the pH_i-g_j curve was steepest near normal pH_i. With slight acidifications from pH 7, g_j was significantly reduced between cardiac cells (Spray et al., 1985a,b; White et al., 1985). In guinea pig ventricular cell pairs, however, g_j was reduced only when pH_i dropped below 6.5 and complete block was not observed until a pH of 5.0 was achieved (Noma and Tsuboi, 1987). Similarly, Pressler (1989) found that longitudinal resistance (r_i) in sheep Purkinje fibers increased only 2.2% per 10 nM increase in intracellular $[H^+]$ (pH 7.8 to 6.9), and suggested that the action of protons on r_i may be subordinate to an intermediate pH-dependent reaction such as a calmodulin-dependent mechanism. It is intriguing that a prolonged depolarizing step to -30 mV in frog muscle results in an immediate intracellular acidification of 0.3–0.4 pH units that lasts for several minutes (Abercrombie and Roos, 1983). Thus, a change in either pH_i or Ca_i could mediate a voltage-induced fall in g_j, by different mechanisms.

Regulation by Protein Kinases

Junctional permeability is modulated by phosphorylation (see Loewenstein, 1985, 1987 for review). Cyclic AMP and phosphodiesterase (PDE) inhibitors increase the junctional permeability of mammalian cells (Loewenstein, 1985; DeMello, 1986a; DeMello and van Loon, 1987). This process occurs over a period of minutes or hours and apparently requires the formation of new channels (Saez et al., 1986). Conversely, calmodulin-dependent protein kinases and protein kinase C have been implicated in reducing junctional permeability (Peracchia and Girsch, 1985; Gainer and Murray, 1985; Verselis et al., 1986; Yada et al., 1985). The concept that junctional permeability is regulated by kinase-mediated phosphorylation is supported by evidence that gap junction protein is a substrate for all three protein kinases (Saez et al., 1986; Takeda et al., 1987). Whether this phosphorylation affects channel gating directly or indirectly remains to be determined.

REGULATION OF g_j AT THE SINGLE CHANNEL LEVEL IN EMBRYONIC HEART CELLS

Measurement of g_j

With independent voltage clamp circuits applied to each member of a cell pair, Veenstra and DeHaan (1986a, 1988a) routinely held cell 1 constant at $V_1 = -40$ mV and measured the current passing through each electrode (I_1 and I_2) in response to application of rectangular voltage clamp steps from -40 to -80 mV applied to cell 2. Thus, V_j (defined as $V_1 - V_2$) was alternated between 0 and 40 mV (Fig. 1A). With both cells at -40 mV ($V_j = 0$), junctional current (I_j) was zero. In response to the step to -80 mV in V_2, which applied a 40 mV positive V_j, I_j was outward from cell 1 and into its

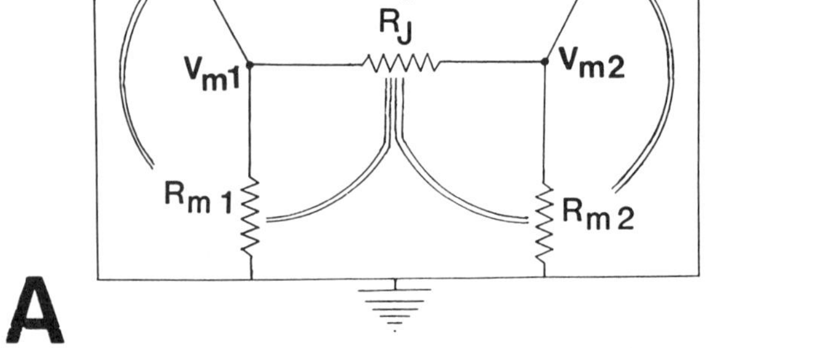

Figure 1. Measurement of macroscopic junctional current and junctional conductance. A. Equivalent circuit of the two-electrode patch clamp. Each patch electrode has an access resistance to the cell interior (R_{e11}, R_{e12}) and a seal resistance (R_{s1}, R_{s2}) between the cell interior and external reference. The membrane resistance of each cell is R_{m1}, R_{m2}, while R_j is the junctional resistance between the cells. Membrane potential of each cell (V_{m1}, V_{m2}) is controlled separately by two patch-clamp circuits, represented by amplifiers 1 and 2. Typical values for named resistances are: $R_{el} = 5$–15 MΩ, $R_s =$ 5–50 GΩ, $R_j = 0.05$–5 GΩ ($g_j = 0.2$–20 nS).

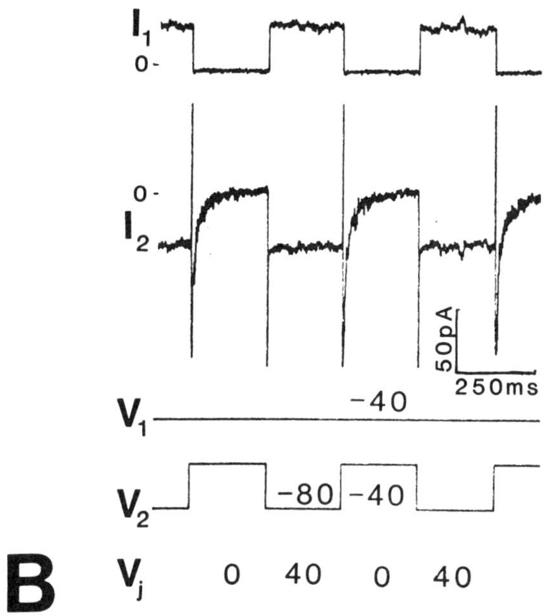

Figure 1B. I_1 and I_2 are whole-cell current records from cell 1 and cell 2, obtained when V_j was stepped repeatedly from 0 to 40 mV. V_1 was held constant at −40 mV while 250 ms rectangular steps from −40 to −80 mV were applied to V_2. $I_j = I_1(-40) - I_1(-80)$; $g_j = I_j/V_j$. In the example shown, $g_j = 0.79 \pm 0.05$ nS (mean ± S.D. averaged over 12 pulses). (Adapted from Veenstra and DeHaan, 1988a).

more negative neighbor. Thus, the current recorded at each electrode was:

$$I_1 = (V_1 - V_2)g_j = I_j \quad [1]$$

$$I_2 = -[(V_1 - V_2)g_j + V_2/R_{in2}] = -(I_j + I_{in2}) \quad [2]$$

where g_j = junctional conductance = I_j/V_j, R_{in2} is the parallel sum of the resistances of the electrode seal on cell 2 and the nonjunctional membrane of cell 2, and I_{in2} is the current crossing R_{in2}. At the end of each pulse the depolarizing step from −80 to −40 mV in V_2 brought V_j back to 0, and also caused an outward capacitive transient and a slowly inactivating inward membrane current (I_m) in cell 2 (Fig. 1B). Because V_1 was held constant, these currents across the nonjunctional membrane of cell 2 were not sensed by electrode 1. As shown in eq.1, I_1 included only current across the junction: that is, to a close approximation, $I_1 = I_j$, and $g_j = I_j/V_j$. Among 26 cell pairs, g_j varied greatly from one preparation to the next. When measured 1–3 min after both membrane patches were ruptured, it ranged from 0.15 nS to 35 nS (mean = 6.20 ± 9.12 nS, N = 26).

Do Regulators of g_j Affect N, γ_j, or P_o?

Total junctional conductance is determined by the number of channels in the junction (N), the single-channel conductance (γ_j), and the probability (P_o) that a channel is in the open state: $g_j = N\gamma_j P_o$. We noted above that slow increases in g_j brought about over periods of many minutes or hours by shifts in intracellular cAMP levels, appeared to be associated with an increase in N (Saez et al., 1986). In our original work with embryonic heart cells (Veenstra and DeHaan, 1988a,b) we found that g_j and P_o were reduced in parallel over a period of several minutes by elevated Ca_i and by octanol, but γ_j was unaffected by these agents. In these experiments, the voltage dependence of g_j was tested by varying V_j in 5 mV steps from −80 mV to 80 mV, with a low-calcium, unbuffered pipette-filling solution. In this condition, the g_j-V_j relation was almost flat between −60 mV and 60 mV, and channel gating fluctuated in a voltage-independent manner.

Gap Junction Channels have Multiple Conductance States

In our initial experiments, we measured γ_j from spontaneous channel open-close events that occurred in the steady state with V_j held constant for many minutes at 40 mV. Currents through single junctional channels (i_j) were seen in the two electrodes as symmetrical signals of equal size and opposite polarity (Veenstra and DeHaan, 1986a; 1988a). These were readily distinguishable from nonjunctional currents (ion channels in the peripheral membrane or seal currents), because the latter were seen with the same polarity and different magnitudes in the two electrodes. From measurements of over 15,000 channel events with V_j = 40 mV, we recorded two readily distinguishable conductance levels, near 80 and 160 pS (Veenstra and DeHaan, 1988a), and less frequent openings to near 40 and 240 pS (Chen and DeHaan, 1989). Recent measurements of γ_j from other cell-pair preparations confirm that channel proteins may be able to take on multiple open-state configurations. The junctional channels between pairs of neonatal rat heart cells had two conductance levels near 30 and 60 pS (Rook et al., 1988). In pairs of rat lacrimal gland cells, Neyton and Trautmann (1986a) measured γ_j of about 90 pS, and channels of about the same conductance were observed during development of electrical coupling between embryonic amphibian muscle cells (Chow and Young, 1987). Somogyi and Kolb 1988a) measured discrete levels of γ_j in pairs of mouse pancreatic acinar cells of 130 and 27 pS, and five reproducible levels between 22 and 120 pS in CHO cells. The value of γ_j for hepatic channels was 140–150 pS (Spray et al., 1986b; Young et al., 1987), and for isolated bovine lens junctional channels, about 200 pS (Hall and Zampighi, 1985). These data are consistent with a pore that can fluctuate between different open states, but which, when fully open, has a diameter of about 1.5 nm as indicated by permeability and structural studies (DeHaan, 1988; Bennett et al., 1988). Alternatively, one may postulate a special cooperativity among groups of channels, or a multi-barrelled channel with a common gate, similar to that conceived by Hunter and Giebisch (1987).

Embryonic Cardiac Gap Junctions are Voltage-dependent

To determine the dependence of g_j on V_j, in our initial experiments (Veenstra and DeHaan, 1988a), V_1 was held constant at -40 mV while V_2 was stepped sequentially from -100 to 20 mV in 5 mV, 300 msec steps, thereby varying V_j from 60 to -60 mV. The pipettes were filled with Ca-free solution (IPS 59) unbuffered with EGTA, to allow Ca_i to fluctuate normally. Over the voltage range tested, mean g_j was constant in each cell pair from -15 to 60 mV, but declined by about 30% between -15 and -60 mV. Since standard errors of the means of data from pooled cell pairs were as large as 0.5 nS, this slight voltage dependence was not significant. In these experiments, voltage-sensitive components of g_j might have been masked by the small size and brief duration of the increments in V_j. Therefore, a new clamp-step protocol (R41) was applied that imposed progressively larger steps from $V_j = 0$, as follows: cell 1 was held constant at -40 mV; V_2 was stepped from -40 mV to -30 mV for 1.6 sec before returning to -40 mV for 1 sec. This produced a 1.6 sec period of $V_j = -10$ mV, and a rectangular pulse of inward (downward) current recorded in electrode 1 (Fig. 2A). After 1 sec of

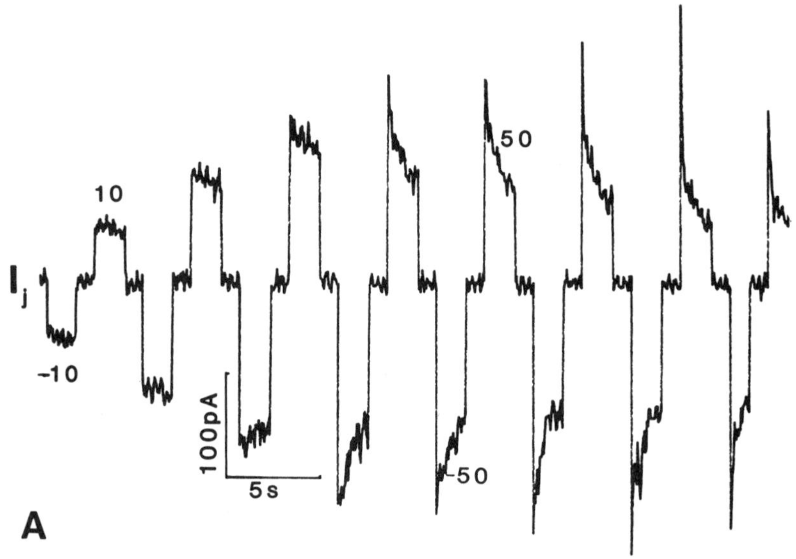

Figure 2. Effect of magnitude and polarity of V_j on g_j. A. Record of I_1 in response to voltage sequence R41. V_1 is held constant at -40 mV, while V_j is stepped through a series of 1.6 second pulses at ± 10, 20 . . . 80 mV, with each voltage step separated from the next by a 1 second-period during which $V_1 = V_2 = -40$ mV; $V_j = 0$.

$V_j = 0$, V_2 was stepped to -50 mV, for a 1.6 sec pulse of $V_j = 10$ mV. This pattern was then repeated with alternating pulses of $V_j = \pm 20$, 30, 40, 50, 60, 70, and 80 mV, with each step separated from the next by 1 sec of $V_j = 0$. Steps in V_2 from -40 mV to more negative membrane potentials produce positive potentials across the junction and outward junctional current (seen as upward-going steps in Fig. 2A). It should be emphasized again that since V_1 was held constant while V_j was changed, the current labeled I_j ($= I_1$) in Fig. 2 is virtually uncontaminated by nonjunctional currents or passive membrane time dependencies. From simple inspection of Fig. 2A it is apparent that I_j, and therefore g_j, show both time and voltage dependence. At each voltage step greater than about ± 20 mV, the current is largest initially and then decays. The rapidly decaying spike is particularly pronounced at $V_j = \pm 50$ mV and greater. But neither the initial nor the final current increases linearly with V_j, indicating that g_j changes with V_j. As shown in Fig. 1B, both the

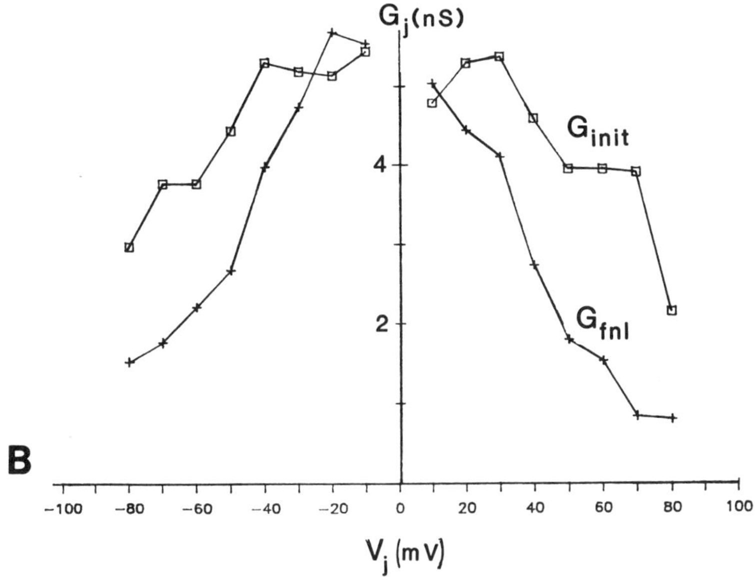

Figure 2B. The g_j–V_j relation shows a dramatic decline of both initial (box) and final (+) junctional conductance as V_j is increased, which, moreover, is slightly asymmetric. Both electrodes contained IPS57 with free Ca_i buffered to 10^{-6} M with 5 mM EGTA. (Pair 101387)

initial (peak) conductance and that at the end of the 1.6 sec pulses decline sharply with V_j. Moreover, the voltage dependence is not completely symmetrical. Junctional conductance is influenced not only by the magnitude of V_j, but by its polarity. The decline in end conductance is steeper and greater for positive current than for negative. An average of four repeated sequences confirmed that the junction rectifies at V_j steps beyond ±40 mV, passing more current from the pulsed cell into the one held constant, than in the other direction.

Is the Rapidly Decaying Spike of I_j Due to an Activation-inactivation Sequence?

The asymmetric bell-shape of the g_j-V_j curves in Fig. 2B suggests that g_j has a substantial resting value at $V_j = 0$. Is the large spike of current that follows a 40–80 mV step in V_j (Fig. 2A) due to the rapid activation of an increase in conductance from the resting state just prior to the applied potential, which then rapidly inactivates? Or does it merely reveal the steady-state resting conductance, before the applied V_j causes its inactivation? Two lines of evidence indicate that the decaying current spikes reflect a voltage-dependent inactivation of resting g_j, rather than activation of an increased conductance. Activated currents normally show time-dependence, i.e., they reach a peak with a finite delay. With very fast membrane currents, such as the excitatory sodium current, the time to peak may be less than 1 msec, but with adequate recording electronics, the delay is readily measurable (Fujii et al., 1988). Careful measurement of peak I_j records, recorded on VCR tape at 20 kHz indicated that they are virtually instantaneous, reaching their peak value in <300 μsec. This suggests that the current measured in the first few milliseconds after a voltage step reflects the steady-state conductance of the resting junction just before the voltage step. The second argument in support of this contention comes from direct measurements of g_j during the period of $V_j = 0$. This was accomplished by holding V_1 at -80 mV, while applying 5-sec steps from -80 mV to 0 mV in V_2. Superimposed on these alternating 5-sec periods of 0 mV and 80 mV V_j, were 10 mV, 100 msec test pulses, repeated every 500 msec. The test pulses gave an accurate measure of g_j without being large enough or long enough to cause inactivation themselves. The result of this test was clear: the peak current recorded immediately after an 80 mV step in V_j was close to, but never larger than, eight times that measured during a 10 mV step at the end of the previous period at $V_j = 0$ mV. After 5 sec at $V_j =$ 0 mV, a 10 mV step and an 80 mV step revealed virtually the same conductance. The difference between the two potentials was that 10 mV applied across the junction caused no change in g_j, whereas application of an 80 mV V_j resulted in a rapid shutdown of junctional channels, and a fall in g_j to about 20% of its value at the beginning of that step. Thus, applied potentials have only an inactivating effect on g_j; they do not activate it.

Inactivation of g_j Depends on Polarity

The inactivation of I_j following an 80 mV step in V_j was best fit by a tri-exponential curve with time-constants of about 50 msec, 500 msec, and 60 sec, suggesting that the current decay is a complex

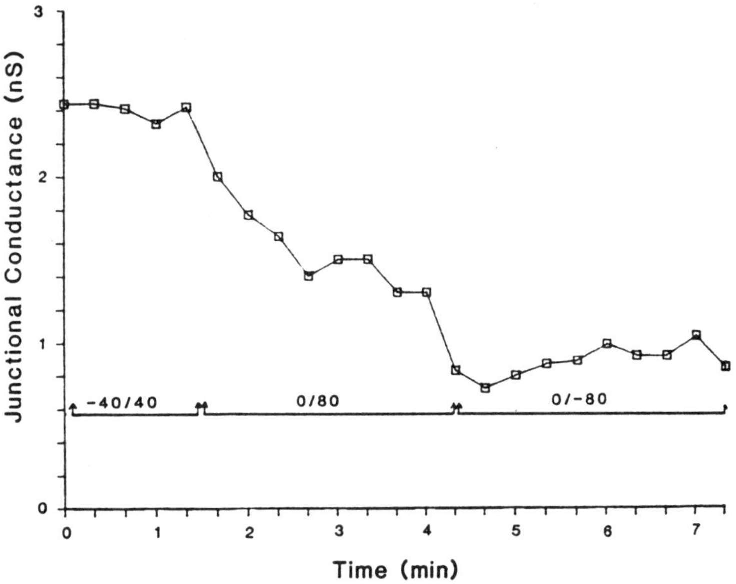

Figure 3. The effect of the polarity of repeated V_j pulses on g_j while running voltage sequence R40. During a period of 7.3 minutes, V_2 was alternated between 0 mV and −80 mV, in 5 second-steps. V_1 was held at −40 mV for the first 80 seconds, 0 mV for the next 180 seconds, and −80 mV for the last 170 seconds. g_j was sampled every 20 seconds; it remains stable when V_j is stepped repeatedly from 40 to −40 mV; it declines steadily while V_j alternates from 0 to 80 mV; and it becomes stable again when V_j switches between 0 to −80mV (Cell pair 121687, IPS66).

phenomenon with several component processes. An experiment designed to test the cumulative effect of repeated long positive or negative currents confirmed the existence of a slow component with a time-constant of many seconds. In this experiment, V_1 was maintained at −40, 0 or −80 mV for 2–3 minutes each, while stepping V_2 back and forth between 0 and −80 mV every 5 sec. The results on one cell pair are shown in Fig. 3. With this protocol running, g_j (measured as I_{jfnl}) remained constant for 80 sec at about 2.4 nS, while V_1 was at −40 mV and V_j alternated between 40 and −40 mV. When V_1 was shifted to 0 mV for 3 minutes, causing V_j to switch every 5 sec between 0 and 80 mV, g_j declined steadily. As soon as V_1 was clamped at −80 mV, with V_j alternating between 0 and −80 mV, g_j again stabilized and began to recover. We interpret this result, tentatively, as follows: alternating periods of ± 40 mV V_j had little cumulative effect, suggesting that in this preparation, the voltage threshold for g_j inactivation was greater than ± 40 mV. With V_1 held at 0 mV (V_j alternating between 0 and 80 mV), application of the first pulse of 80 mV across the junction caused a marked inactivation of g_j, which then failed to recover fully during the next 5-sec period of 0 V_j. The second period of 80 mV V_j therefore started at a lower g_j but caused an equal degree of inactivation. Again, recovery was incomplete during the period of 0 mV. Thus, with each subsequent pulse to 80 mV, g_j would fall to progressively lower levels, yielding the continuous 3-minute decline seen in Fig. 3. When V_1 was held at -80 mV (V_j alternating between 0 and -80 mV), the effect is quite different. With a negative polarity of V_j, the g_j-inactivation caused by each -80 mV pulse was more than completely reversed during the subsequent period of 0 V_j, leading to the beginning of a slow recovery of g_j, seen in the last 3 minutes of the experiment. A simple model that could account for these results is that of a positively charged blocking ion induced by the prolonged period of depolarization in cell 1, that would be driven into the channels by a positive V_j.

Models of Voltage Dependence and Rectification in Gap Junctions

Contingent Gating

The rectifying synapses of the crayfish and other nervous systems are characterized by an asymmetric anatomy of the neurons on the two sides of the synaptic junction, and probably by an asymmetry in response of the pore-forming channels or *connexons* to an applied electric field (Giaume et al., 1987; Brink et al., 1988). In contrast, there is no apparent physical asymmetry in pairs of frog blastomeres or chick ventricle cells. Moreover, at least at the ultrastructural level, the junctional channels that join vertebrate hepatic and cardiac cells appear to be formed from structurally identical connexons (reviewed in DeHaan, 1988b). To explain the time- and voltage- dependence they observed in amphibian blastomeres, Harris et al. (1981) have postulated a model based on *contingent gating*. In these cells, g_j had a mono-exponential decline to a steady-state non-zero value in response to a step change in V_j. However, when the polarity of V_j was reversed, g_j underwent a transient overshoot before decaying back to the same steady-state value. In their two-state model of the g_j channels, the transition between the open and closed configuration is controlled by conventional voltage-dependent rate constants, α and β. However, they proposed that each connexon gate senses a local field only in its own pore, and that the gates have zero conductance when closed. In the presence of a voltage that closes one gate, the entire transjunctional potential drop is developed across that gate, and the voltage across the open gate is near zero. The model explains the overshooting behavior by assuming that channels must pass through an open state before closing. When both gates are open, the voltage across each is approximately half the transjunctional potential drop. When the connexon at the more positive end of the channel closes, it experiences the entire voltage drop. Upon reversal of the polarity, the closed gate must first open before the open one can close, resulting in the transient overshoot of the conductance. This portion of the model, in which only one connexon of each apposed pair is closed at a time, can account for the time-dependence of the response to a voltage step. The model explains the decrease in g_j with increasing V_j by assuming that the opening rate, α, saturates for moderate voltages.

Charged Blocking Particle

The voltage sequence applied in Fig. 3, in which V_1 was held constant for 2–3 minutes at one of three levels (-40, 0, or -80 mV) while V_2 was stepped every 5 sec back and forth between 0 and -80 mV, resulted first in a series of alternating 5 sec periods of $V_j = 40$ mV or -40 mV. The conditions, however, were not symmetrical. With each step from -80 mV to 0 mV in V_2, to yield $V_j = -40$ mV, I_{Ca} was activated in cell 2, and the direction of I_j was from cell 2 across the junction to cell 1. That is, during the transient increase in Ca_i induced by I_{Ca} (Lee and Clusin, 1987), the potential difference across the junction would tend to drive Ca ions from cell 2 into the g_j channels, and transiently reduce g_j. In contrast, at $V_j = 40$ mV when V_2 is stepped to -80 mV there is no Ca-transient, and I_j flows from cell 1 (being held constant at -40 mV) into the more negative cell 2. Ca in cell 1 is at a low steady-state level, presumably below the concentration needed to close the g_j channels. If beat-to-beat fluctuations in Ca_i cause transient rhythmic reductions in g_j, then the rate of Ca extrusion and resequestration should determine if g_j returns to a basal level at the end of each beat. In the intact heart, in conditions of even slight Ca load or tachycardia, Ca_i might increase with each beat in a staircase effect (Lee and Clusin, 1987) to levels that would compromise AP propagation and lead to heart failure. The long-term effect seen in Fig. 3 might also be explained in terms of pH_i. An extended period of depolarization to 0 mV in cell 1 would tend to drive Na out of the cell because of the sharp decrease in driving force on that ion. Efflux of Na would activate the Na^+/H^+ exchange pump, which is active in embryonic chick heart cells (Piwnica-Worms et al., 1985), and cause a reduction in pH_i, as shown in skeletal muscle preparations (Abercrombie and Roos, 1983).

The voltage-dependence of cell-to-cell conductance in other embryonic systems is apparently not polarity-dependent. The fall in steady-state junctional conductance in amphibian blastomeres was perfectly symmetrical in the positive and negative directions, forming a bell-shaped g_j-V_j relation (Spray et al., 1981). Our results with embryonic heart cells (Chen et al., 1988b), show that embryonic cardiac junctions rectify in the sense that g_j is not only dependent on the magnitude but also on the polarity of V_j. As noted above, this could be accounted for if the rectification in embryonic heart cells resulted from a depolarization-induced change in the channels when they pass current into the more negative cell. One mechanism might invoke a blocking Ca or Mg ion that functions like Mg in causing the rectification of I_{K1} (Matsuda et al., 1987). However, from what is known about the size of the g_j channel pore, it would not be occluded by a single Ca or Mg ion (DeHaan, 1988). A variation on the model would visualize one or more Ca (or proton) binding sites which, when occupied, would close the channel. If these were deep enough in the pore to be affected by the voltage drop within the channel, a voltage sensitivity would result. As noted above, in many cell systems, intracellular acidification reduces g_j. By bathing pairs of amphibian blastomeres in CO_2-equilibrated saline, Bennett et al. (1988) caused graded levels of cytoplasmic acidification and reported well-behaved titration curves of g_j *vs.* V_j. However, unilateral acidification affected voltage dependence asymmetrically, inducing an apparent rectification in the junctions reminiscent of that seen in Fig. 2.

THE ROLE OF JUNCTIONAL VOLTAGE DEPENDENCE IN AP PROPAGATION

Are our findings of junctional voltage-dependence in embryonic chick ventricle cells relevant to the adult mammalian heart? Perhaps not to the normal healthy ventricle. Even when substantial voltages were applied across the junctions between adult ventricle cells under voltage-clamp control, g_j was unaffected (Kameyama, 1983; Weingart, 1986; Noma and Tsuboi, 1987). However, the electrical properties of embryonic ventricular cells bear a closer resemblance to adult pacemaker cells than to adult ventricular myocytes (DeHaan, 1980), and in both adult sinoatrial [SA] (Jalife, 1984) and atrioventricular [AV] (Paes de Carvalho et al., 1969) nodes, appreciable propagation delays and voltage gradients may appear across the cell junctions with each beat. Moreover, within 5 minutes after the onset of acute myocardial ischemia in adult ventricular tissue, longitudinal resistance increases dramatically, propagation velocity falls, and conduction block ensues (Kleber et al., 1986). With pairs of cardiac myocytes isolated in culture under double voltage clamp, the role of junctional resistance (R_j) in conduction of the AP can be distinguished from other parameters such as extracellular resistance and excitability of the cells. Cell-to-cell impulse transfer depends both on the amount of current that crosses the junction (determined by V_j/R_j) and on the electrical load, i.e., the input resistance (R_{in}) of the cell or cells into which I_j flows (Clapham et al., 1980; Joyner et al., 1984). The ratio, R_j/R_{in}, is therefore a useful parameter for assessing the conductive state of a multicellular tissue like the heart. In earlier work, DeHaan and coworkers found that AP transfer occurred between pairs of embryonic heart cell aggregates when R_j/R_{in} was in the range of 1–12 (R_j = 1–20 MΩ, R_{in} = 1.5 MΩ; Clapham et al., 1980; Veenstra and DeHaan, 1986b). With good coupling (R_j/R_{in} = 1–4), APs arose virtually simultaneously in the two aggregates. At the upper end of the R_j/R_{in} range, however, conduction delays of 40–100 msec were seen (Clapham et al., 1980; Veenstra and DeHaan, 1986b). In good agreement, Weingart and Maurer

(1988) recently found instantaneous AP transfer between coupled pairs of adult rat or guinea pig ventricular cells with R_j/R_{in} up to 5, propagation with delays to 7.5, and conduction block at $R_j/R_{in} >$ 15. Modeling single cells as cellular domains, Joyner and van Capelle (1986) found succesful transmission with R_j/R_{in} ratios up to 10. In terms of cable theory, this means that the longitudinal resistance of a one-dimensional fiber can increase about 100-fold before conduction fails. In ischemia or conditions of elevated Ca_i (Hofmann, 1985; Kleber et al., 1986; 1987; Maurer and Weingart, 1987), the slowing and ultimate failure of AP propagation that lead to conduction block and arrhythmias result from an increase of R_j/R_{in} beyond that threshold. Under such conditions of discontinuous propagation, where electrical interactions are dominated by junctional conductance, and transjunctional voltages of 20–50 mV can occur (Cole et al., 1988), voltage-dependent junctions would have profound effects. The fact that voltage-dependent junctions with properties similar to those in embryonic chick ventricle cells have recently been seen in pairs of neonatal rat heart cells (Rook et al., 1988) confirms the relevance of this behavior to the mammalian heart. But additional work on postnatal changes in gap junction behavior is needed to understand the transition from the voltage-dependent neonatal condition to the voltage-independence of the adult heart.

ARE THERE DEVELOPMENTAL CHANGES IN g_j?

The differences between adult and embryonic junctional channels were strikingly demonstrated when Dahl et al. (1987) produced functional liver junctional channels in a Xenopus oocyte expression system. Oocytes injected with cDNA prepared from adult mammalian liver would form coupling junctions when pressed together in pairs. However, the properties of these newly expressed liver junctions differed from those that normally couple Xenopus blastomeres. Conductance of the endogenous embryonic channels was sensitive to V_j; was only weakly affected by changes in Ca_i, but was sharply reduced by cytoplasmic acidification. In contrast, the cDNA-directed channels had properties like those of adult liver: they were voltage-insensitive; closed by small increases in Ca_i, but were relatively unaffected by even pronounced cytoplasmic acidification.

As noted above, in the adult heart junctional conductance is a critical parameter in regulating propagation of the AP. Conduction velocities ranging from 0.4 to 2 m/sec in different regions ensure that the AP propagates throughout the organ in a fraction of a second, i.e., at a rate that is optimal for the hemodynamic pumping of blood through the organ. In both mammals and birds (Sturkie, 1986), it takes about 15 msec for the excitation wave to spread from the base of the interventricular septum through the apex and distal walls of the ventricle, with a velocity of about 1 m/sec. In the chick embryo, as soon as differentiation has proceeded far enough that cardiac myocytes are able to generate electrical activity, the cells are connected by low-resistance junctions that support AP propagation. In the 28–30 hour embryo, the heart tube is less than 0.5 mm long and consists entirely of about 3,000 cells that comprise the conus and rostral ventricle (reviewed in DeHaan, 1989b). Using a multiple-site optical recording system and a voltage-sensitive dye, Komuro et al. (1985) recorded the early spontaneous APs from 25 locations simultaneously in the early chick heart. Action potentials originated in the caudal-most differentiated part of the left side of the conoventricular tube, and propagated rostrally with a linear conduction velocity of about 1 mm/sec; it took 200–300 msec for the excitation wave to propagate throughout the heart. Measuring by total cell number, the heart increases in size by more than 1,000-fold during embryogenesis (DeHaan, 1989b), while the time required for the spread of excitation decreases. Propagation outpaces the increasing size of the early heart because the conduction velocity increases dramatically in the ventricle. For example, AP propagation through the 2d, 3d, and 4d chick ventricle was 17, 45 and 93 mm/sec, respectively (Arguello et al., 1986). That is, conduction velocity in the ventricle increases roughly 100 times between 30 hours and 4 days, and another 10-fold throughout the rest of development.

The velocity of AP propagation through a multicellular tissue is determined by at least three parameters in addition to g_j: the dimensions of the individual cells, the external (intercellular cleft) resistance, and the shape of the AP upstroke (Fozzard, 1979). All of these parameters change with development in the embryonic heart. Therefore, the magnitude of the contribution that junctional conductance makes to the developmental change in conduction velocity needs to be determined with more precise observations.

CONCLUSIONS

The steady-state conductance of the gap junctions that join embryonic heart cells is highest when V_j is less than ± 20 mV. Upon application of a larger transjunctional potential step, junctional conductance falls rapidly to a lower level with no sign of a transient additional activation. The kinetics and magnitude of the inactivation depend on both the size and polarity of V_j. The current decay induced by an 80 mV potential across the junction is best fit by a tri-exponential curve, suggesting that g_j inactivation is a multi-component process. It is not clear if inactivation results from a direct closing effect of a transjunctional electric field on gap junction channels, or is mediated by a voltage-induced change in the intracellular milieu of one or the other member of the cell pair, such as Ca_i or pH_i. Maintenance of junctional conductance is crucial for action potential propagation in both the embryonic and adult heart. The slow conduction velocity in the embryonic heart may result, in part, from junctional inactivation caused by a steep transjunctional potential gradient at the action potential wave front. Gap junctions in the normal adult heart are voltage-insensitive. However, an interesting question that arises from the work discussed here is whether conditions of ischemia that foster conduction block might also cause cardiac gap junctions to revert to an embryonic-like state in which they are voltage-dependent.

BIBLIOGRAPHY

Abercrombie RF, Roos A. The intracellular pH of frog skeletal muscle: its regulation in hypertonic solutions. *J Physiol* (London) 345:189–204, 1983.

Aickin CC. Intracellular pH regulation by vertebrate muscle. *Ann Rev Physiol* 48:349–361, 1986.

Arguello C, Alanis J, et al. Electrophysiological and ultrastructural study of the atrioventricular canal during the development of the chick embryo. *J Mol Cell Cardiol* 18:499–504, 1986.

Bargiello TA, Saez L, et al. The Drosophila clock gene per affects intercellular junctional communication. Nature 328:686–88, 1987.

Bennett MVL, Verselis V, et al. Gap junctional conductance: gating. In: Hertzberg EL, Johnson RG, eds. *Gap Junctions*. New York, NY:Alan R. Liss; 287–304, 1988.

Blinks JR. Intracellular [Ca^{2+}] measurements. In: Fozzard HA, et al., eds. *The Heart and Cardiovascular System*. New York, NY: Raven Press; 671–701, 1986.

Brink PB, Jaslove SW, et al. Voltage clamp studies of gap junctions. In: Hertzberg EL, Johnson RG, eds. *Gap Junctions.* New York, NY: Alan R. Liss; 321–334, 1988.

Cannell MB, Berlin JR, Lederer WJ. Effect of membrane potential changes on the calcium transient in single rat cardiac muscle cells. *Science* 238:1419–1423, 1987.

Chen Y, DeHaan RL. Cardiac gap junction channels shift to lower conductance states when temperature is reduced. *Biophys J* 55, 152a, 1989.

Chen Y, Penrod RL, DeHaan RL. Conductance of gap junctions in embryonic heart cells is voltage-dependent. Int Conf on Cell Biology, Montreal, 1988.

Chow I, Young SH. Opening of single gap junction channels during formation of electrical coupling between embryonic muscle cells. *Dev Biol* 122:332–337, 1987.

Clapham DE, Shrier A, DeHaan RL. Junctional resistance and action potential delay between embryonic heart cell aggregates. *J Gen Physiol* 75:633–654, 1980.

Cole WC, Picone JB, Sperelakis N. Gap junction uncoupling and discontinuous propagation in the heart. A comparison of experimental data with computer simulations. *Biophys J* 53:809–818, 1988.

Dahl G, Isenberg G. Decoupling of heart muscle cells: correlation with increased cytoplasmic calcium activity and changes of nexus ultrastructure. *J Membr Biol* 53:63–75, 1980.

Dahl G, Miller T, et al. Expression of functional cell-cell channels from cloned rat liver gap junction complementary DNA. *Science* 236:1291–1293, 1987.

DeHaan RL. Dynamic behavior of gap junction channels. In: Hertzberg E, Johnson R, eds. *Gap Junctions.* New York, NY: Alan R. Liss; 305–320, 1988.

DeHaan RL. Embryonic origin of the heartbeat. In: Hurst JW, et al., eds. *The Heart.* 7th ed. New York, NY: McGraw-Hill; 72–76, 1989.

DeHaan RL. Modulation of cell electrical properties by peptide hormones. In: Nathan R, ed. *Cardiac Muscle: Regulation of Excitation and Contraction.* New York, NY: Academic Press; 129–170, 1986.

DeHaan RL, Williams EH, Ypey DL, Clapham DE. Intercellular coupling of embryonic heart cells. In: Pexieder T, ed. *Perspectives in Cardiovascular Research.* Vol. 5, *Mechanisms of Cardiac Morphogenesis and Teratogenesis.* New York, NY: Raven Press; 299–316, 1981.

DeMello WC. Increased spread of electrotonic potentials during diastolic depolarization in cardiac muscle. *J Mol Cell Cardiol* 18:23–29, 1986a.

DeMello WC. Interaction of cyclic AMP and Ca^{2+} in the control of electrical coupling in heart fibers. *Biochim Biophys Acta* 888:91–99, 1986b.

DeMello WC, van Loon P. Influence of cyclic nucleotides on junctional permeability in atrial muscle. *J Mol Cell Cardiol* 19:83–94, 1987.

Fozzard H. Conduction of the action potential. In: *Handbook of Physiology.* Vol.1, *The Heart.* Bethesda, MD: Am Physiol Soc; 335–356, 1979.

Fujii S, Ayer RK Jr, DeHaan RL. Development of the fast sodium current in early embryonic chick heart cells. *J Membr Biol* 101:209–233, 1988.

Gainer H St. C, Murray AW. Diacylglycerol inhibits gap junctional com-

munication in cultured epidermal cells: evidence for a role of protein kinase C. *Biochem Biophys Res Commun* 126:1109–1113, 1985.
Giaume C, Kado RT, Korn H. Voltage-clamp analysis of crayfish rectifying synapse. *J Physiol* 386:91–112, 1987.
Hall JE, Zampighi GE. Protein from purified lens junctions induces channels in planar lipid bilayers. In: Bennett MVL, Spray DC, eds, *Gap Junctions.* Cold Spring Harbor, NY: Cold Spring Harbor Lab; 177–189, 1985.
Harris AL, Spray DC, Bennett MVL. Kinetic properties of a voltage-dependent junctional conductance. *J Gen Physiol* 77:95–117, 1981.
Hofmann H. Interaction between normoxic and a hypoxic region of guinea pig and ferret papillary muscles. *Circ Res* 56:876–883, 1985.
Hunter M, Giebisch G. Multi-barrelled K-channels in renal tubules. *Nature* 327:522–524, 1987.
Imanaga I, Kameyama M, Irisawa H. Cell-to-cell diffusion of fluorescent dyes in paired ventricular cells. *Am J Physiol: Heart* 252:H223-H232, 1987.
Jalife J. Mutual entrainment and electrical coupling as mechanisms for synchronous firing of rabbit sino-atrial pacemaker cells. *J Physiol* 356:221–243, 1984.
Johnston MF, Simon SA, Ramon F. Interaction of anesthetics with electrical synapses. *Nature* 286:498–500, 1980.
Joyner RW, van Capelle FJL. Propagation through electrically coupled cells. How a small SA node drives a large atrium. *Biophys J* 50:1157–1164, 1987.
Joyner RW, Veenstra R, Rawling D, Chorro A. Propagation through electrically coupled cells: effects of a resistive barrier. *Biophys J* 45:1017–1025, 1984.
Kameyama M. Electrical coupling between ventricular paired cells isolated from guinea-pig heart. *J Physiol* 336:345–357, 1983.
Kleber AG, Janse MJ, Wilms-Schopmann FJG, Wilde AAM, Coronel R. Changes in conduction velocity during acute ischemia in ventricular myocardium of the isolated porcine heart. *Circ* 73:189–198, 1986.
Kleber AG, Riegger CB, Janse MJ Electrical uncoupling and increase of extracellular resistance after induction of ischemia in isolated, arterially perfused rabbit papillary muscle. *Circ Res* 61:271–279, 1987.
Komuro H, Hirota A, Yada T, et al. Effects of calcium on electrical propagation in early embryonic precontractile heart as revealed by multiple-site optical recordings of action potentials. *J Gen Physiol* 85:365, 1985.
Lee HC, Clusin WT. Cytosolic calcium staircase in cultured myocardial cells. *Circ Res* 61:934–939, 1987.
Loewenstein WR. Junctional intercellular communication: the cell-to-cell membrane channel. *Physiol Rev* 61:829–913, 1981.
Loewenstein WR. Regulation of cell-to-cell communication by phosphorylation. *Biochem Soc Symp* 50:43–58, 1985.
Loewenstein WR. The cell-to-cell channel of gap junctions. *Cell* 48:725–726, 1987.
Matsuda H, Saigusa A, Irisawa H. Ohmic conductance through the inwardly rectifying K channel and blocking by internal Mg^{2+}. *Nature* 325:156–159, 1987.

Maurer P, Weingart R. Cell pairs isolated from adult guinea pig and rat hearts: effects of $[Ca^{2+}]_i$ on nexal membrane resistance. *Pflug Arch* 409:394–402, 1987.

Metzger P, Weingart R. Electric current flow in cell pairs isolated from adult rat hearts. *J Physiol* (London) 366:177–195, 1985.

Moolenaar WH. Effects of growth factors on intracellular pH regulation. *Ann Rev Physiol* 48:363–376, 1986.

Nathan RD, DeHaan RL. Voltage clamp analysis of embryonic heart cell aggregates. *J Gen Physiol* 73:175–198, 1979.

Neyton J, Trautmann A. Acetylcholine modulation of the conductance of intercellular junctions between rat lacrimal gland cells. *J Physiol* (London) 377:283–295, 1986b.

Neyton J, Trautmann A. Physiological modulation of gap junction permeability. *J Exp Biol* 124:93–114, 1986a.

Noma A, Tsuboi N. Dependence of junctional conductance on proton, calcium and magnesium ions in cardiac paired cells of guinea-pig. *J Physiol* (London) 382:193–211, 1987.

Obaid AL, Socolar SL, Rose B. Cell-to-cell channels with two independently regulated gates in series: analysis of junctional conductance modulation by membrane potential, calcium, and pH. J. *Membr Biol* 73:69–89, 1983.

Paes de Carvalho A, Hoffman BF, Carvalho MP. Two components of the cardiac action potential. I. Voltage time course and the effects of acetylcholine on atrial and nodal cells of the rabbit heart. *J Gen Physiol* 54:607–635, 1969.

Page E, Manjunath CK. Communicating junctions between cardiac cells. In: Fozzard HA, et al., eds. *The Heart and Cardiovascular System.* New York, NY: Raven Press; 573–600, 1986.

Peracchia C. Calmodulin-like proteins and communicating junctions. Electrical uncoupling of crayfish septate axons is inhibited by the calmodulin inhibitor W7 and is not affected by cyclic nucleotides. *Pflug Arch* 408:379–385, 1987.

Peracchia C, Girsch SJ. An in vitro approach to cell coupling: permeability and gating of gap junction channels incorporated into liposomes. In: Bennett MVL, Spray DC, eds. *Gap Junctions.* Cold Spring Harbor, NY: Cold Spring Harbor Lab; 191–203, 1985.

Piwnica-Worms D, Jacob R, Horres RC, Lieberman M. Na/H exchange in cultured chick heart cells. pH_i regulation. *J Gen Physiol* 85:43–64, 1985.

Powell TD, Terrar A, Twist VW. Electrical properties of individual cells isolated from adult rat ventricular myocardium. *J Physiol* (London) 303:131–153, 1980.

Pressler ML. Intracellular pH and cell-to-cell transmission in sheep Purkinje fibers. *Biophys J* 55:53–65, 1989.

Ramon F, Zampighi GA, Rivera A. Control of junctional permeability. In: Bennett MVL, Spray DC, eds. *Gap Junctions.* Cold Spring Harbor, NY: Cold Spring Harbor Lab; 155–166, 1985.

Reverdin EC, Weingart R. Electrical properties of the gap junctional membrane studied in rat liver cell pairs. *Am J Physiol: Cell* 23:C226-C234, 1988.

Rook MB, Jongsma HJ, van Ginnekin ACG. Properties of single gap junction channels between isolated neonatal rat heart cells. *Am J Physiol: Heart* 255:H770-H782, 1988.

Rose B, Yada T, Loewenstein WR. Downregulation of cell-to-cell communication by the viral src gene is blocked by TMB-8 and recovery of communication is blocked by vanadate. *J Membr Biol* 94:129–142, 1986.

Saez JC, Spray DC, Nairn AC, Hertzberg EL, Greengard P, Bennett MVL. cAMP increases junctional conductance and stimulates phosphorylation of the 27-kDa principal gap junction polypeptide. *Proc Nat Acad Sci (USA)* 83:2473–2477, 1986.

Simpson I, Rose B, Loewenstein WR. Size limit of molecules permeating the junctional membrane channels. *Science* 195:294–296, 1977.

Somogyi R, Kolb HA. Cell-to-cell channel conductance during loss of gap junctional coupling in pairs of pancreatic acinar and chinese hamster ovary cells. *Pflug Arch*412:54–65, 1988.

Spray DC, Bennett MVL. Physiology and pharmacology of gap junctions. *Ann Rev Physiol* 47:281–303, 1985.

Spray DC, Campos de Carvalho A, Bennett MVL. Sensitivity of gap junctional conductance to H ions in amphibian embryonic cells is independent of voltage sensitivity. *Proc Nat Acad Sci (USA)* 83:3533–3536, 1986a.

Spray DC, Ginsberg RD, Morales EA, Gatmaitan Z, Arias IM. Electrophysiological properties of gap junctions between dissociated pairs of rat hepatocytes. *J Cell Biol* 103:135–144, 1986c.

Spray DC, Harris AL, Bennett MVL. Equilibrium properties of a voltage-dependent junctional conductance. *J Gen Physiol* 77:77–93, 1981.

Spray DC, Nerbonne J, Campos de Carvalho A, Harris AL, Bennett MVL. Substituted benzyl acetates: a new class of compounds that reduce gap junctional conductance by cytoplasmic acidification. *J Cell Biol* 99:174–179, 1984a.

Spray DC, Saez JC, Brosius D, Bennett MVL, Hertzberg EL. Isolated liver gap junctions: gating of transjunctional currents is similar to that in intact pairs of rat hepatocytes. *Proc Nat Acad Sci (USA)* 83:5494–5497, 1986b.

Spray DC, White RL, Campos de Carvalho A, Harris AL, Bennett MVL. Gating of gap junction channels. *Biophys J* 45:219–230, 1984b.

Spray DC, White RL, Mazet F, Bennett MVL. Regulation of gap junctional conductance. *Am J Physiol: Heart* 248:H753-H764, 1985a.

Spray DC, White RL, Verselis V, Bennett MVL. General and comparative physiology of gap junction channels. In: Bennett MVL, Spray DC, eds. *Gap Junctions*. Cold Spring Harbor, NY: Cold Spring Harbor Lab; 139–153, 1985b.

Sturkie PD. Heart: contraction, conduction and electrocardiography. In: Sturkie PD, ed. *Avian Physiology*. New York, NY: Springer-Verlag; 67–190, 1986.

Takeda A, Hashimoto E, Yamamura H, Shimazu T. Phosphorylation of liver gap junction protein by protein kinase C. *FEBS Letters* 210:169–172, 1987.

Veenstra RD, DeHaan RL. Cardiac gap junction channel activity in embryonic chick ventricle cells. *Am J Physiol: Heart* 254:H170-H180, 1988a.

Veenstra RD, DeHaan RL. Electrotonic interactions between aggregates of chick embryo cardiac pacemaker cells. *Am J Physiol: Heart* 250:H453-H463, 1986b.

Veenstra RD, DeHaan RL. Measurement of single channel currents from cardiac gap junctions. *Science* 233:972–974, 1986a.

Veenstra RD, DeHaan RL. Regulation of single channel activity in cardiac gap junctions. In: Cole WC, Sperelakis N, eds. *Cell Interactions and Gap Junctions*. Vol.II. Boca Raton, FL: CRC Press; 65–83, 1988b.

Verselis V, White RL, Spray DC, Bennett MVL. Gap junctional conductance and permeability are linearly related. *Science* 234:461–464, 1986.

Weingart R. Electrical properties of the nexal membrane studied in rat ventricular pairs. *J Physiol* 370:267–284, 1986.

Weingart R, Maurer P. Action potential transfer in cell pairs isolated from adult rat and guinea pig ventricles. *Circ Res* 63:72–80, 1988.

White RL, Spray DC, Campos de Carvalho A, Wittenberg BA, Bennett MVL. Some electrical properties of gap junctions between adult ventricular myocytes. *Am J Physiol: Cell* 249:C447-C455, 1985.

Wier WG, Cannell MB, Berlin JR, Marban E, Lederer WJ. Cellular and subcellular heterogeneity of $[Ca^{2+}]i$ in single heart cells revealed by Fura-2. *Science* 235:325–328, 1987.

Wittenberg BA, White RL, Ginzberg RD, Spray DC. Effect of calcium on the dissociation of the mature rat heart into individual and paired myocytes: electrical properties of cell pairs. *Circ Res* 59:143–150, 1986.

Wojtczak JA. Electrical uncoupling induced by general anesthetics: a calcium-independent process? In: Bennett MVL, Spray DC, eds. *Gap Junctions*. Cold Spring Harbor, NY: Cold Spring Harbor Lab; 13–22, 1985.

Yada T, Rose B, Loewenstein WR. Diacylglycerol downregulates junctional membrane permeability. *J Membr Biol* 88:217–232, 1985.

Young JD-E, Cohn ZA, Gilula NB. Functional assembly of gap junctional conductance in lipid bilayers: demonstration that the major 27 kd protein forms the junctional channel. *Cell* 48:733–743, 1987.

Chapter 3

Influence of Non-Homogeneous Tissue on Normal and Abnormal Conduction

Madison S. Spach
Paul C. Dolber
J. Francis Heidlage
C. Frank Starmer

In the past, mechanisms that influence the shape of the upstroke of the cardiac action potential have been attributed to differences in the membrane ionic properties (channels) that alter the magnitude of the depolarizing currents (Schmitt and Erlanger, 1928; Wiedmann, 1955). Several years ago, however, we presented evidence that the anisotropic passive properties of cardiac muscle have an independent role in determining the shape of the upstroke of propagating action potentials depending upon the direction of propagation with respect to the orientation of the fibers (Spach et al., 1981; 1982). Fast upstrokes were associated with slow conduction (in a direction transverse to the long cell axis) and slow upstrokes with fast conduction (in the direction of the long cell axis). The usual association of high velocity and high safety factor for propagation is reversed by this anisotropic mechanism: propagation at a low velocity (transverse) is more resistant to decreases in the membrane

Hondeghem, Luc (ed): Molecular and Cellular Mechanisms of Antiarrhythmic Agents, Futura Publishing Company, Inc., Mount Kisco, NY, © 1989.

ionic currents than is propagation at a higher velocity (longitudinal). Consequently, this new phenomenon represents a major digression from traditional mechanisms that cause differences in the shape of the upstroke, excitability, and the safety factor of the cardiac action potential.

To account for this previously unrecognized direction-dependent behavior of depolarization, we proposed the term *anisotropic discontinuous propagation* as a descriptor of the following general hypothesis: In addition to the classical influence of the membrane ionic properties on conduction, the anisotropic structural complexities have an independent role in determining the functional electrical properties of cardiac muscle. We further suggested that recurrent discontinuities of effective axial resistivity affect the membrane ionic currents during propagating depolarization in association with the changes in shape of the upstroke when the direction of propagation is altered (Spach et al., 1981). The occurrence of notches at the peak of the depolarization phase of action potentials when propagation occurs in the transverse direction suggests that propagation is discontinuous in that direction. Notches might be expected when the intracellular current has to pass through localized regions (cell junctions) of high resistance relative to the cytoplasm. Such junctions would separate active membrane into patches loosely coupled to each other during transverse propagation, each patch generating action potentials that would be more like membrane action potentials than those propagating at uniform velocity in a continuous structure.

The Problem

Thus far, however, computer simulations by ourselves and by others have failed to explain the above anisotropic behavior of the upstroke of the cardiac action potential. For example, a discretized one-dimensional cable has been used to represent the discrete pattern of electrical coupling between cells. This model uses a large spatial increment (i.e., large size for each isopotential patch of membrane) with a high value of internal resistance to increase dV/dt_{max} above that of a continuous cable (Joyner, 1982; Spach, 1983). Similar theoretical results are produced by a cable model of cylindrical cardiac cells interconnected by an intercalated disc structure (Diaz et al., 1983). Although dV/dt_{max} increases, the foot of the action potential is prolonged, just the opposite of the change observed experimentally. Thus, both discretization and a recurrent disc structure are quite incomplete models of anisotropic discontinuous propagation (Spach et al., 1987a). Another possible mechanism for the directional differences in the shape of the upstroke is that of directional differences in axial impedance, which could result from the presence of a capacitance in parallel with the internal resistance at the intercalated disc (Freygang and Trautwein, 1970). We performed simulations to determine the effect of differences in internal impedance versus a pure internal resistance by adding a capacitance in parallel with the resistance of the nexus: the added capacitance had no effect on the shape of the action potential (Spach and Dolber, 1989).

A two-dimensional model based on the distribution of cellular connections was proposed by Geselowitz and Miller (1982). They suggested that during transverse propagation "each cell will be excited by colliding waves moving in opposite directions along the cell axis" (thus increasing maximum dV/dt). Our simulations and experiments, however, failed to justify a model of collisions at a microscopic level. With a real collision, the foot of the upstroke does not change, and the shape of the phase-plane plot of dV_m/dt versus V_m of a collision does not fit that of an action potential measured during transverse propagation (Spach et al., 1987a). That is, during a collision the rate of rise of the upstroke does not increase until approximately the time of turn-on of the sodium current (Paes de Carvalho et al., 1982; Spach and Kootsey, 1985) whereas during transverse propagation the rate of rise increases from the onset of the foot.

The above evidence suggests that models based solely on the nonhomogeneous distribution of the cellular connections do not account for the anisotropic behavior of the upstroke of the cardiac action potential. We have found, however, by repeated computer simulations and experimental measurements of propagating action potentials that the direction-dependent upstroke shape differences behave as though there is a directional difference in the *effective* membrane capacitance.

Since the time course of the sodium conductance and the sodium current cannot be measured directly during a propagating action potential, we obtained simulation results to demonstrate theoretically how the different shapes of depolarization are associated with differences in the magnitude of the inward sodium current. These differences describe a relationship between the magnitude of the sodium current and dV/dt_{max} for multidimensional (anisotropic) propagation that is diametrically opposite to the classical relationship for one-dimensional homogeneous propagation where dV/dt_{max} decreases in association with a decrease in the magnitude of the sodium current in proportion to the square of the conduction velocity (Hodgkin and Katz, 1949).

This chapter reviews our experimental-theoretical evidence that illustrates the behavior of anisotropic propagation when the takeoff potential is changed and shows that a quite simplified cable model of directional differences in effective membrane capacitance, along with directional differences in effective axial resistivity, produces an excellent fit of the experimental data. A more extensive analysis is presented in recent publications (Spach et al., 1987b; 1988). Also, experimental evidence is presented that the same alterations in the available sodium conductance by early premature beats and by sodium channel-binding drugs result in different propagation responses depending on the anisotropic passive properties of the muscle bundle.

METHODS

Experiment

Atrial specimens were studied from human subjects whose ages varied between 1 and 72 years. These age ranges provided preparations with both uniform and nonuniform anisotropic electrical properties, dependent primarily on the age of the patient (Spach and Dolber, 1986). To make certain that the results had general applicability (i.e., they were not species specific), atrial and ventricular specimens from adult dogs were also studied.

Each specimen was rapidly pinned to the floor of a tissue bath (4 cm × 5 cm) and maintained at 35° C. The composition of the perfusate, in mM, was: NaCl, 128; KCl, 4.69; $MgSO_4$, 1.18; NaH_2PO_4, 0.41; $NaHCO_3$, 20.1; $CaCl_2$, 2.23; and dextrose 11.1. The solutions were gassed in a reservoir with a mixture of 95% O_2-5% CO_2 and perfused through a cannula to produce a very high flow rate. Particularly important experimental procedures involved: (1) the use of extracellular electrodes made of flexible tungsten wire, 50 μm in diameter, and insulated, except at the tip, to detect changes in the excitation sequence at the microscopic level; and (2) a dissecting microscope equipped with a Nikon F250 35-mm camera to document all recording positions. Separate reference electrodes for each extracellular and intracellular electrode were located 7 cm away from the recording area. To measure directional differences in the shape of the upstroke of premature action potentials, one stimulus electrode was positioned to produce propagation in the longitudinal direction and another to produce transverse propagation at the microelectrode impalement site.

A pacemaker stimulus of 1.0 msec in duration and 1.5 times threshold was applied to the endocardial surface of each muscle bundle at a basic cycle length varying between 250 and 1000 msec. A PDP-11/44 computer system controlled the rate and synchronized the stimuli with the data recording. The computer stored the data and displayed the waveforms concurrently on a display unit with a persistent screen. After each experiment, appropriate waveforms were selected and transferred to a HP-9000 computer for automatic plotting of the waveforms and their derivatives, as well as for constructing digital phase-plane plots (Jenerick, 1963). The transmembranc potential V_m was calculated by subtracting the extracellular potential from the intracellular potential as described previously (Spach et al., 1981).

Theory

The goal of the theoretical analysis was to determine if a simplified cable model based on differences in the membrane capacitance could predict the observed directionally-dependent shape of the upstroke in response to modification of the sodium conductance by changing the hold (takeoff) potential. For the purpose of this study, the model does not include the details of discontinuities of resistance that produce notches at the peak of the upstroke during transverse propagation (Spach et al., 1981); rather, it represents an averaged description of the tissue.

The problem was simplified by using a single transient sodium current mechanism with the equivalent electrical circuit of a continuous cable. As noted in a recent analysis (Spach and Dolber, 1986), models in the form of the Hodgkin-Huxley equations for the macroscopic sodium current (Hodgkin and Huxley, 1952) were considered most appropriate because of the small time-scale they describe and fit. The Ebihara-Johnson description of the fast sodium current was used because it is based on voltage clamp data in cardiac muscle under normal conditions (Ebihara and Johnson, 1980).

For one-dimensional propagation along a uniform structure, the time course of V_m is governed by the cable equation:

$$I_m = (a/2R_i)(\partial^2 v_m/\partial x^2) = c_m \partial v_m/\partial t + I_{ion}, \quad [1]$$

where a is the radius of the cylinder (in cm), R_i is the internal resistivity (Ohm-cm), and C_m is the specific membrane capacitance ($\mu F/cm^2$). The ionic current I_{ion} ($\mu A/cm^2$) during the depolarization phase of the action potential was approximated by the fast transient sodium current in parallel with a leakage (repolarizing) current:

$$I_{ion} = g_{Na}(v_m - v_{Na}) + g_L(v_m - v_L), \quad [2]$$

where g_{Na} is the sodium conductance (mS/cm^2), g_L is the leakage conductance (mS/cm^2), and V_{Na} and V_L are the sodium and leak equilibrium potentials respectively.

The sodium conductance g_{Na} per unit area was given by:

$$g_{Na} = G_{Na}\, m^3 h, \quad [3]$$

where G_{Na} is the maximum sodium conductance and the dimensionless activation and inactivation variables m and h were assumed to follow the kinetics described by Ebihara and Johnson (1980).

For the results to be presented here, a value of 33.4 mV was chosen for V_{Na}. There were no qualitative differences in the results when V_{Na} was varied from 25 mV–76 mV, a range consistent with observations following changes in internal sodium concentration in ventricular muscle (Glitsch et al., 1970) and in Purkinje fibers (Fozzard and Wasserman, 1985). g_L was maintained constant at 0.05 mS/cm^2 and V_L was adjusted to each value of the resting potential; i.e., the leakage current was zero at the hold potential. To mimic early premature action potentials, G_{Na} was maintained constant at a value of 35 mS/cm^2 and the hold potential was varied between −80 mV and −50 mV.

To evaluate the effects of differences in membrane capacitance, a membrane capacitance of 1.0 $\mu F/cm^2$ and an internal resistivity of 190 Ohm-cm were used in a continuous cable to represent the longitudinal direction. Another cable with values of 0.5 $\mu F/cm^2$ and 4990 Ohm-cm for C_m and R_i respectively were used to represent the transverse direction. The longitudinal R_i value was selected from experimental results available from other species and preparations

(Weidmann, 1952; Lieberman et al., 1975). There is no appropriate model to base an extraction of R_i values in the transverse direction; therefore, transverse R_i values were selected to produce the appropriate low conduction velocities in that direction (Clerc, 1976; Spach et al., 1979).

Equation 1 was solved numerically for a cylinder with a length of 3.6 mm (greater than 15 resting space constants) and a radius of 5 μm (approximate to a cell diameter). The time course of V_m, g_{Na}, I_{Na}, as well as the conduction velocity, were computed at the midpoint of the cable where there was uniform conduction (i.e., no end effects). The ordinary differential equations for m and h were solved by the predictor-corrector or modified Euler method (e.g., Gerald, 1970) with a time increment of 2 μsec. Equation 1 (the cable equation) was solved by the Crank-Nicolson implicit method (1947) using a length increment (Δx) of 0.014 resting space constants (Spach and Kootsey, 1985).

The total sodium conductance and the total sodium current were obtained from the areas of the curves by numerical integration. Phase-plane graphs were made of dV_m/dt versus V_m and the trajectorics of g_{Na} and I_{Na} were plotted as a function of V_m.

RESULTS

To facilitate comparison of the initial experimental and theoretical results for altering the available sodium conductance (Cohen et al., 1984) by changing the takeoff potential, typical changes in the experimentally measured upstrokes are presented with the corresponding simulation results for two theoretical cables. One was assigned a C_m value of 1 $\mu F/cm^2$ to mimic longitudinal propagation (C_m1) and the other a C_m value of 0.5 $\mu F/cm^2$ to mimic transverse propagation ($C_m.5$).

The experimental results presented here were obtained from human preparations; no species differences were found. Also, the changes in the shape of the upstroke were similar in both uniform and nonuniform anisotropic atrial preparations. The terms *uniform* and *nonuniform* anisotropic properties are used in the context of our past descriptions for propagation at a microscopic level (Spach and Dolber, 1985; 1986). In uniform anisotropic cardiac muscle there is tight electrical coupling between groups of fibers in all directions; the advancing wavefront of propagation in a direction transverse to the long axis of the fibers is smooth and the associated extracellular potential waveforms are also smooth. In the nonuniform anisotropic type, we have presented further evidence that there is tight electrical coupling between cells in the longitudinal direction. However, transversely there are areas in which there is absence of side-to-side electrical coupling of adjacent groups of parallel fibers; here propagation transverse to the long fiber axis is interrupted such that adjacent groups of fibers are excited in a markedly irregular sequence that results in extracellular depolarization waveforms that are polyphasic with multiple small deflections (Spach and Dolber, 1986).

Uniform anisotropic properties characterized atrial preparations from patients less than 29 years old, and the preparations from patients between 43 and 68 years of age all demonstrated nonuniform anisotropic properties. The lowest takeoff potential (least negative value) that produced a propagated response was −63 mV. Thus, we considered the mechanism of depolarization of the most rapid component of all action potentials to be the fast sodium current. *TP* is used to mean propagation in the direction along an axis transverse to the long axis of the fibers and *LP* is used to mean propagation along the longitudinal axis of the fibers.

Anisotropic Differences in the Shape of the Upstroke of the Action Potential and the Associated Effects on g_{Na} and I_{Na}

Figure 1A shows a typical experimental result from a single cell impalement during longitudinal and transverse propagation. The rate of rise and amplitude of the upstroke were greater during transverse propagation than during longitudinal propagation, as expected (Spach et al., 1981). Also, initial repolarization was more rapid with transverse propagation in association with the larger amplitude of the upstroke (panel A1). The phase-plane plots of the measured upstrokes (panel A3) show that the slope of the initial trajectory of dV_m/dt was greater with transverse than with longitudinal propagation; that is, the rate of the rise of the foot of the action potential was greater with transverse than with longitudinal propagation. An initial linear trajectory of the phase-plane plot (dashed lines in panel A3) indicates an exponential process (Jenerick, 1963). However, in most preparations there were small devia-

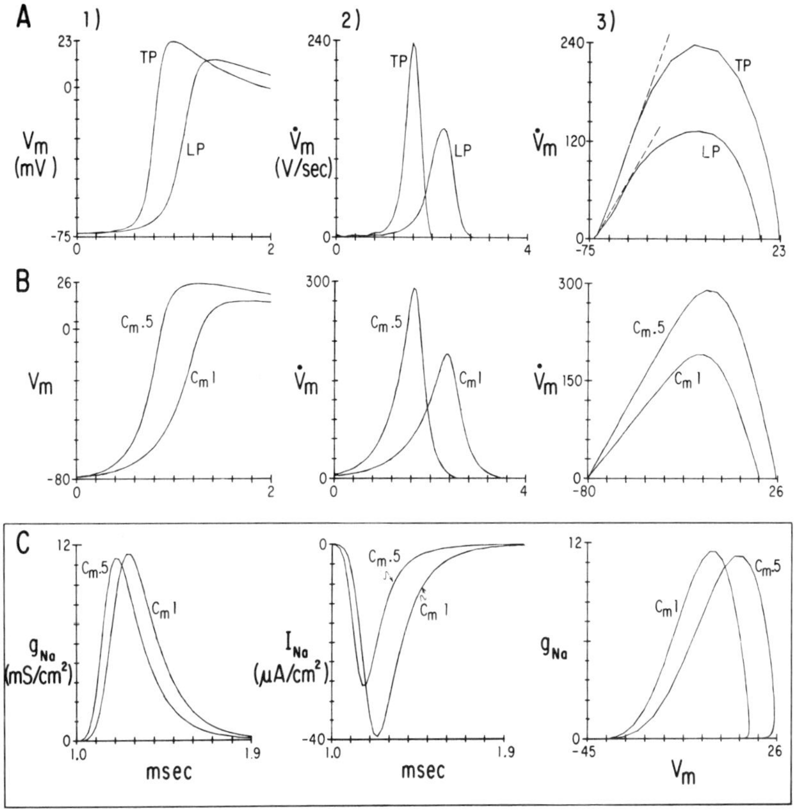

Figure 1. (A) Typical experimentally measured upstrokes of V_m during longitudinal and transverse propagation; (B) computed upstrokes for two theoretical cables which were identical except for different membrane capacitances of 1 and 0.5 $\mu F/cm^2$; (C) influence of the different shapes of the upstroke on the sodium conductance and sodium current. In A and B, the time course of V_m is shown in column 1 and of dV_m/dt in column 2, and phase-plane plots of dV_m/dt vs. V_m are shown in column 3. LP = longitudinal propagation; TP = transverse propagation. In C, columns 1 and 2 show the time course of the sodium conductance and sodium current, and the trajectory of g_{Na} as a function of V_m is shown in column 3. The action potentials in A were measured in an atrial bundle from a 49-year-old subject. (Reproduced from *Circ Res* 60:206–219, (1987), by permission of the American Heart Association, Inc.)

tions (concavity up) from a straight line during longitudinal propagation (see LP in Figure 1A3). During transverse propagation small deviations were occasionally found but the initial phase plane trajectory was characteristically a straight line. As yet, we have no simulation result to provide a mechanism for this deviation from an exponential rise of the foot, a deviation we have measured frequently during longitudinal propagation in ventricular and atrial muscle but not in Purkinje fibers. Its significance is that there is no uniform continuous propagation of the upstroke during longitudinal propagation, indicating that discontinuities exist along the long axis of the fibers in some bundles.

The simulation results for the upstrokes and the associated time course of the sodium conductance and sodium current are shown in panels B and C of Figure 1. The experimental directional difference of τ_{foot}, dV/dt_{max}, V_{amp}, and the initial phase of repolarization were reproduced by the computed action potentials of the two theoretical cables with different values of the membrane capacitance (Fig. 1B). The more rapid initial repolarization of cable $C_m.5$ was due to the greater repolarization current I_R that occurred with the more positive peak of the upstroke. That is, $(V_m - V_L)$ was greater during initial repolarization when the maximum value of the upstroke was more positive.

Figure 1C shows the influence of the different shapes of the upstroke on g_{Na} and I_{Na}, variables that are not measurable in a propagated action potential. Although the peak values of g_{Na} were almost the same, the area of the g_{Na} curve was 16% greater for the slower upstroke (C_m1 in panel C1). Also, in shifting from cable C_m1 to cable $C_m.5$, the increase in dV/dt_{max} was associated with a *decrease* in peak I_{Na} (↓ 27%) and in the area of the I_{Na} curve (↓ 44%), (panel C2). This relationship between the sodium current and dV/dt_{max} is diametrically opposite of the classical one; i.e., decreases in the sodium current are generally considered to be associated with decreases in dV/dt_{max} (Weidmann, 1955), such as occur with ischemia, drugs, and premature beats.

The phase-plane plots of dV_m/dt versus V_m (Fig. 1, A3 and B3) and the trajectory of g_{Na} as a function of V_m (panel C3) provide insight to the mechanism of the differences in the time-course of the internal membrane variables. The major difference was that the total electrical load in cable C_m1 was greater than in cable $C_m.5$. That is, the sodium current in cable C_m1 had to discharge a greater local as well as a greater downstream capacitance through local circuit currents (electrotonus). Thereby, the area of the I_{Na} curve serves as an index of the total capacitance (local and downstream) discharged by the sodium current (Spach and Kootsey, 1985). Panel C3 shows that although the maximum values achieved by g_{Na} were nearly the same for the two upstrokes, the difference between V_{Na} and V_m for any given value of g_{Na} was less with the more rapid rise of the upstroke (cable C_m.5). Because the instantaneous magnitude of I_{Na} (equation 2) is determined by the product of g_{Na} and (V_m − V_{Na}), the considerable decrease in peak I_{Na} and in the total sodium current was due largely to the decrease in the driving force for the sodium current during the more rapid upstroke.

Anisotropic Response of the Shape of the Upstroke to Changes in the Takeoff Potential

Typical anisotropic changes in dV/dt_{max} due to changes in the takeoff potential are shown in Figure 2A for premature action potentials. The results in the figure are presented to show different comparisons (the original measured and computed values for LP and TP, normalized curves, and ratios to emphasize conditions where the directional differences are most important). At all takeoff potentials, dV/dt_{max} was greater with transverse propagation than with longitudinal propagation. As the takeoff potential became less negative, the normalized values of dV/dt_{max} decreased slightly more with longitudinal than with transverse propagation (Fig. 2A2). Large changes in the takeoff potential produced small changes in the dV/dt_{max} TP/LP ratio at takeoff potentials more negative than −74 mV. However, small positive shifts of the takeoff potential at less negative values produced large increases in the dV/dt_{max} TP/LP ratio, and the increases became more pronounced as the takeoff potential approached the value at which propagation ceased (Fig. 2A3). The least negative takeoff potential that produced longitudinal propagation was −65 mV; however, transverse propagation continued at takeoff potentials between −64 and −63 mV in the absence of propagation in the longitudinal direction (Fig. 2A1) in the preparations with nonuniform anisotropic properties.

The simulation results (Fig. 2B) reproduced all of the features of the experimentally measured directional differences in dV/dt_{max} discussed previously: (1) dV/dt_{max} was greater in cable C_m.5 than in cable C_m1 at all takeoff potentials. (2) The decrease in the normal-

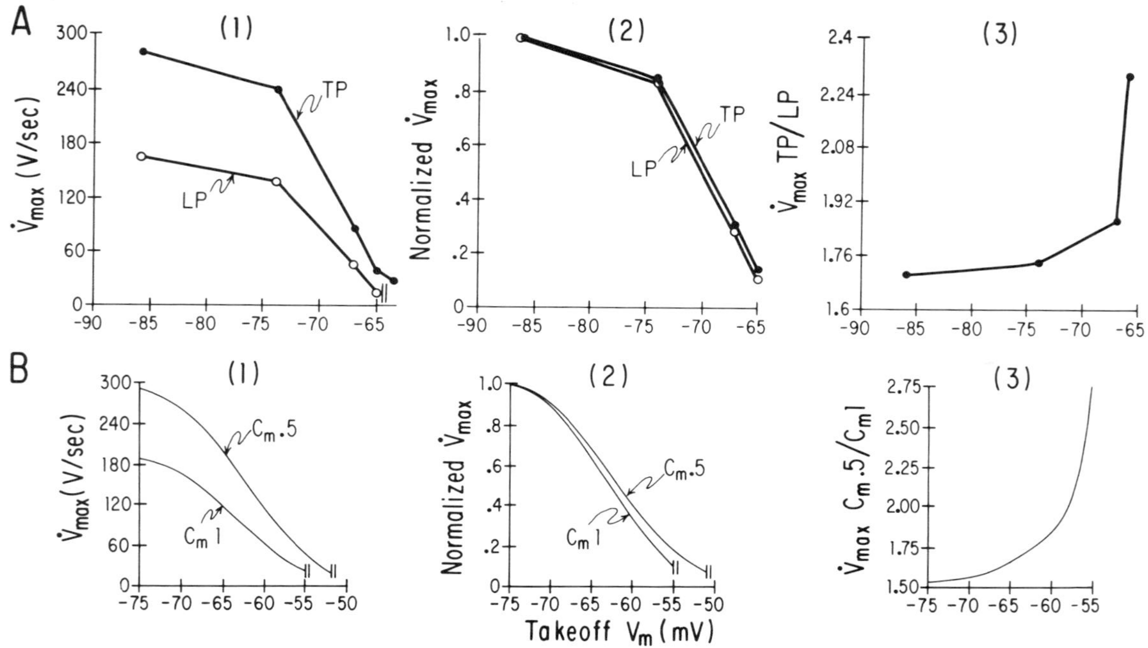

Figure 2. Anisotropic changes in dV/dt_{max} secondary to changes in the takeoff potential: Experimental results (A) with corresponding theoretical predictions based on directional differences in C_m (B). Panel A shows the effects of changes in the takeoff potential on the absolute (1) and normalized (2) values of dV/dt_{max} during longitudinal and transverse propagation, as well as the effect on the ratio of the dV/dt_{max} values (3). The experimental results were obtained in an atrial preparation from a 43-year-old subject. Panel B shows the theoretically predicted changes in dV/dt_{max} as a function of the takeoff potential in the two cables with different values of C_m (changing R_i had no effect on dV/dt_{max}). (Reproduced from *Circ Res* 60:206–219, (1987), by permission of the American Heart Association, Inc.)

ized values of dV/dt_{max} was greater in the cable with the inherently slower upstroke (C_m1 in Fig. 2B2). (3) The slope of the curve of the dV/dt_{max} $C_m.5/C_m1$ ratio versus takeoff potential was small between -75 and -65 mV, becoming quite steep at -55 mV. (4) Propagation did not occur in cable C_m1 at takeoff potentials less negative than -55 mV, but stable propagation continued in cable $C_m.5$ at more positive takeoff potentials. In the theoretical curves, the takeoff potential was 10–12 mV more positive than in the experimental data. This likely reflects a shift in the voltage dependence of the kinetic parameters of the membrane model from the preparation in which they were originally measured (cultured chick embryonic heart cells; Ebihara and Johnson, 1980).

Figure 3 shows a similar experimental-theoretical test of the time constant of the foot of the upstroke for the same action potentials analyzed in Figure 2. At all takeoff potentials the time constant of the foot was greater with longitudinal than transverse propagation (Fig. 3A1). At values more negative than -74 mV, large changes in the takeoff potential produced little change in the normalized values of τ_{foot} and in the τ_{foot} LP/TP ratio. However, at takeoff potentials less negative than -74 mV, small positive shifts in the takeoff potential produced greater increases in the normalized values of τ_{foot} with longitudinal propagation than with transverse propagation (panel A2). Further, the τ_{foot} LP/TP ratio increased progressively as the takeoff potential approached the value at which propagation failed (panel A3).

The fit of experimental results by the computed values of τ_{foot} are shown in Figure 3B. (1) At all takeoff potentials τ_{foot} was greater in the cable with the greater membrane capacitance. (2) The relative values of τ_{foot} of the action potentials of either theoretical cable demonstrated little change in response to large changes in the takeoff potential at values more negative than -65 mV. (3) The slope of the τ_{foot} $C_m1/C_m.5$ ratio versus takeoff potential increased at more positive takeoff potentials, becoming quite steep as the takeoff potential approached the value at which propagation failed.

Figure 4 shows a final test of the simplified model of directional differences of C_m for the amplitude of the upstroke of premature action potentials. At all takeoff potentials the amplitude was greater with transverse propagation than with longitudinal propagation (panel A1). As the takeoff potential became more positive the normalized values of V_{amp} decreased more with longitudinal than with transverse propagation. As occurred with dV/dt_{max} and τ_{foot}, large

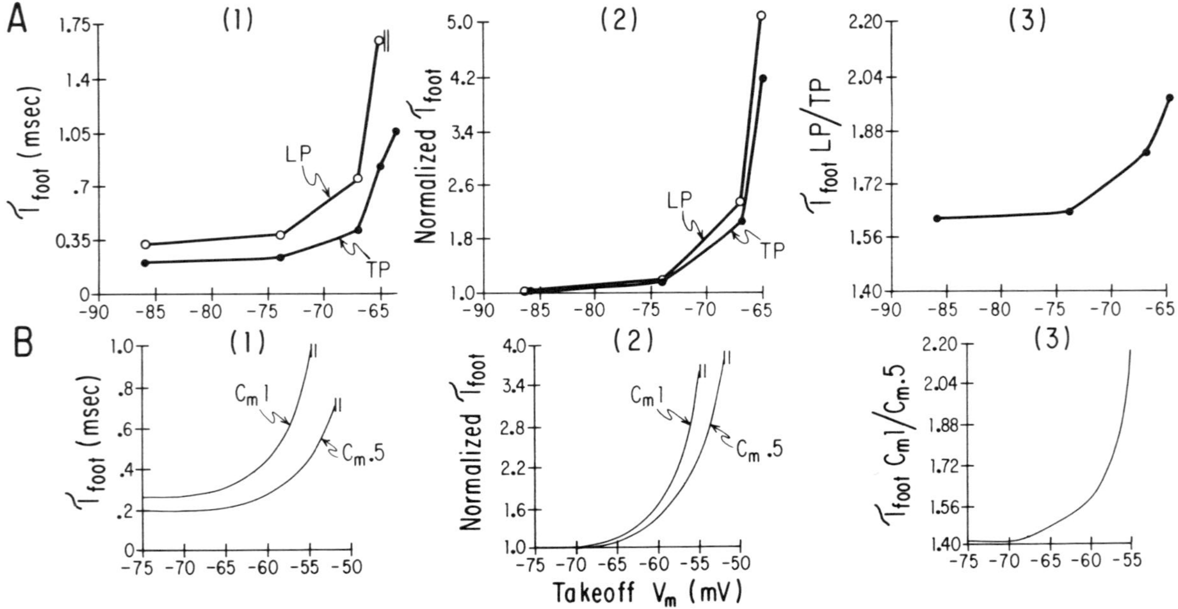

Figure 3. Directionally different effects of altering the takeoff potential on the foot of the action potential. Panel A shows the experimental results during longitudinal and transverse propagation with the absolute (1) and normalized (2) values of the time constant of the foot, along with the ratio of the τ_{foot} values (3). The τ_{foot} values were measured from the action potentials analyzed in Figure 2. Panel B shows the computed changes in τ_{foot} as a function of the takeoff potential in the two theoretical cables with different values of C_m. (Reproduced from *Circ Res* 60:206–219, (1987), by permission of the American Heart Association, Inc.)

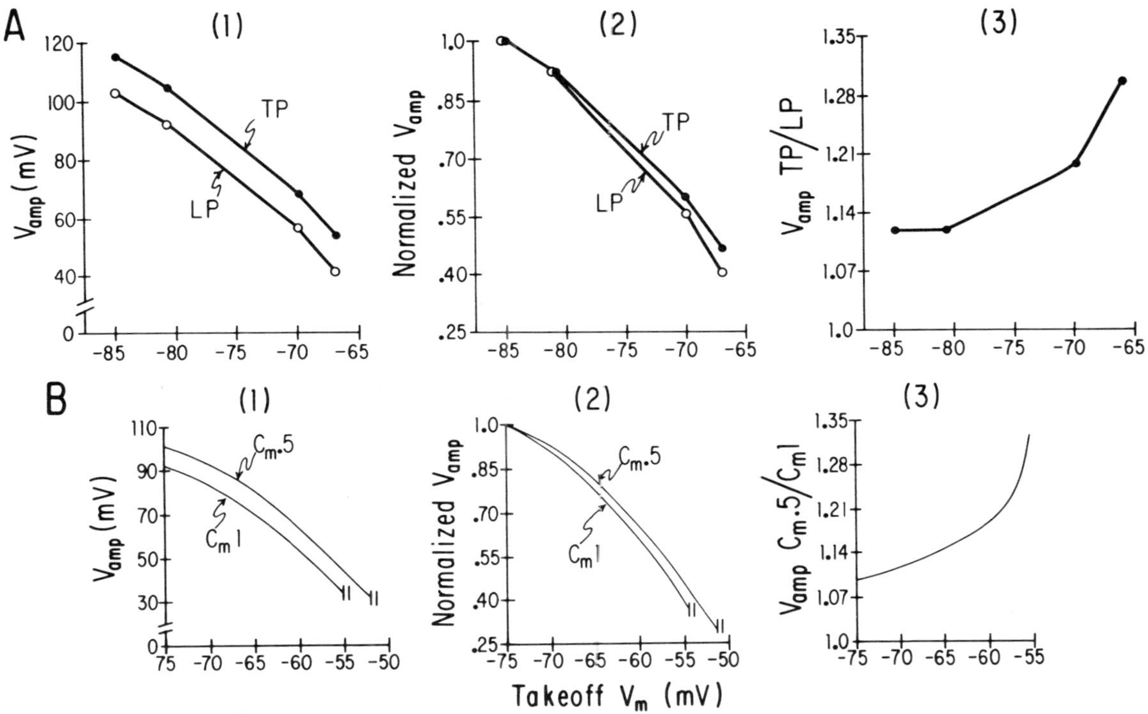

Figure 4. Anisotropic differences in the amplitude of the upstroke as a function of the takeoff potential. The experimental results obtained during longitudinal and transverse propagation in an atrial preparation with uniform anisotropic properties from a two-year-old subject are shown in Panel A with the absolute (1) and normalized (2) values of the amplitude (V_{amp}), plus the ratio of the V_{amp} values (3). Panel B shows the computed changes in V_{amp} as a function of the takeoff potential in the two theoretical cables with different values of C_m. (Reproduced from *Circ Res* 60:206–219, (1987), by permission of the American Heart Association, Inc.)

shifts in the takeoff potential at more negative values produced little change in the relative difference in the V_{amp} values. At less negative values, however, the V_{amp} TP/LP ratio increased progressively at more positive takeoff potentials (Fig. 4A3). In this preparation, which was characterized by uniform anisotropic properties, longitudinal and transverse propagation failed at the same takeoff potential (−67 mV); i.e., there was no unidirectional longitudinal propagation failure as occurred in the nonuniform anisotropic preparations.

The fit of the simulation results of the experimentally measured changes in V_{amp} is shown in Figure 4B: (1) At all takeoff potentials the amplitude of the upstroke was less in the action potential with the inherently slower upstroke (C_m1 in Fig. 4B1). (2) A given shift of the takeoff potential to a more positive value produced a greater decrease in the normalized values of V_{amp} of the action potential with the slower upstroke (C_m1 in Fig. 4B2). (3) The slope of the relationship between the V_{amp} $C_m.5/C_m1$ ratio and the takeoff potential increased with more positive takeoff potentials, again becoming quite steep as the takeoff potential approached the value at which propagation failed.

Influence of the Passive Anisotropic Properties on the Propagation Response to Modification of the Sodium Conductance

The above evidence indicates that the passive anisotropic properties of cardiac muscle bundles have significant effects on the shape of the upstroke of the action potential and, in turn, the directional differences in shape are associated with differences in the kinetics of the membrane ionic channels and the ionic currents for the same available sodium conductance at different takeoff potentials. This suggests that any complete theory of cardiac conduction disturbances leading to re-entry, as well as drug action on reentrant arrhythmias, should include the anisotropic passive properties of cardiac muscle. At present, however, the fundamental limitation to the development of such a model is that there is practically no information available about the role of anisotropy as an independent influence on excitability and the safety factor of propagation. We therefore investigated the effects of modifying the sodium conductance in preparations with uniform versus nonuniform anisotropic properties. Premature action potentials were used as before to alter the takeoff potential and quinidine gluconate (10 mg/L) was used to produce use-dependent blockade of the sodium channels.

Progressive shortening of the premature interval produced different types of propagation responses dependent upon the presence of uniform versus nonuniform anisotropic properties of the individual muscle bundles. Figure 5A shows a typical result in a young uniform anisotropic bundle with the pattern of excitation spread and the extracellular waveforms of normal action potentials on the left and early extrasystoles on the right. As the premature interval was shortened, the extracellular waveforms maintained the same general shape with a smooth contour; however, the peak-to-peak amplitude decreased relatively more with longitudinal than transverse propagation. The conduction velocity of premature action potentials also decreased relatively more in the longitudinal than in the transverse direction, producing isochrones with a blunted shape (Figure 5A, 345 msec). The shape and the smooth contour of the extracellular waveforms indicated that the propagation of premature action potentials continued in all directions at a microscopic level as a spatially smooth process with near-synchronous firing of adjacent groups of fibers.

In the older, nonuniform anisotropic bundles, however, premature action potentials produced two types of propagation response involving an abnormality of longitudinal conduction that did not occur in uniform anisotropic bundles. In the first type, progressive shortening of the premature interval resulted in the abrupt occurrence of unidirectional decremental conduction to block in the longitudinal direction (Figure 5B1, positions 3 and 4, 327 msec). When the premature interval was decreased further, slow transverse propagation continued in the absence of longitudinal propagation until the absolute refractory period was reached. This result is consistent with the results of Figures 2 and 3, which show that unidirectional propagation failure can occur at a single low take-off potential if there are directional differences in the effective membrane capacitance.

With the second type of response in the nonuniform anisotropic older bundles, shortening of the premature interval produced drastic changes in the sequence of excitation spread along the long axis of the fibers. The large smooth biphasic deflection of the extracellular waveform of longitudinal propagation suddenly changed to a complex waveform with numerous small deflections that occurred dur-

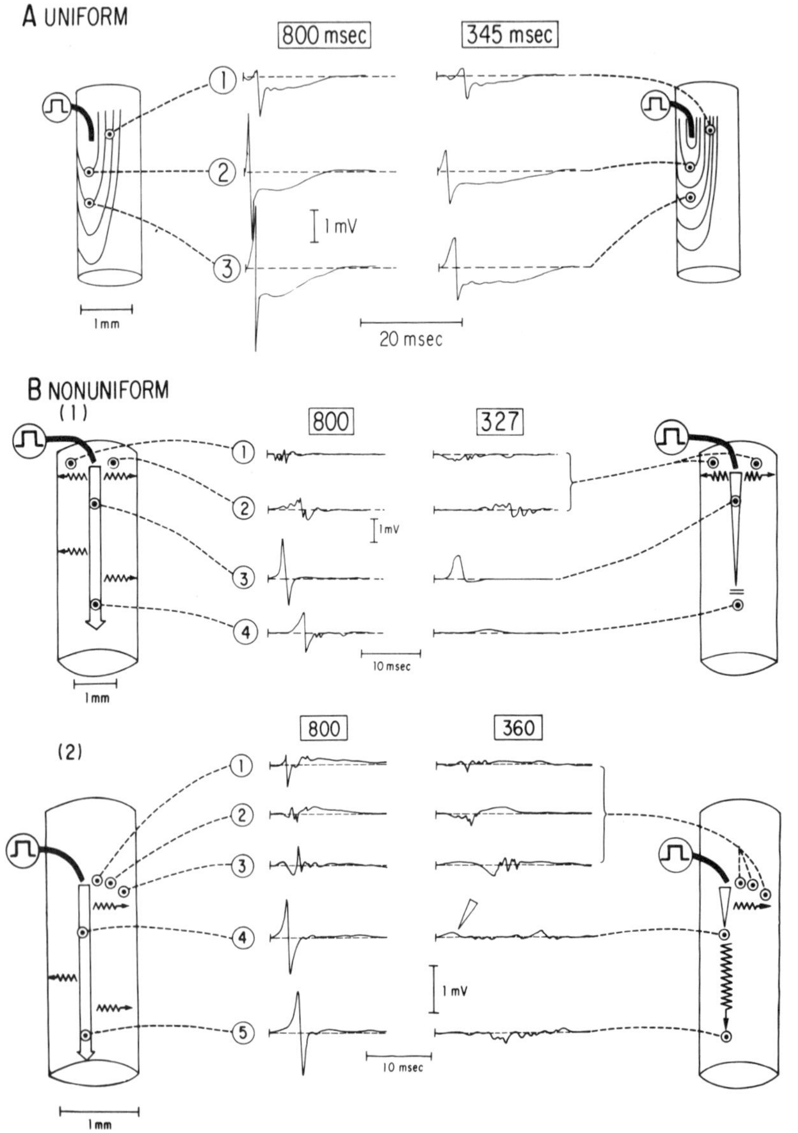

Figure 5. Propagation of normal and premature action potentials in bundles with uniform (A) and nonuniform (B) anisotropic properties. In each panel, the excitation sequence and selected extracellular waveforms are shown for normal (left) and early premature beats. The interstimulus interval in msec is shown within the boxes above each group of waveforms. Panel A: The

(*continued on next page*)

ing an interval of 15—40 msec (Figure 5B2, positions 4 and 5). Within the narrow 100 μm to 200 μm zone of longitudinal conduction intracellular-extracellular microelectrode measurements at multiple sites confirmed that there was asynchronous firing of adjacent groups of parallel-oriented fibers as depolarization of early premature action potentials progressed longitudinally in a *zigzag* manner along the long axis of the bundle. With normal action potentials there was synchronous excitation at sites along an axis perpendicular to the long axis of the fibers (time difference of dV/dt_{max}: 0–0.4 msec). On the other hand, early premature action potentials produced during the same impalements resulted in marked differences in the time of depolarization at sites only 10 μm to 50 μm apart (time difference of dV/dt_{max}: 3–15 msec). Also, different premature intervals produced different durations and shapes of the complex polyphasic extracellular waveforms, an indication of changes in the complex pattern of excitation spread at a microscopic level for different magnitudes of the depolarizing sodium current. Despite the marked changes in longitudinal propagation produced by early premature action potentials, stable conduction continued in the transverse direction with much less change from normal (Figure 5B2, positions 1–3).

This new type of dissociated *zigzag* longitudinal propagation (LP-dz) was not species specific; we subsequently encountered it frequently in nonuniform anisotropic canine atrial bundles. Also, it was not due to a large magnitude of the stimulus current (as we were able to demonstrate by strength-interval curves in dog atrial muscle bundles), rather the dissociated *zigzag* longitudinal conduction was due to the decrease in takeoff potential during the relative refractory period (Spach et al., 1988).

(*Figure 5 cont.*)
bundle was from a 12-year-old subject. The isochrones represent a time difference of 1 msec. Panel B: The excitation sequences were so complex that it was not possible to construct isochrones. In the normal sequences, the elongated open arrow represents the narrow region of fast conduction along the longitudinal axis of the fibers; the *saw-tooth* curves indicate an irregular course of excitation spread. On the right, the elongated triangles represent decremental conduction. The bundle in Panel B1 was from a 64-year-old subject and the bundle in Panel B2 was from a 52-year-old subject. (Reproduced from *Circ Res* 62: 811–832, (1988), by permission of the American Heart Association, Inc.)

Effects of Quinidine on Multidimensional Propagation in Preparations with Different Anisotropic Properties

Drug Effects Common to Uniform and Nonuniform Anisotropic Bundles

Classical Wenckebach cycles developed in bundles exposed to quinidine in preparations with either uniform or nonuniform anisotropic properties. A typical experimental result is shown for a uniform anisotropic bundle (dog papillary muscle) in Figure 6. Considerable use-dependent drug block of the sodium channels was produced initially by stimulating the preparation at a frequency of 100/min during exposure to quinidine gluconate (10 mg/L), which was associated with a decrease in dV/dt_{max} from 133 V/sec to 72 V/sec during longitudinal propagation. Repeated Wenckebach cycles developed with propagation failure (dropped beat) every 5th stimulus when the stimulus frequency was increased from 100/min to 120/min. In Figure 6A, the action potential with the earliest excitation time followed the dropped beat, and the next 3 action potentials occurred at progressively later times with prolongation in the local excitation times of LP and TP being greatest with the second beat. The increment of delay was progressively less for each subsequent action potential until propagation failure occurred simultaneously in all directions (classical Wenckebach cycles).

Wenckebach periodicity also characterized dV/dt_{max} of the transmembrane potential as well as the maximum negative derivative of the extracellular potential waveform during longitudinal and transverse propagation (Fig. 6). For each of these variables, the maximum value of each of the derivatives occurred with the first beat after the pause of the dropped beat, the greatest decrease occurred with the second beat, and the subsequent decreases in magnitude occurred with less decrement until propagation failed. The recurrent Wenckebach cycles disappeared immediately when the stimulus frequency was returned to the original lower value of 100/min, and recurred when the stimulus frequency was increased back to 120/min. The normal rest potential showed no change during quinidine exposure, as previously demonstrated by Hondeghem and Katzung (1980), even with drug blockade to the point of propagation failure (Figure 6A).

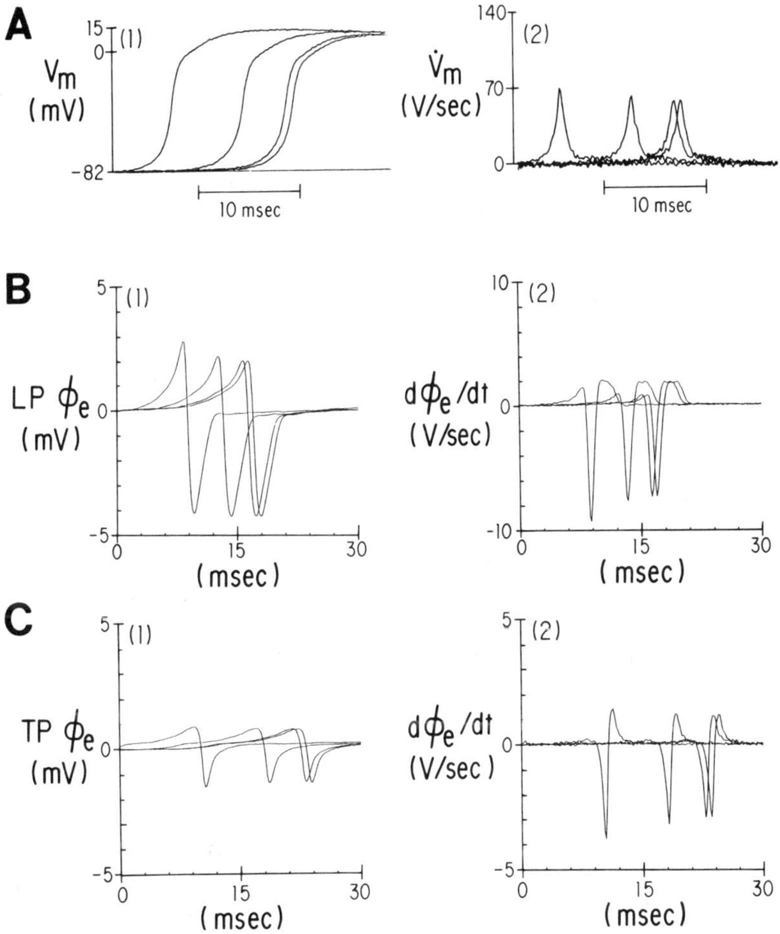

Figure 6. Quinidine-induced Wenckebach periodicity of anisotropic conduction. V_m during longitudinal propagation (A) and the extracellular potential waveforms during longitudinal (B) and transverse (C) propagation (LP ϕ_e and TP ϕ_e, respectively) were measured in dog papillary muscle (uniform anisotropic properties). The results were obtained at a stimulus rate of 120/min during exposure to quinidine gluconate 10 mg/L. (Reproduced from *Circ Res* 62: 811–832, (1988), by permission of the American Heart Association, Inc.)

Drug Effects Dependent on the Anisotropic Passive Properties

With progressive drug blockade in the uniform anisotropic bundles, the extracellular waveforms and their derivatives decreased in amplitude but maintained the same general shape and a smooth contour up to the point of simultaneous propagation failure in all directions (Figure 6). This response was the same as that produced by premature action potentials in the uniform anisotropic bundles; i.e., propagation continued as a spatially smooth process in all directions without changes in the sequence of excitation spread (cf. Figure 5A). However, when the older, nonuniform anisotropic bundles were exposed to quinidine, dissociated *zigzag* longitudinal propagation developed, just as occurred with premature action potentials (Figure 5B2).

Figure 7A shows the use-dependent effects of quinidine gluconate (10 mg/L) on the longitudinal conduction velocity and the associated extracellular waveforms in a nonuniform anisotropic preparation. At a stimulus frequency of 75/min, quinidine produced a steady-state longitudinal velocity of 0.25 m/sec. Following an increase in frequency to 85/min (arrow in Figure 7A), the velocity decreased exponentially with time. The velocity decrease was associated with a decrease in the magnitude of the extracellular waveform and its derivative, both of which changed from a single large biphasic smooth deflection to a fragmented waveform with an increasing number of small deflections typical of dissociated *zigzag* longitudinal propagation.

After 2 minutes at the higher stimulus rate of 85/min (basic cycle length of 700 msec), recurrent Wenckebach cycles developed with successive beat-to-beat changes from regular to dissociated *zigzag* longitudinal propagation as the velocity decreased with each beat up to the point of propagation failure (Fig. 7B). After the pause produced by the dropped beat, the initial action potential of the next Wenckebach cycle was associated with a submaximal increase in velocity (still with fragmented waveforms). The largest biphasic extracellular waveform of smooth contour and maximum velocity occurred with the second beat of the series, following which an approximately exponential decay in velocity occurred with progressive fragmentation and loss of amplitude of the extracellular waveforms (Figure 7B). The failure of the maximum velocity and amplitude of the extracellular waveform to occur immediately after the pause suggests that the drug process affecting the propagation sequence

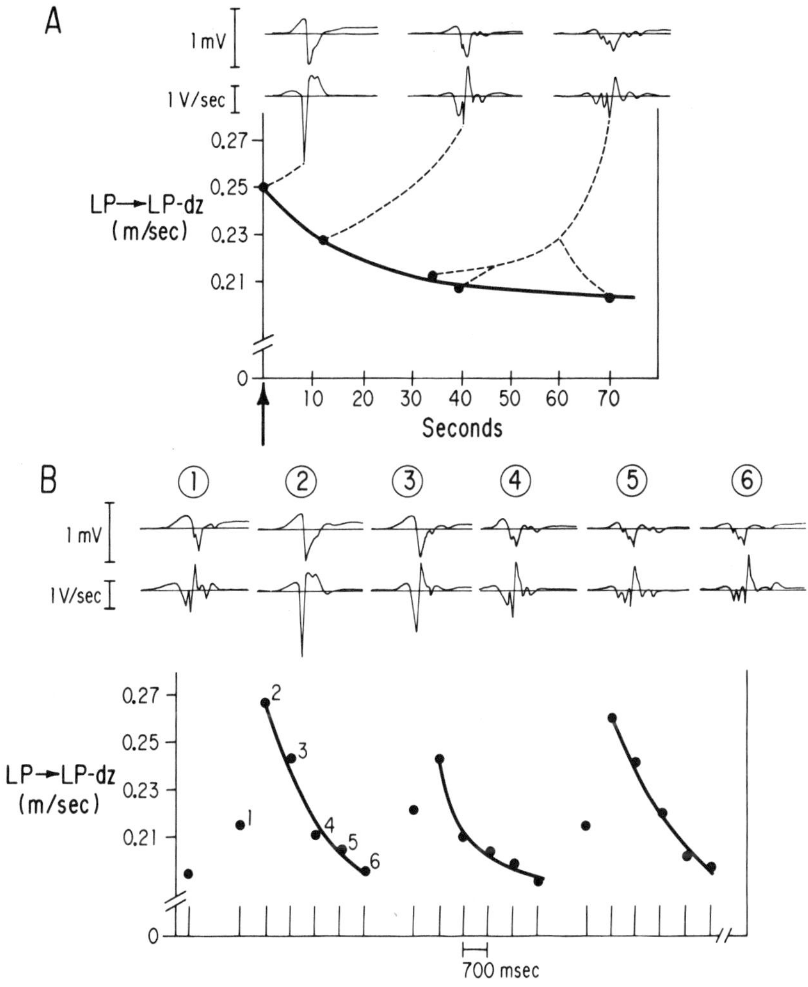

Figure 7. Use-dependent dissociated zigzag longitudinal conduction in a nonuniform anisotropic preparation during exposure to quinidine gluconate (10 mg/L). Prior to obtaining the results shown, the longitudinal velocity decreased from 0.4 to 0.25 m/sec at a stimulus rate of 70/min during quinidine exposure. Panel A: Arrow at time zero indicates the time at which the stimulation rate was increased from 70–85/min. The single extracellular waveform and its derivative at the right were the same for each data point connected by the single interrupted line. Panel B: Wenckebach cycles with beat-to-beat changes in the shape of the extracellular waveform indicative of changes from regular to dissociated zigzag longitudinal conduction in association with decreasing velocity (lower part of B). The preparation was from a 66-year-old subject. (Reproduced from *Circ Res* 62: 811–832, (1988), by permission of the American Heart Association, Inc.)

was prolonged. In the young, uniform anisotropic bundles with Wenckebach periodicity secondary to quinidine exposure, there were no changes in the excitation sequence and maximum velocity occurred with the first beat of each Wenckebach cycle.

DISCUSSION

The results show that the anisotropic passive properties of cardiac muscle highly determine the propagation response of action potentials at a microscopic level when interventions modify the available sodium conductance. The directional differences in shape of the upstroke behave as though there are directional differences in the effective membrane capacitance to be filled by the upstroke of propagating action potentials. Due to the shape differences during longitudinal versus transverse propagation, the relationship between the magnitude of the sodium current and dV/dt_{max} is the opposite of the classical relationship where decreases in dV/dt_{max} occur secondary to decreases in the magnitude of the sodium current (Hunter et al., 1975). Thereby, in multidimensional cardiac muscle an increase in dV/dt_{max} for propagating depolarization can be associated with either an increase or a decrease in the magnitude of the sodium current. The association depends on the relative contributions of 1) primary modification of the sodium conductance (changes in the inactivation variable h and in G_{Na}); and 2) changes in the direction of propagation with respect to the fiber orientation (changes in the effective membrane capacitance to be discharged).

It is well known that in one-dimensional homogeneous structures, changes in dV/dt_{max} as a function of the available sodium conductance is not linear (Cohen et al., 1984), although both variables increase or decrease together (see Chapter 1). However, differences in dV/dt_{max} secondary to changes in the direction of propagation result in a diametrically opposite relationship between dV/dt_{max} and the sodium current. This makes it necessary during experiments to verify that at a microscopic level there are no changes in the direction of propagation at the microelectrode impalement site when dV/dt_{max} is used to evaluate the kinetics of I_{Na} during interventions, such as use-dependent drug blockade of sodium channels. Our results especially emphasize the importance of monitoring the extracellular potential waveforms at the site of intracellular potential measurements because the extracellular waveforms provide a simple but sensitive index of changes in the sequence of excitation at a small size scale.

Thus far we have used the simplest possible model of directional differences in *effective* membrane capacitance, which is clearly an oversimplification of the actual tissue structure, to account for the directional differences in shape of the upstroke. More realistic models will be necessary in the future. As yet we have no simulation to answer the major question as to how the effective membrane capacitance can be different when the direction of propagation is altered. However, the results indicate that directional differences in effective membrane capacitance, or its equivalent, will be necessary (in addition to directional differences and discontinuities of effective axial resistivity) for a full accounting of anisotropic propagation. Our studies indicate that collagen per se is not a contributor to the anisotropic difference in the shape of the upstroke. However, in both uniform and nonuniform anisotropic muscle there are multiple regions of restricted extracellular space. In working atrial and ventricular fibers, these regions are located primarily at intercalated discs. Indeed, nearly a third of the total plasmalemma faces restricted extracellular space at the discs (Page, 1978). Since the transmembrane potential of membrane facing restricted extracellular space may deviate significantly from the potential of other membrane (Sommer and Johnson (1968), it will be necessary to explicitly include these regions in electrical models of anisotropic propagation.

A major conclusion from the results is that at a microscopic level the propagation behavior of individual cardiac muscle bundles is highly determined by the presence of uniform versus nonuniform anisotropic properties. For example, the results indicate that with increasing age and hypertrophy there is progressive electrical uncoupling of the side-to-side connections between small groups of fibers and, thereby, propagation events differ in an age-and-condition related manner in response to the same change in the sodium conductance.

Thus far all of the anisotropic propagation phenomena we have found in response to premature action potentials and to drug blockade of the sodium channels further support an emerging theory of anisotropic discontinuous propagation (Spach et al., 1981, 1982). The breakdown of longitudinal propagation to decremental conduction with block, or the abrupt change to dissociated *zigzag* conduction is consistent with the excitability and safety factor of propagation being greater during transverse than longitudinal propagation. With use-dependent drug blockade in nonuniform anisotropic preparations, transverse propagation remained stable while longitudinal propagation shifted to a slow dissociated *zigzag* type of conduction, similar to transverse propagation (Spach et al., 1988). These results suggest that when quinidine reduces the depolarization current to near threshold levels, preparations with sparse cell-to-cell coupling between adjacent fibers switch to a safer type of disorganized longitudinal conduction before propagation fails.

In conclusion, the results indicate that the anisotropic passive properties and the number of available sodium channels provide interactive mechanisms that determine the propagation response in the presence of drug blockade of the channels and with variations in the takeoff potential.

BIBLIOGRAPHY

Clerc L. Directional differences of impulse spread in trabecular muscle from mammalian heart. *J Physiol (Lond)* 255:335–346, 1976.

Cohen CJ, Bean BP, Tsien RW. Maximal upstroke velocity as an index of available sodium conductance. Comparison of maximal upstroke velocity and voltage clamp measurements of sodium current in rabbit Purkinje fibers. *Circ Res* 54:636–651, 1984.

Crank J, Nicolson P. Practical method for numerical evaluation of solutions of partial differential equations of the heat-conduction type. *Proc Cambridge Phil Soc* 43:50–67, 1947.

Diaz PJ, Rudy Y, Plonsey R. Intercalated discs as a cause for discontinuous propagation in cardiac muscle: a theoretical simulation. *Ann Biomed Eng* 11:177–189, 1983.

Ebihara L, Johnson EA. Fast sodium current in cardiac muscle. A quantitative description. *Biophys J* 32:779–790, 1980.

Fozzard HA, Wasserstrom JA. Voltage dependence on intracellular sodium and control of contraction. In: Zipes DP, Jalife J, eds. *Cardiac Electrophysiology and Arrhythmias* Orlando, Fla: Grune & Stratton, Inc.; 51–57, 1985.

Freygang WH, Trautwein W. The structural implications of the linear electrical properties of cardiac Purkinje strands. *J Gen Physiol* 55:524–547, 1970.

Gerald CF. *Applied Numerical Analysis.* Reading, Mass: Addison-Wesley Publishing Co; 250–288, 1970.

Geselowitz DB, Miller WT III. Active electrical properties of cardiac muscle. *Bioelectromagnetics* 3:127–132, 1982.

Glitsch HD, Reuter H, Scholtz H. The effect of the internal sodium concentration on calcium fluxes in isolated guinea-pig auricles. *J Physiol (Lond)* 209:25–43, 1970.

Hodgkin AL, Huxley AF. A quantitative description of the membrane current and its application to conduction and excitation in nerve. *J Physiol (Lond)* 117:500–544, 1952.

Hodgkin AL, Katz B. The effect of sodium ions on the electrical activity of the giant axon of the squid. *J Physiol (Lond)* 108:37–77, 1949.

Hondeghem L, Katzung BG. Test of a model of antiarrhythmic drug action. Effects of quinidine and lidocaine on myocardial conduction. *Circulation* 61:1217–1226, 1980.

Hunter PJ, McNaughton PA, Noble D. Analytical models of propagation in excitable cells. *Prog Biophys Mol Biol* 30:99–144, 1975.

Jenerick H. Phase-plane trajectories of the muscle spike potential. *Biophys J* 3:363–377, 1963.

Joyner RW. Effects of the discrete pattern of electrical coupling on propagation through an electrical syncytium. *Circ Res* 50:192–200, 1982.

Lieberman M, Sawanobori T, Kootsey JM, Johnson EA. A synthetic strand of cardiac muscle: Its passive electrical properties. *J Gen Physiol* 65: 527–550, 1975.

Page E. Quantitative ultrastructural analysis in cardiac membrane physiology. *Am J Physiol* 235:C147-C158, 1978.

Paes de Carvalho A, Saldena TA, Garcia EAC, Campos de Carvalho AC, Tashiro T, de Paula Carvalho M. Homogeneous and nonhomogeneous conduction of impulses in heart and other excitable tissues. In: Paes de Carvalho A, et al, eds. *Normal and Abnormal Conduction in the Heart.* New York, NY: Futura Publishing Co.; 117–143, 1982.

Schmitt FO, Erlanger J. Directional differences in the conduction of the impulse through heart muscle and their possible relation to extrasystolic and fibrillary contractions. *Am J Physiol* 87:326–347, 1928.

Sommer JR, Johnson EA. Cardiac muscle: A comparative study of Purkinje fibers and ventricular fibers. *J Cell Biol* 36:497–526, 1968.

Spach MS. The discontinuous nature of electrical propagation in cardiac muscle. Consideration of a quantitative model incorporating the membrane ionic properties and structural complexities. *Ann Biomed Eng* 11:209–261, 1983.

Spach MS, Dolber PC. Anisotropic discontinuous propagation: Directional differences in the distribution of gap junctions and in the effective membrane capacitance of cardiac muscle. In: Sperelakis N, Cole WB, eds. *Cell Interactions and Gap Junctions.* Boca Raton, Fla: CRC Press, Inc.; 95–121, 1989.

Spach MS, Dolber PC. Relating extracellular potentials and their derivatives to anisotropic propagation at a microscopic level in human cardiac muscle. Evidence for electrical uncoupling of side-to-side fiber connections with increasing age. *Circ Res* 58:356–371, 1986.

Spach MS, Dolber PC. The relation between discontinuous propagation in anisotropic cardiac muscle and the "vulnerable period" of reentry. In: Zipes Dp, Jalife J, eds. *Cardiac Electrophysiology and Arrhythmias.* Orlando, Fla: Grune & Stratton; 241–252, 1985.

Spach MS, Dolber PC, Heidlage JF. Influence of the passive anisotropic properties on directional differences in propagation following modification of the sodium conductance in human atrial muscle. A model of reentry based on anisotropic discontinuous propagation. *Circ Res* 62:811–832, 1988.

Spach MS, Dolber PC, Heidlage JF. Use of computer simulations for combined experimental-theoretical study of anisotropic discontinuous propagation at a microscopic level in cardiac muscle. In: Sideman S, ed. *Electromechanical Activation, Metabolism, and Perfusion of the Heart—Simulation and Experimental Models* Boston, Mass: Martinus Nijhoff Publishers; 3–27, 1987a.

Spach MS, Dolber PC, Heidlage JF, Kootsey JM, Johnson EA. Propagating depolarization in anisotropic human and canine cardiac muscle: apparent directional differences in membrane capacitance. *Circ Res* 60:206–219, 1987b.

Spach MS, Kootsey JM. Relating the sodium current and conductance to the shape of transmembrane and extracellular potentials by simulation: effects of propagation boundaries. *IEEE Trans Biomed Eng BME* 32:743–755, 1985.

Spach MS, Miller WT III, Dolber PC, Kootsey JM, Sommer JR, Mosher CR Jr. The functional role of structural complexities in the propagation of depolarization in the atrium of the dog. Cardiac conduction disturbances due to discontinuities of effective axial resistivity. *Circ Res* 50:175–191, 1982.

Spach MS, Miller WT III, Geselowitz DB, Barr RC, Kootsey JM, Johnson EA. The discontinuous nature of propagation in normal canine cardiac muscle. Evidence for recurrent discontinuities of intracellular resistance that affect the membrane currents. *Circ Res* 48:39–54, 1981.

Spach MS, Miller WT III, Miller-Jones E, Warren RB, Barr RC Extracellular potentials related to intracellular action potentials during impulse conduction in anisotropic canine muscle. *Circ Res* 45:188–204, 1979.

Weidmann S. The effect of the cardiac membrane potential on the rapid availability of the sodium-carrying system. *J Physiol (Lond)* 127: 213–224, 1955.

Weidmann S. The electrical constants of Purkinje Fibers. *J Physiol (Lond)* 118:348–360, 1952.

Chapter 4

Direct G Protein Gating of Cardiac K^+ and Ca^{2+} Channels

Arthur M. Brown
Atsuko Yatani
Juan Codina
Lutz Birnbaumer

INTRODUCTION

Recently it has been shown that guanine nucleotide binding, or G proteins, directly couple muscarinic and β-adrenoreceptors to K^+ and Ca^{2+} channels, respectively, in heart. In this chapter the evidence on which this concept is based will be reviewed. Direct coupling has not actually been proven; what has been established is that the coupling is membrane delimited and does not involve cytoplasmic second messengers.

The concept is shown in Figure 1. G proteins are generally thought to couple receptors to ionic channels via cytoplasmic mediators such as cGMP in the case of retinal rods, cAMP in the case of olfactory cells, and the cAMP cascade in the case of cardiac myocytes. The membrane delimited pathway has only recently been uncovered and is exemplified best by the atrial muscarinic receptor (mAChR) and the K^+ channel to which it is coupled, K^+[ACh]. Here

Hondeghem, Luc (ed): Molecular and Cellular Mechanisms of Antiarrhythmic Agents, Futura Publishing Company, Inc., Mount Kisco, NY, © 1989.

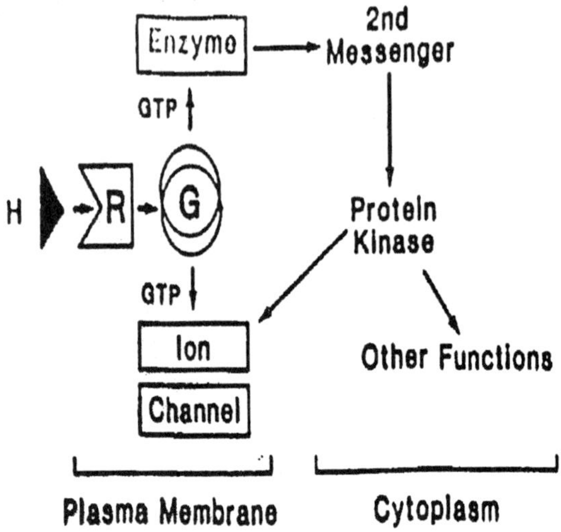

Figure 1. Effector function may be under dual control: directly by a G protein and indirectly by a G protein-regulated second messenger.

the latency after ACh application is about 50 msec (Purves, 1976; Glitsch and Pott, 1978; Hartzell, 1980; Osterrieder et al., 1982; Pott, 1983), much longer than the 1 msec latency of the nicotinic acetylcholine receptor where the receptor and the ionic channel are the same protein. The rate-limiting step was not agonist occupancy (Nargeot et al., 1983) and possible second messengers such as cGMP (Nawrath, 1977; Trautwein et al., 1982; Nargeot et al., 1983), cAMP (Trautwein et al., 1982; Nargeot et al., 1983) and Ca^{2+} (Trautwein et al., 1982) were ruled out. The second messenger concept was also excluded on theoretical grounds (Osterrieder et al., 1982). Then it was shown that ACh applied outside a cell-attached patch of membrane could not activate K^+ channels whereas ACh in the patch pipette could (Soejima and Noma, 1984). It was known that mAChR's were linked to G proteins in the heart from binding studies and that PTX substrates were present in atrial tissues (Rosenberger et al., 1979; Hazeki and Ui, 1981; Kurose and Ui, 1983; Halvorsen and Nathanson, 1984). The link with electrophysiological changes such as the ACh-activated inwardly rectifying whole cell current (Pfaffinger et al., 1985) and resting membrane potential (Endoh et al., 1985; Sirota et al., 1985) was established when block by PTX was shown along with, in the case of the whole cell current experiments, a requirement for intracellular GTP. Furthermore, the non-hydrolyzable GTP analog, GppNHp, disconnected the currents from ACh control (Breitwieser and Szabo, 1985). These experiments were not definitive because a non-PTX sensitive phosphoinositide pathway (Brown and Brown, 1984), which contributes an inward current, is also present in atrial cells and contaminates whole cell current or membrane potential measurements (Tajima et al., 1987). A most revealing set of experiments then showed that GTPγ S applied to the cytoplasmic face of an inside-out membrane patch activated a specific set of inwardly rectifying single K^+ channel currents that were the same as those activated by ACh and did so in a Mg-dependent manner (Kurachi et al., 1986a; 1986b). To this point the particular G proteins involved had not been specified nor had the exact mechanism been determined. Thus, a membrane-associated G protein effect such as PKC activation could have affected the single channel results. Our contribution was to apply specific G proteins to inside-out patches and observe their effects. In addition we tested whether PKC activation could be involved.

RESULTS AND DISCUSSION

We found that a specific G protein purified from human red blood cell (hrbc) membranes and preactivated with GTPγS activated the K^+[ACh] channels at picomolar concentrations (Fig. 2; Yatani et al., 1987a). The effect was concentration-dependent. Phorbol ester, ATP, and the non-hydrolyzable ATP analog, AppNHp, had no effect on the response so PKC involvement could be excluded. The other G protein present in hrbc membranes, G_s, had no effect even at nanomolar concentrations. G proteins are heterotrimers, and since these two proteins share the same $\beta\gamma$ dimer we concluded that the α subunit was the mediator. This was tested directly (Codina, 1987) and the α subunit was equipotent to the holomeric G protein (Fig. 2).

The experiments to this point dealt with reconstitution of the response using exogenous G proteins and it was desirable to examine the coupling process under more physiological conditions using specific G protein probes, which modify function by reacting with a specific site, requirements that monoclonal antibodies (mAb) with functional effects satisfy. We have used mAbs generated by α_t of

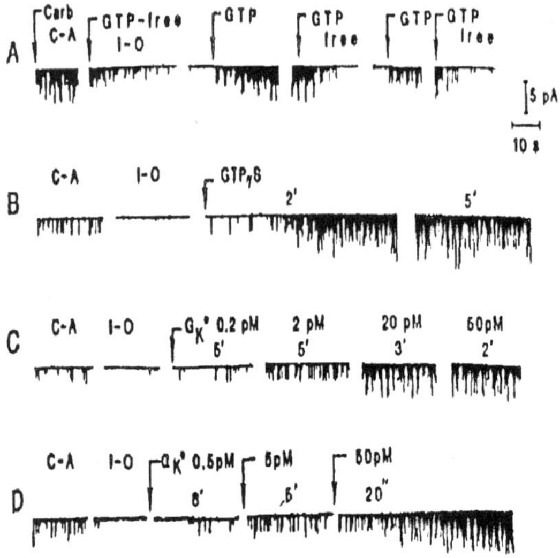

Figure 2. Activation of atrial K^+[ACh] currents in inside-out membrane patches by carbachol and GTP (A), GTPγS (B), and GTPγS-treated, PTX-sensitive G protein G_k^* from human erythrocytes (C), GTPγS-treated α subunit of G_k, α_k^* (D). Single channel K^+ currents from atrial membrane patches were recorded in symmetrical isotonic K^+ solutions at −80 mV, first in the cell-attached (C-A) mode and then after patch excision under cell-free inside-out (I-O) conditions both before and after addition to the bathing media of (A) 50 μM GTP, (B) 50 μM GTPγS, (C) increasing concentrations of activated G_k^*, (D) increasing concentrations of activated α_k^*. Times on top of each trace are minutes elapsed between the last addition and the recording of the trace shown. In (A), five minutes elapsed between C-A and I-O; the remainder is a continuous record with 5 sec gaps.

frog transducin; these antibodies cross-react with α_k. One of them, mAb 4A, has functional effects whereas another, mAb 4H, does not.

mAb 4A blocked carbachol-activated K^+ channels in inside-out membrane patches of guinea pig atrium while mAb 4H had no effect (Yatani et al., 1988b). The data suggested that mAb 4A blocked the K^+ channel currents by binding to either the activated holo-G protein or its dissociated α subunit. In the first case G_k^* and its mediator subunit, either α_k or βγ, must be equipotent. This is true for G_k^* and α_k^* which are effective at picomolar concentrations, but not for βγ which is effective at nanomolar concentrations (Yatani et al.,

1987a). In the second case, mAb blocks by binding to dissociated endogenous α subunit. Either case leads to the conclusion that α_k is the physiological mediator of muscarinic activation of atrial K^+ channels.

K^+ channels are not the only ionic channels coupled directly to G proteins and G_k is not the only G protein that gates ionic channels. G_s, the stimulatory regulator of adenylyl cyclase purified from hrbc and preactivated with GTPγS, at picomolar concentrations directly activates Ca^{2+} channels in cardiac sarcolemma (Yatani et al., 1987b; Fig. 3). The effect is mediated by the α subunit and the latter is equipotent with the holoprotein; the $\beta\gamma$ dimer is ineffective. Unlike the atrial K^+[ACh] channels, G protein activation is not obligatory but is modulatory. The Ca^{2+} channels will not open unless the cell membrane is depolarized and G_s increases the frequency of opening. The cardiac experiments on excised patches required that the β-agonist Isoproterenol (Iso) be present in the patch pipette and GTPγS be present in the bath. In order to have more stable recording conditions, we used the method of incorporating vesicles into planar lipid bilayers. It was also necessary to use the 1,4-dihydropyridine agonist Bay K 8644 to obtain a reasonable opening frequency at the potentials where the single channel currents were detectable. Nevertheless, this activity still decreased with time and the G_s effect may have been to stabilize rather than to modulate the channel. In skeletal muscle it was possible to demonstrate a stimulatory effect of G_s in the absence of BAY K 8644 or Iso (Yatani et al., 1988a). The G_s effects were independent of cAMP stimulation and occurred in the presence of ADPβS at 100 μM, 0 cAMP and 0 ATP.

The physiological importance of direct G_s gating of calcium channels in muscle remains to be determined since the cAMP cascade, which indirectly modulates the channel, is activated by the same G protein. It is probably related to the fact that the direct pathway is faster than the second messenger pathway. The significance at present rests more with the fact that by identifying Ca^{2+} channels as direct targets for G proteins, we have another indication that the phenomenon of direct G protein gating of ionic channels is likely to be widespread.

Thus, we have a third major category to be added to the categories of ligand- and voltage-gated channels, the G protein-gated channels.

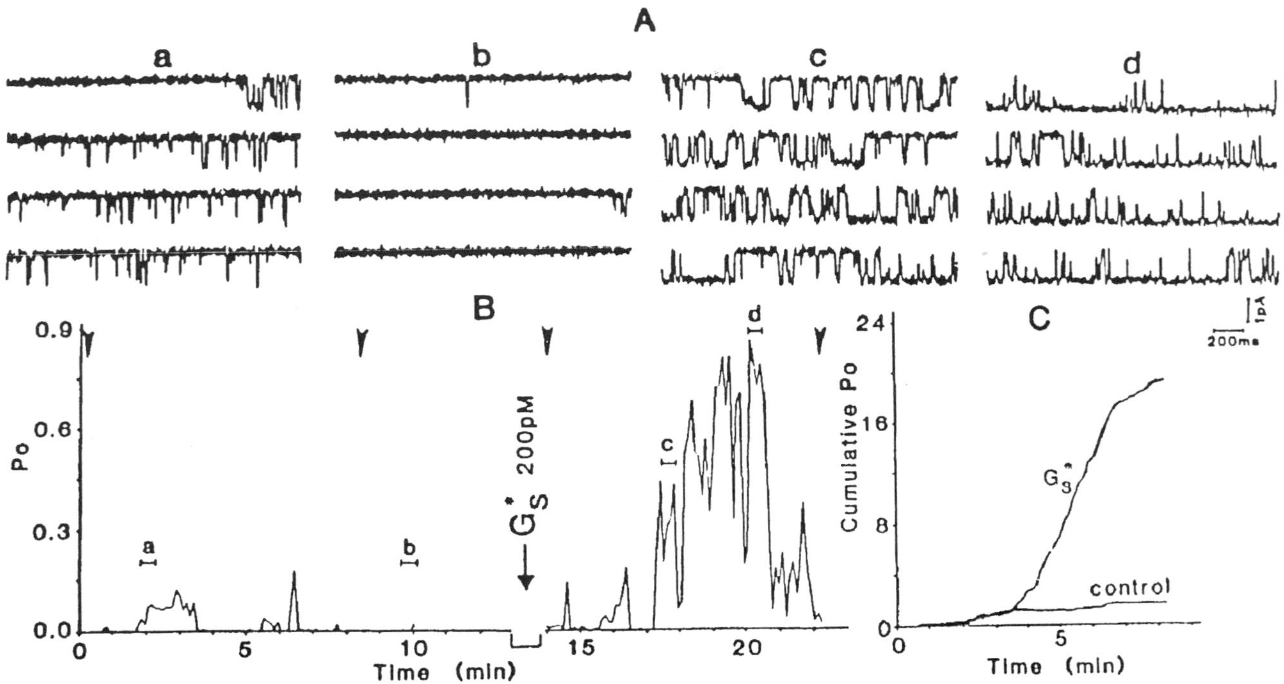

Figure 3. Effects of G_s^* on single cardiac Ca^{2+} channels incorporated into a planar lipid bilayer. The number of functional Ca^{2+} channels incorporated into the bilayer was usually less than three and often one. As originally reported, cardiac sarcolemmal Ca^{2+} channels incorporated into this type of bilayer had properties similar to those of high-threshold or L-type cardiac Ca^{2+} channels. (*continued on opposite page*).

BIBLIOGRAPHY

Breitwieser GE, Szabo G. Uncoupling of cardiac muscarinic and beta-adrenergic receptors from ion channels by a guanine nucleotide analogue. *Nature* 317:538–540, 1985.

Brown JH, Brown SL. Agonists differentiate muscarinic receptors that inhibit cycle AMP formation from those that stimulate phosphoinositide metabolism. *J Biol Chem* 259:3777–3781, 1984.

Codina J, Yatani A, Grenet D, Brown AM, Birnbaumer L. The alpha subunit of G_k opens atrial potassium channels. *Science* 236:442–445, 1987.

Endoh M, Maruyama M, Iijima T. Attenuation of muscarinic cholinergic inhibition by islet-activating protein in the heart. *Am J Physiol* (*Heart Circ Physiol 18*) 249:H309–H320, 1985.

Glitsch HG, Pott L. Effects of acetylcholine and parasympathetic nerve stimulation on membrane potential in quiescent guinea-pig atria. *J Physiol* (*Lond*) 279:655–668, 1978.

Halvorsen SW, Nathanson NM. Ontogenesis of physiological responsiveness and guanine nucleotide sensitivity of cardiac muscarinic receptors during chick embryonic development. *Biochemistry* 23:5813–5321, 1984.

Hartzell HC. Distribution of muscarinic acetylcholine receptors and presynaptic nerve terminals in amphibian heart. *J Cell Biol* 86:6–20, 1980.

Hazeki O, Ui M. Modification by islet-activating protein of receptor-mediated regulation of cAMP accumulation in isolated rat heart cells. *J Biol Chem* 256:2856–2862, 1981.

Kurachi Y, Nakajima T, Sugimoto T. Acetylcholine activation of K^+ channels in cell-free membranes of atrial cells. *Am J Physiol* (*Heart Circ Physiol* 20) 251:H681–H684, 1986.

Kurachi Y, Nakajima T, Sugimoto T. Role of intracellular Mg^{2+} in the activation of muscarinic K^+ channels in cardiac atrial cell membrane. *Pfluegers Arch* 407:572–574, 1986.

(*Figure 3 cont.*) In the presence of BAY K 8644 and with 100 mM Ba^{2+} as the charge carrier, the conductance between −50 and +20 mV was ~20 pS. The channel opened in bursts, and the probability of opening was voltage-dependent. Brief openings that dominate under control conditions could not be detected at the recording bandwidth, and the mean open times were fit to an exponential distribution ($\tau \sim 12 \pm 3$ msec, n = 9, at test potentials between 0 and +20 mV). The values are consistent with those obtained for BAY K 8644-stimulated channels in cell-attached patches. Current traces produced by depolarizing clamp steps to 0 mV from a holding potential of −40 mV are shown in (A) before (1 and 2) and after (3 and 4) addition of G_s^*. Pulses were applied every 30 seconds for 20 seconds. Leakage and capacitive currents were subtracted. Traces 1 to 4 were taken at the times indicated in (B) and are 2-second segments from the 20-second pulses. (B) The entire experimental record. Note the decrease in activity with time in control in (B) before addition of G_s^* (100 pM) to the trans chamber. The ordinate is given as P_o because N was 1 in this experiment. (C) Cumulative P_o's obtained between the arrows in (B). Cum $P_o(G_s^*)$/cum P_o (control) 11. Reprinted from *Science* with permission.

Kurose H, Ui M. Functional uncoupling of muscarinic receptors from adenylate cyclase in rat cardiac membranes by the active component of islet-activating protein, pertussis toxin. *J Cyclic Nucleotide and Protein Phosphorylation Res* 9:305–318, 1983.

Nargeot J, Nerbonne JM, Engels J, Lester HA. Time course of the increase in the myocardial slow inward current after a photochemically generated concentration jump of intracellular cAMP. *Proc Natl Acad Sci USA* 80:2395–2399, 1983.

Nawrath H. Does cyclic GMP mediate the negative inotropic effect of acetylcholine in the heart? *Nature* 267:72–74, 1977.

Osterrieder W, Yang Q-F, Trautwein W. Mode of action of acetylcholine on the rabbit SA node cell. In: Bouman LN, Jongsma HT, eds. *Cardiac Rate and Rhythm.* Boston, MA: Martinus Nijhoff; 485–505, 1982.

Pfaffinger PJ, Martin JM, Hunter DD, Nathanson NM, Hille B. GTPbinding proteins couple cardiac muscarinic receptors to a K channel. *Nature* 317:536–538, 1985.

Pott L. Effects of fast and slowly acting antagonists on the times course of the muscarinic response in guinea-pig atrial muscle. *Pflugers Arch* 399:35–41, 1983.

Purves RV. Function of muscarinic and nicotinic acetylcholine receptors. *Nature* 261:151–159, 1976.

Rosenberger LB, Roeske WR, Yamamura HI. The regulation of muscarinic cholinergic receptors by guanine nucleotides in cardiac tissue. *Eur J Pharmacol* 56:179–180, 1979.

Sirota S, Tsuji Y, Pappano A. Pertussis toxin blocks muscarinic hyperpolarization and action potential shortening in chick atrium. *Fed Proc* 44:729, 1985. Abstract.

Soejima M, Noma A. Mode of regulation of the ACh-sensitive K-channel by muscarinic receptor in rabbit atrial cells. *Pflugers Arch* 400:424–431, 1984.

Tajima T, Tsuji Y, Brown JH, Pappano AJ. Pertussis Toxin-insensitive phosphoinositide hydrolysis, membrane depolarization, and positive inotropic effect of carbachol in chick atria. *Circ Res* 61(3):436–445, 1987.

Trautwein W, Taniguchi J, Noma A. The effect of intracellular cyclic nucleotides and calcium on the action potential and acetylcholine response of isolated cardiac cells. *Pflugers Arch* 392:307–314, 1982.

Yatani A, Codina J, Brown AM, Birnbaumer L. Direct activation of mammalian atrial muscarinic potassium channels by GTP regulatory protein G_k. *Science* 235:207–211, 1987a.

Yatani A, Codina J, Imoto Y, Reeves JP, Birnbaumer L, Brown AM. A G protein directly regulates mammalian cardiac calcium channels. *Science* 238:1288–1292, 1987b.

Yatani A, Hamm HE, Codina J, Birnbaumer L, Brown AM. Monoclonal antibody 4A to the α-subunit of transducin blocks activation of mammalian atrial K^+ channels. *Faseb J* 2(5):A1278, 1988b. Abstract.

Yatani A, Imoto Y, Codina J, Hamilton SL, Brown AM, Birnbaumer L. The stimulatory G protein of adenylyl cyclase, G_s, also stimulates dihydropyridine-sensitive Ca^{2+} channels. Evidence for direct regulation independent of phosphorylation by cAMP-dependent protein kinase or stimulation by a dihydropyridine agonist. *J Biol Chem* 263(20):9887–9895, 1988a.

Chapter 5

Modified Single Sodium Channel Gating in Excised Membrane Patches from Neonatal Rat Ventricular Myocytes

G. E. Kirsch

INTRODUCTION

Excitation of cardiac muscle is critically dependent on the operation of voltage-dependent sodium (Na^+) channels. Both the rapid upstroke and part of the plateau phase are generated by transient and sustained components of the inward Na^+ current, respectively, as demonstrated by their sensitivity to tetrodotoxin block (Baer et al., 1976; Attwell et al., 1979; Gintant et al., 1984). From single channel studies we know that the transient component originates from channels that open briefly at the beginning of a step depolarization and quickly close into an inactivated state, whereas slower components arise from late reopenings of non-inactivated channels (Kunze et al., 1985; Starmer and Grant, 1987). Recently, several investigators have reported the infrequent occurrence of long-lasting bursts of single channel activity, which have the kinetic features appropriate to a sustained component of membrane Na^+ current (Patlak and Ortiz, 1986; Grant and Starmer, 1987; Kolhardt et al.,

Hondeghem, Luc (ed): Molecular and Cellular Mechanisms of Antiarrhythmic Agents, Futura Publishing Company, Inc., Mount Kisco, NY, © 1989.

1987; and Clark and Giles, 1987). In this chapter we describe experimental conditions that potentiate sustained bursting and show that such activity can be explained by a decrease in the transition rate from open to inactivated states.

METHODS

Solutions and Drugs

Experiments were performed in a chamber placed on a temperature-controlled microscope stage and filled with 0.6 ml external or internal solution, depending on the recording mode. Extracellular solution for patch recording consisted of mammalian Tyrode's (mM): NaCl 137, KCl 5.4, $MgCl_2$ 1.0, $CaCl_2$ 1.8, glucose 10, HEPES 5; pH 7.4. Depolarizing bath solution for cell-attached patch recording consisted of high-K^+, low-Ca^{++} Tyrode's made by replacing all NaCl with either KCl or KF and replacing Ca^{++} with Mg^{++}. Intracellular solution for outside-out patch recording consisted of (mM): CsF, 120; EGTA, 11; $MgCl_2$, 2; HEPES, 10; pH 7.4. All experiments were performed at 9.5–10.5° C.

Cell Culture

Primary cardiac cell cultures were prepared from hearts of neonatal rats (1–3 days old) as described previously (Yatani and Brown, 1985). Briefly, hearts were removed under sterile conditions, the ventricles cut into pieces and incubated at 37° C for 5 min in Ca^{++}-free Hanks solution containing 0.5% trypsin (T-0134, Sigma, St. Louis, MO). The supernatant was removed and the pelleted cells were added to culture medium, DMEM-10 FCS, to stop enzyme action. Resuspended cells were seeded on glass cover-slips and incubated in culture medium at 37° C in 5% CO_2-95% O_2 atmosphere. Cells were used for recording on days 1–2 after seeding.

Electrophysiological Recording

Patch clamp recording was performed using techniques described previously (Hamill et al., 1981; Lux and Brown, 1984). Single channel Na^+ currents were recorded from membrane patches using

Sylgard-coated micropipettes (Corning 7052 glass) with resistances of 8–15 mΩ connected to a commercial patch clamp amplifier (EPC-7, List Co., Darmstadt, West Germany). Currents evoked by 140 ms depolarizing test pulses were stored on videocassette tape (PCM-1 Medical Systems Inc., New York) at a bandwidth of 16 kHz. The data were later digitized by a PDP-11/73 computer (Digital Equipment Corp., Marlboro, MA) with 12-bit resolution at a sample rate 10 kHz after low-pass filtering at 3.15 kHz (−3dB) using a 4-pole Bessel filter (Ithaco Inc., Ithaca, NY). Digitized records were corrected off-line for linear leakage and capacitative currents by subtracting the average of records lacking single channel activity (null traces), then digitally filtered using a zero-phase 4-pole low pass Bessel filter at 1.4 kHz prior to level detection. Transitions between closed and open levels were determined using a threshold detection program in which opening threshold was set at half-maximum amplitude of single unit opening. Computer-detected openings were confirmed by visual observation and used to generate idealized records from which histograms of amplitude, waiting, closed and open time distributions were constructed. Amplitude histograms were fit by Gaussian functions using a chi-square non-linear regression routine. Single units of less than 0.4 ms duration were excluded from the histogram to avoid truncation error introduced by the limited frequency response of the recording system. Waiting time distributions were obtained by determining the latency between the beginning of each test pulse and the first channel event detected in the record. The distributions were corrected for the number of channels in a patch, estimated from channel overlap at potentials of −20 to −10 mV, by the method of Patlak and Horn (1982). Open time distributions were constructed from data sets in which events consisting of overlapping openings of two or more channels were excluded. Prepulse potentials (100 ms duration) were adjusted to ensure that the fraction of such events was less than 15% of the total events at a given test potential, in order to minimize the bias introduced by excluding overlaps. The sum of the idealized records at a given test potential was used to reconstruct probability of opening (Po) as a function of time. Histograms of open time, closed time, waiting time and burst duration were analyzed by fitting the data to the sum of exponential decay functions using a maximum likelihood estimate. Where appropriate, data are expressed as mean ± standard error. Significance of differences between means was evaluated using a two-tailed Student's t-test ($p < 0.05$).

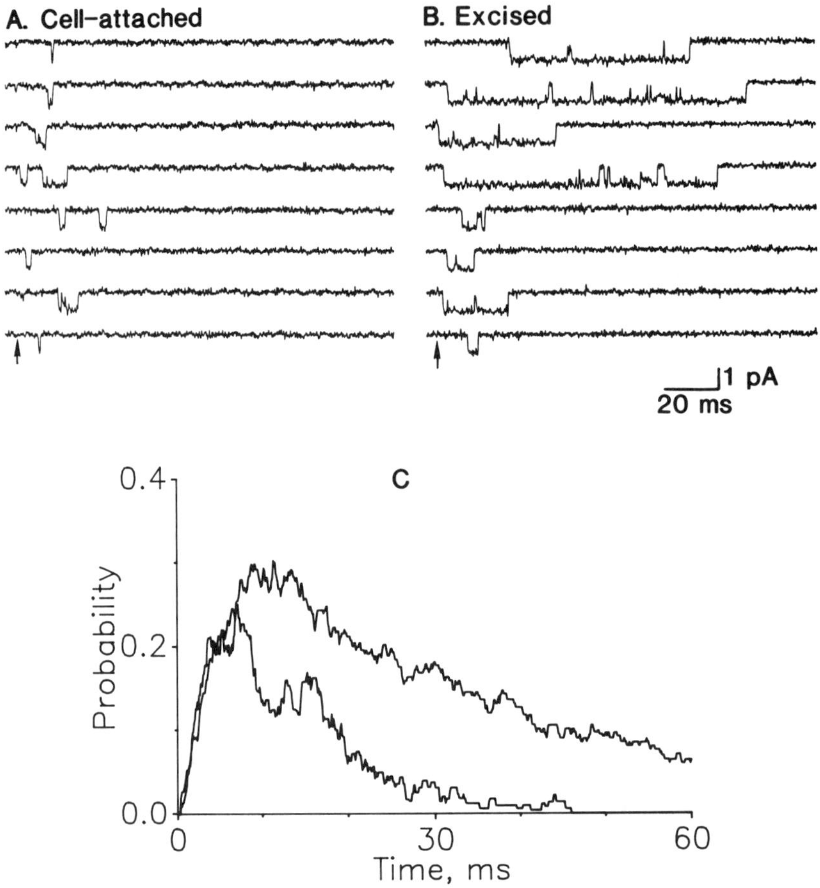

Figure 1. Single Na channel currents in cell-attached (A) and outside-out excised (B) membrane patches from neonatal rat ventricular myocytes. Panels A and B show records evoked by 140 ms test pulses (onset marked by arrow) to a test potential of −60 mV. Channel openings are indicated by downward deflections. The end of the trace coincides with the end of the test pulse. Records were filtered at 1432 Hz. In (A) the cell was bathed in a KCl-depolarizing solution, the pipette contained Tyrode's solution and the holding potential was −110 mV. A prepulse of 100 ms duration to −150 mV was applied to remove resting inactivation. The patch contained 3 channels based on observation of maximum number of overlapping unitary openings. In (B) the extracellular solution was Tyrode's, the pipet solutionm was CsF, and the holding potential was −140 mV. No prepulse was applied. In panel C the probability of single channel opening (Po) as a function of time was calculated by averaging 200 idealized single channel records and cor-

(*continued on next page*)

RESULTS

We recorded single channel currents in 10 cell-attached and 9 excised patches. Detailed analysis of a representative patch of each type is described below.

Typical single channel records obtained from a cell-attached (Fig. 1A) and an outside-out (Fig. 1B) patch at a test potential near threshold (−60 mV) show strikingly different patterns of channel activity. Qualitatively, activity in excised patches displayed two unique characteristics: (1) prolonged duration of individual openings and (2) long-lasting single channel bursts. Thus, under cell-attached conditions openings were brief (about 2 ms) and occurred either singly or in short bursts of 2–3 openings. In excised patches, however, prolonged bursts were often observed and as will be shown later the individual openings were of unusually long duration (>3 ms).

The probability of opening as a function of time (Po-t relationship) was constructed from the average of 200 single channel records as shown in Figure 1C. The superposition of the lower and upper Po curves (obtained from the patches illustrated in Figs. 1A and 1B, respectively) shows that the differences observed in single channel gating result in a marked prolongation of the decay phase with virtually no effect on the rising phase of membrane Na^+ conductance at this test potential.

Based on the maximum number of overlapping openings, the patch illustrated in Fig. 1A contained 3 channels, therefore we cannot be sure whether all of the events in a given trace arise from a single channel; however in Fig. 1B, a total of 1286 traces (excluding null traces) were recorded without a single overlapping event, strongly suggesting that only a single channel was present in this patch. A trace-by-trace diary of activity in this patch should, therefore, reveal whether the channel displays uniform gating behavior over a long period of time. Such a diary is shown in Figure 2 for 260 consecutive traces obtained in a cell-attached (A) and an excised

---

(Figure 1 cont.)
rected for the unitary amplitude and number of channels. The upper and lower curves show Po in the excised patch and cell attached patch respectively. The cell attached Po curve was scaled by a factor of three (determined by comparing the ratio of null traces to those containing openings in cell-attached and excised patch data) to correct for slow inactivation at −110 mV holding potential. Temperature was 10.4°C.

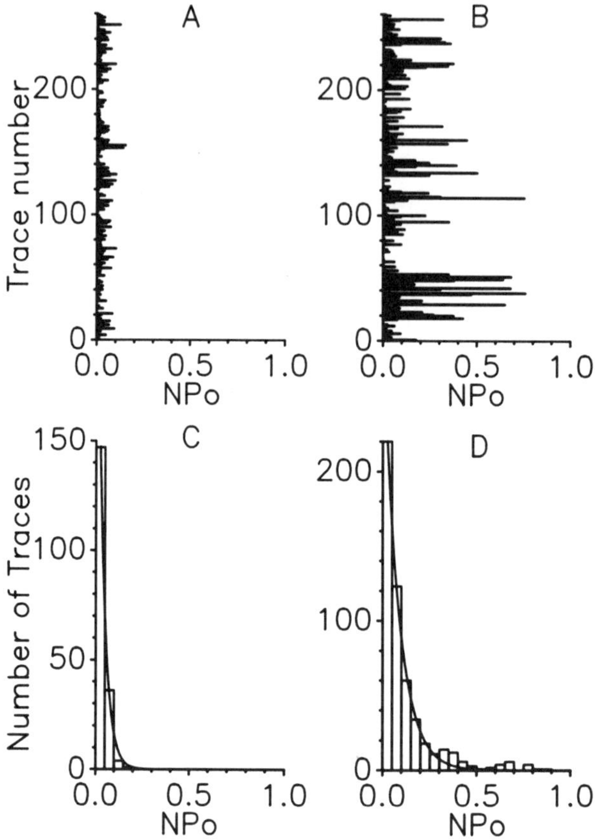

Figure 2. Diary analysis of probability of opening in consecutive traces from cell-attached (A,C) and excised (B,D) patches at a test potential of −60 mV. In panels (A) and (B) the ratio of total open time to pulse duration (NPo where N = number of channels in patch) was calculated for each of 260 consecutive traces and plotted against trace number. These data were binned and histograms of NPo plotted in panels (C-D). The smooth curves are monoexponential fits to the data.

patch (B). The ratio of total open time to test pulse duration (NPo, where N = number of channels) in each trace was plotted against trace number (test pulses were delivered at a frequency of 0.625 Hz) for a total observation period of 2.7 minutes. By comparing Figures 2A and 2B, the marked increase in traces with high Po in excised patch is readily apparent; correcting Fig. 2A for the number of channels in the patch would exaggerate the difference still further. These data were subjected to a runs analysis (Sokal and Rohlf, 1981), in order to determine whether high-Po traces tend to cluster together. At a confidence level of $p < 0.05$ no clustering was detected. Uniform gating behavior in both patches is also indicated by Figures 2C-D in which NPo histograms were constructed from all traces except nulls and fit accurately by single exponential decay curves. From this analysis we conclude that Na^+ channels in cell-attached and excised patches may show markedly different gating behavior, but that within either of these two experimental conditions gating is uniform. In the following sections we analyze in more detail the single channel kinetics of these two patches. Similar results were obtained in the other patches.

Analysis of the amplitude histograms of cell-attached (Fig. 3A) and excised (3B) patches reveals that the mean single channel amplitudes were similar (0.99 and 1.1 pA in 3A and 3B, respectively), but the standard deviation was greater in the cell-attached than in the excised patch. A likely explanation is the greater number of channels in the cell-attached patch. The mean single channel conductance from pooled data was 9.4 ± 0.4 ($n = 10$) and 9.0 ± 0.3 ($n = 9$) pS in cell-attached and excised patches respectively. In the single channel patch of Figure 3B, the small degree of variation in the major peak and the large total number of events reveals a small tail of low amplitude events (50–70% of the mean amplitude) that cannot readily be discerned under other conditions. Events falling within this tail may represent a second type of channel that rarely opens, or a substate of the open channel that occurs rarely. Figure 4 shows representative examples of traces containing low-amplitude events. The solid line represents the mean amplitude of the major peak and the broken line shows the average amplitude of the small events. The small units can occur either as separate events (e.g., last trace) or as part of a burst containing normal-sized units. In the latter case, the transition between small and normal units occurs without a measurable closed period, suggesting that the small amplitude events represent substates (Fox, 1987) rather than independent channels (Scanley and Fozzard, 1987).

Prolonged single channel open time is a consistent attribute of channels recorded in excised patches. This is clearly seen by comparing the open time histograms in Figure 5. The upper histogram (5A, cell-attached) was accurately fit by a single exponential decay with time constant, 2.4 ms, which closely approximates the mean open time (arithmetic mean of all events, 2.6 ms). By contrast the

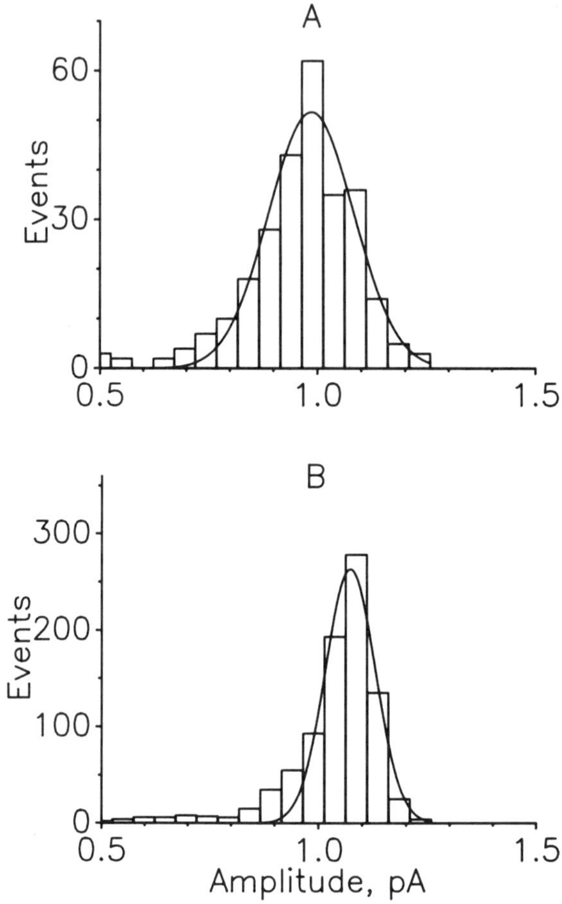

Figure 3. Analysis of single channel amplitude in cell-attached (A) and excised patch at a test potential of −60 mV. Openings less than 0.4 ms in duration were excluded to avoid errors arising from limited frequency response of the recording system. Smooth curves are Gaussian distributions with means of 0.99 and 1.07 pA, respectively in (A) and (B). Same experiment as Fig. 1.

lower histogram (5B, excised) was fit by a decay constant nearly three times as long. The monophasic shape of both histograms suggests that only one kinetically distinct open state exists. Whether the substate referred to above has a different open time cannot be resolved given the rarity of its occurrence. As shown in Figure 6,

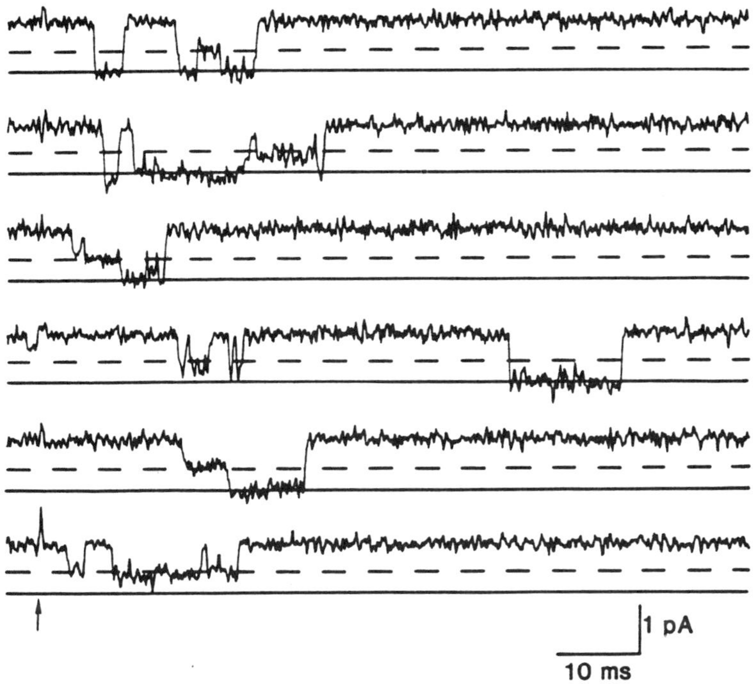

Figure 4. Small amplitude events recorded from an excised patch at test potential –60 mV. Solid horizontal line is 1.1 pA, the mean amplitude of the majority of events. Broken line is 0.55 pA, the mean amplitude of the low conductance events. Vertical arrow in lower left marks the onset of the depolarizing step. Only the first 86 ms of the test pulse is illustrated. Same experiment as Fig. 3B.

open time in the excised patch (open circles) was longer than in the cell-attached patch throughout the potential range −70 to −20 mV. However, the voltage dependence of open time in both patches has a similar inverted-U shape such that open time reaches a peak near −60 mV. Similarly, pooled data from all of the experiments showed that in excised patches mean open time decreased from 4.6 ± 0.8 ms at a test potential of −60 mV to 3.27 ± 0.4 ms at −20 mV, whereas in cell-attached patches the mean open times were 2.5 ± 0.2 ms and 2.0 ± 0.2 ms, respectively at −60 and −20 mV. Thus, patch excision consistently produced a marked increase in mean open time which was especially pronounced at a test potential of −60 mV.

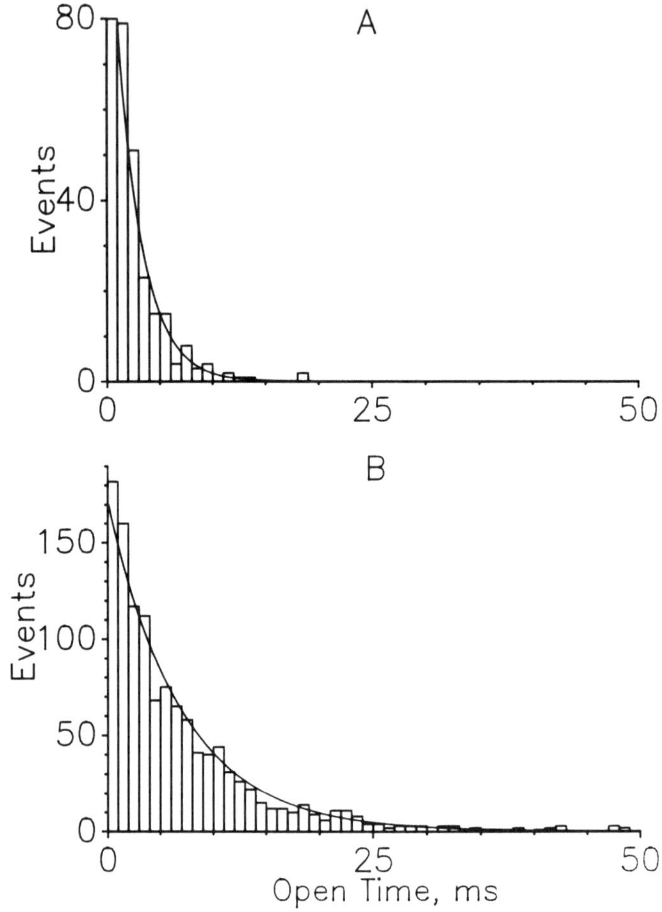

Figure 5. Analysis of open times at −60 mV in a cell-attached (A) and excised (B) patch. Same experiment as Fig. 1. Open time histograms were fit to monoexponential distributions using a Marquardt algorithm and a maximum likelihood estimator. Time constants were 2.4 and 6.9 ms, respectively in A and B. In A events containing overlap of multiple channel openings (less than 5% of the total) were excluded. No overlaps occurred in the experiment of panel B.

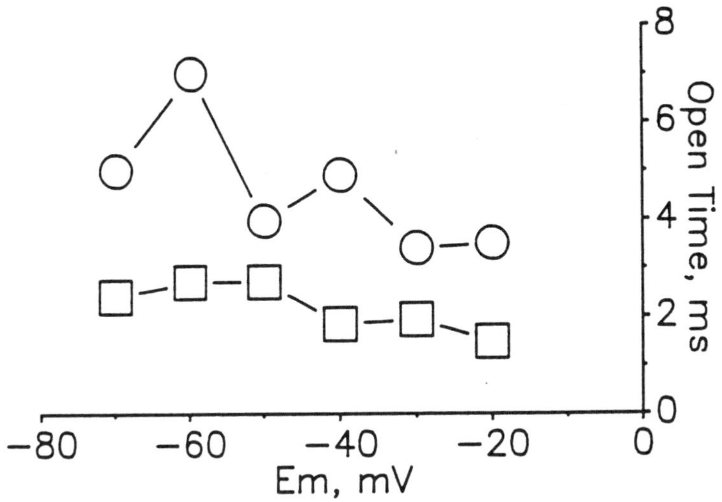

Figure 6. Voltage dependence of mean open time in a cell-attached (squares) and an excised (circles) patch. Same experiments as in Fig. 5. Mean open time obtained from histogram analysis is plotted against test pulse potential.

Comparison of waiting time (latency-to-first opening), in Figure 7 shows that there is little difference between the two patches. Fitting the cumulative waiting time histograms required biexponential functions as expected from the sigmoidal rise of the Po-t relationship (Fig. 1C) and indicative of at least two closed states that preceded opening. Nonetheless, the weighted average latencies were not significantly different at 7.0 and 8.5 ms in Figures 7A and B, respectively. The excision-induced prolongation of the decay phase of Na^+ conductance therefore, cannot be caused by channels that open for the first time late in the pulse. A more likely explanation may be found in the tendency toward prolonged bursting.

In order to analyze bursting behavior in excised patches we first constructed closed time histograms as shown in Figure 8. In both cell-attached (8A) and excised (8B) patches the histograms were accurately fit by a biexponential decay, the fast decay phase corresponding to the closed interval between individual openings within a burst and the slow phase corresponding to the interburst interval. We used the time constants from the closed time histograms to obtain a critical closed duration that would accurately identify bursts by the method of Colquhoun and Sakmann (1985). The analysis of

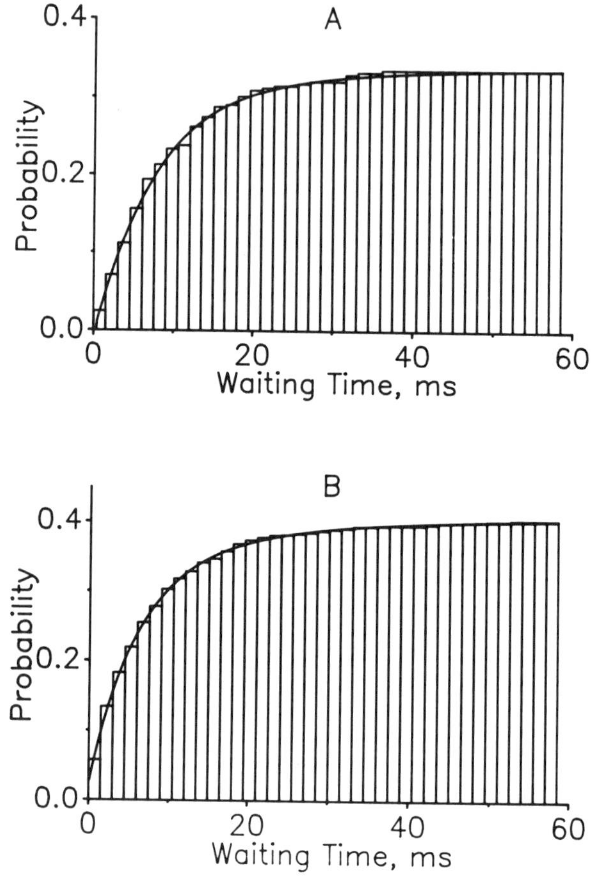

Figure 7. Analysis of waiting times at –60 mV in a cell-attached (A) and an excised (B) patch at a test potential of –60 mV. Frequency distribution of first latencies (waiting times), corrected for the number of channels in the patch by the method of Patlak and Horn (1982) are plotted as cumulative histograms. Smooth curves represent biexponential fits with the following time constants (and weighting factors); (A) 5.2 ms (0.78) and 13.2 ms (0.22); (B) 5.9 ms (0.78) and 17.8 ms (0.22). Same experiments as in Fig. 1.

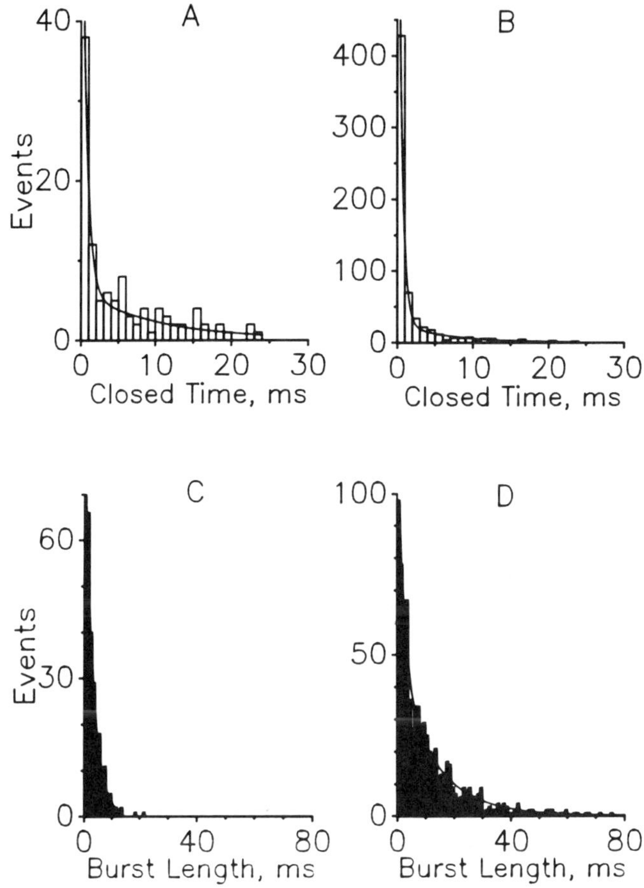

Figure 8. Analysis of bursts in a cell-attached (A,C) and an excised (B,C) patch at test potential –60 mV. Same experiments as Fig. 1. Panels A and B show closed time histograms fit to biexponential decays with time constants (and weighting factors): (A) 0.64 ms (0.4) and 10.54 ms (0.6); (B) 0.7 ms (0.5) and 6.4 ms (0.3). From the two closed time constants and the assumption that the short closed time separates openings within a burst we calculated a critical closed interval which served to identify bursts by the method of Colquhoun and Sakmann (1985). Frequency distributions of burst durations are shown in panels C and D. The smooth curves are fits to sums of exponential distributions with time constants (and weighting factors): (A) 2.9 ms; (B) 2.3 ms (0.23) and 13.3 ms (0.77).

Table I
Kinetic Model Rate Constants

Rate (1/ms)	*Cell-attached*	*Excised*
k_{12}	0.19	0.17
k_{21}	0.60	0.86
k_{23}	0.90	1.00
k_{32}	0.20	0.14
k_{34}	0.26	0.09
k_{24}	0.01	0.01

burst kinetics in Figures 8C-D shows that the mean burst length in the cell-attached patch (8C) was only slightly longer than the mean open time, in the excised patch by contrast, mean burst length was nearly 4 times as long. Mean closed interval within bursts was 0.49 ms. Bursts consisting of more than 1 opening contained on average 3.8 openings.

Long-lasting bursts and long mean open times combine to produce the prolongation of the decay phase of the Po-t curve from the excised patch shown in Figure 1C. These characteristics are consistent with the idea that the inactivation mechanism is modified under cell-free conditions and, at the level of single channel gating, this modification may be explained by a kinetic scheme in which the transition rate from the open to the inactivated state is preferentially reduced in excised patches. From the work of Horn and Vandenberg (1984) we know that single Na^+ channel kinetics can be modelled by a Markov scheme consisting of three interconnected states: closed, open, and inactivated. In the following section we use a similar model to describe a plausible modification in channel gating that can explain the changes caused by patch excision.

The kinetic model consists of two closed states (C_1 and C_2), a single open state (O_3) and a single absorbing inactivated state (I_4) interconnected as shown in the inset of Figure 9. The model rate constants (Table I) were obtained for the excised patch data by fitting the experimentally determined Po-t curve using an iterative method with the following constraints: k_{12} was fixed at 0.16 ms^{-1} since it corresponds to 1/(mean interburst interval) from the closed time histogram; k_{23} was not allowed to exceed 1/(mean closed time within the burst) from the closed time histogram; k_{32} and k_{34} were not

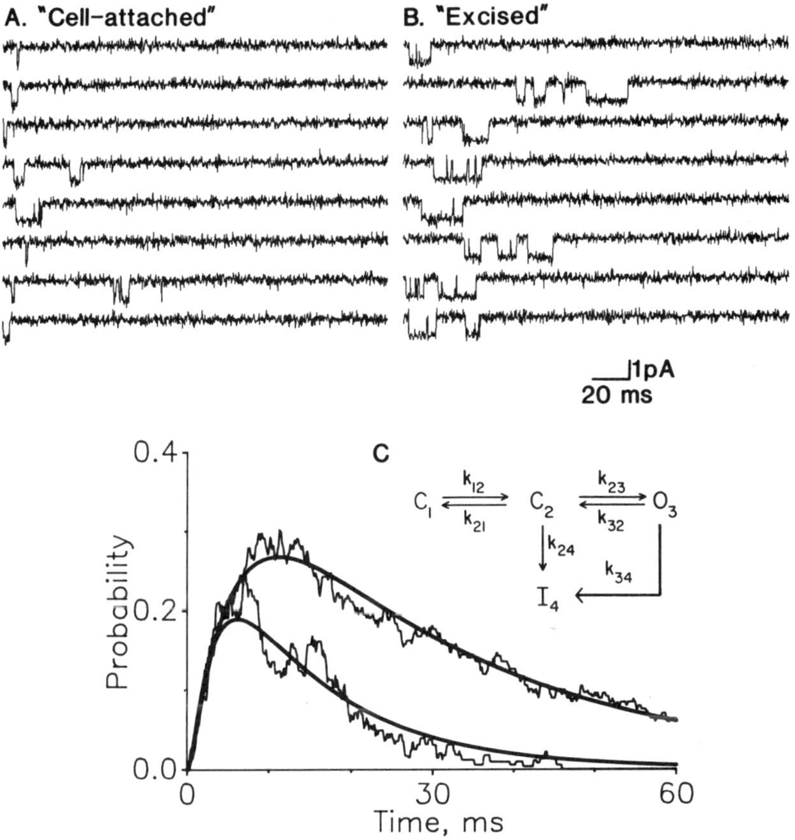

Figure 9. Model simulation of the effects of patch excision on single Na channel gating kinetics at a test potential of −60 mV. Panels A and B show simulated single channel data from the model shown in the inset of C. Noisy curves in C show Po-t relationships obtained experimentally as described in Fig. 1. Smooth curves shown are predicted by the model shown in the inset. Values for rate constants (Table I) were chosen by fitting the experimental Po curves by an iterative procedure.

allowed to exceed 1/(mean open time). Rate constants from the excised patch model were used as initial guesses for fitting the model to the cell-attached Po-t curve with the result that a close super position of model and experimental Po-t curves was obtained by tripling k_{34}. Figure 9A and 9B show that the chosen rate constants can produce single channel events which closely simulate the real data. The close correspondence between real and simulated data therefore demonstrates that the excision-induced changes in Na^+ channel gating can be explained almost entirely by a three-fold decrease in the rate of transit of channels from the open to the inactivated state.

DISCUSSION

The main conclusion from the present study is that cardiac Na^+ channels in excised membrane patches open repetitively in long-lasting bursts consisting of relatively long opening (>3 ms) separated by brief (<1 ms) closed intervals, the result of which is a prolongation of the inactivation phase of membrane Na^+ conductance. A marked reduction in the rate constant leading from open to inactivated states provides a plausible explanation for this effect.

The excision-induced effects on inactivation cannot be explained by a negative shift in the voltage dependence of Na^+ channel gating that has been shown to occur in membrane patches excised from heart cells (Cachelin et al., 1984). Fernandez et al. (1984) has shown that this shift results in an acceleration of the decay phase both in internally dialyzed whole cells and in excised patches at test potentials more negative than −10 mV. A clear distinction between the two types of effects is also evident from the observation that Na^+ channels in excised patches from cortical neurons undergo a negative shift without the appearance of prolonged bursting or long mean open time (Kirsch and Brown, 1989).

Prolonged bursting in excised heart membrane patches at test potentials near threshold may correspond to a slowly inactivating component of membrane Na^+ current recorded in whole cells (Gintant et al., 1984). A similar type of bursting has been observed previously in cell-attached patches from heart cells under a variety of recording conditions, but its occurrence is quite rare (Patlak and Ortiz, 1986; Grant and Starmer, 1987; Kolhardt et al., 1987; Clark and Giles, 1987). Under experimental conditions similar to ours, Patlak and Ortiz (1986) reported bursting in adult rat heart in less than 0.1% of their records. Nonetheless, the characteristic features of such *ultra-slow* Na^+ currents resemble those that predominate in excised patches described here. In the work of Patlak and Ortiz the mean open time of such events was 4–10 ms at a temperature of 10°C and test potentials −50 to −30 mV, which is comparable to the data reported here. Mean closed times within bursts were longer than those reported here, but this may be partially explained by the better time resolution of our measurement (0.1 ms *vs.* 1.0 ms sampling interval in Patlak and Ortiz, 1986). Patlak and Ortiz attribute the ultra-slow currents to the appearance of a spontaneous mode of gating that may be defined as a shift in the rate constants that govern transitions out of the open state. We show that this is the normal mode for channels in excised patches in which the intracellular surface has been exposed to a CsF-rich medium. In nerve, Cs^+ has been implicated as the cause of slow inactivation of Na^+ currents in intracellularly perfused nerve axons (Oxford and Yeh, 1985; Goldman, 1986). Although we cannot rule out a Cs^+ effect, we have found similar bursting to occur in patches exposed to KF-rich solutions as well. Fluoride ions, which reversibly slow the activation of K^+ currents in intracellularly perfused squid axon (Adams and Oxford, 1983; Kirsch et al., 1986) and reversibly activate muscarinic K^+ channels in atrial myocytes by a GTP-binding protein mechanism (Kurachi and Nakajima, 1987), may also contribute to this phenomenon. Patlak and Ortiz (1986) also observed that the slow components of Na^+ channel gating were suppressed by holding potentials as negative as -140 mV, whereas this was not true in the excised patches described here (e.g., Fig. 1). An interesting possibility is that cardiac Na^+ channel gating is modulated by a voltage-dependent, intracellular mechanism that is lost when channels are recorded in cell-free patch conditions. Such modulation would have important physiological consequences since the depolarizing effects of maintained inward Na^+ current have a profound effect on cardiac rhythmicity and may also play a role in the use-dependent block of cardiac Na^+ channels by local anesthetics (Hondeghem and Katzung, 1977). Unravelling the cellular mechanism responsible for modulation would be an important step in elucidating the molecular mechanisms that control electrical activity in the heart.

Acknowledgments: We thank Dr. A. VanDongen for making available the rate-fitting program used for kinetic modelling.

This work was supported by an American Heart Association grant 876197 and by National Heart, Lung and Blood Institute grants HL-5143 and HL-33662 to Dr. A.M. Brown.

BIBLIOGRAPHY

Adams DJ, Oxford GS. Interaction of internal anions with potassium channels of the squid giant axon. *Biophys J* 82:429–448, 1983.

Attwell D, Cohen I, Eisner D, Ohba M, Ojeda C. The steady-state TTX-sensitive ("window") sodium current in cardiac Purkinje fibres. *Pflugers Arch* 379:137–142, 1979.

Baer M, Best PM, Reuter H. Voltage-dependent action of tetrodotoxin in mammalian cardiac muscle. *Nature* 263:344–345, 1976.

Cachelin AB, DePeyer JE, Kokubun S, Reuter H. Sodium channels in cultured cardiac cells. *J Physiol* (*Lond*) 340:389–401, 1983.

Clark RB, Giles W. Sodium current in single cells from bullfrog atrium: voltage dependence and ion transfer properties. *J Physiol* (*Lond*) 391:235–265, 1987.

Colquhoun D, Sakmann B. Fast events in single-channel currents activated by acetylcholine and its analogues at the frog muscle end-plate. *J. Physiol* (*Lond*) 369:501–557, 1985.

Fernandez JM, Fox AP, Krasne S. Membrane patches and whole-cell membranes: a comparison of electrical properties in rat clonal pituitary (GH) cells. *J Physiol* (*Lond*) 356:565–585, 1984.

Fox JA. Ion channel subconductance states. *J Memb Biol* 97:1–8, 1987.

Gintant GA, Datyner NB, Cohen IS. Slow inactivation of a tetrodotoxin-sensitive current in canine cardiac Purkinje fibers. *Biophys J* 45:509–512, 1984.

Goldman L. Internal cesium and the sodium inactivation gate in Myxicola giant axons. *Biophys J* 50:231–238.

Grant AO, Starmer CF. Mechanisms of closure of cardiac sodium channels in rabbit ventricular myocytes: single-channel analysis. *Circ Res* 60:897–913, 1987.

Hamill OP, Marty A, Sakmann B, Sigworth FJ. Improved patch-clamp techniques for high-resolution current recording from cells and cell-free membrane patches. *Pflügers Arch* 391:85–100, 1981.

Hondeghem LM, Katzung GB. Time- and voltage-dependent interactions of antiarrhythmic drugs with cardiac sodium channels. *Biochim Biophys Acta* 472:373–398, 1977.

Horn R, Vandenberg CA. Statistical properties of single sodium channels. *J Gen Physiol* 84:505–534, 1984.

Kirsch GE, Brown AM. Kinectic properties of single sodium channels in rat heart and rat brain. *J Gen Physiol* 93:85, 1989.

Kirsch GE, Yeh JZ, Oxford GS. Modulation of aminopyridine block of potassium currents in squid axon. *Biophys J* 50:637–644, 1986.

Kohlhardt M, Frobe U, Herzig JW. Properties of normal and non-inactivating single cardiac Na^+ channels. *Proc Roy Soc Ser B* 232:71–93, 1987.

Kunze DL, Lacerda AE, Wilson DL, Brown AM. Cardiac Na currents and the inactivating, reopening and waiting properties of single cardiac Na channels. *J Gen Physiol* 86:691–719, 1985.

Kurachi Y, Nakajima T. Intracellular fluoride activation of muscarinic K channel in atrial cell membrane. Circulation 76:105, 1987. Abstract.

Lux HD, Brown AM. Patch and whole cell calcium currents recorded simultaneously in snail neurons. *J Gen Physiol* 83:727–750, 1984.
Oxford GS, Yeh JZ. Interactions of monovalent cations with sodium channels in squid axons. I. Modification of physiological inactivation gating. *J Gen Physiol* 85:583–602, 1985.
Patlak J, Horn R. Effect of N-bromoacetamide on single sodium channel currents in excised membrane patches. *J Gen Physiol* 79:333–351, 1982.
Patlak JB, Ortiz M. Slow currents through single sodium channels of adult rat heart. *J Gen Physiol* 86:89–104, 1986.
Scanley BE, Fozzard HA. Low conductance sodium channels in canine cardiac Purkinje cells. *Biophys J* 52:489–495, 1987.
Sokal RR, Rohlf FJ. *Biometry.* 2nd ed. San Francisco, CA: W.H. Freeman and Co; 624–629, 1981.
Yatani A, Brown AM. The calcium channel blocker nitrenidipine blocks sodium channels in neonatal rat cardiac myocytes. *Circ Res* 57:868 – 875.

Chapter 6

Types of Calcium Channels in Heart Muscle

Bruce P. Bean

Experiments in a number of laboratories over the last 4 years have shown the existence of two distinct types of calcium channels in cardiac muscle cells (Nilius et al., 1985; Bean, 1985; Mitra and Morad, 1986; Bonvallet, 1987; Hagiwara et al., 1988). This chapter reviews the evidence for two different channel types—which by now is overwhelming—and discusses the differences between them.

KINETICS AND VOLTAGE-DEPENDENCE

In recording macroscopic currents from some types of myocardial cells, two components of current can be distinguished. One component is present only if fairly negative holding potentials are used; this component of current is activated by relatively small depolarizations, to potentials of −60 to −50 mV or so, and inactivates fairly quickly (time-constant 5–30 msec) regardless of whether the current-carrying ion is Ca or Ba. This component has been variously referred to as *fast, transient, low-threshold,* and *low-voltage-activated* Ca current. I will follow the terminology originating from the Tsien laboratory and call this T (for transient) current (Nilius et al., 1985).

Hondeghem, Luc (ed): Molecular and Cellular Mechanisms of Antiarrhythmic Agents, Futura Publishing Company, Inc., Mount Kisco, NY, © 1989.

The second component of current is present at all holding potentials negative to about −20 mV; it is activated by depolarizations to potentials positive to about −30 mV and, at least with Ba as the charge carrier, it inactivates relatively slowly. This component has been called *slow, long-lasting, high-threshold,* and *high-voltage-activated* Ca current. In this chapter it will be referred to as the L current. Although the name was given partly because of the *long-lasting* (i.e., slowly-inactivating) nature of the component, it is important to emphasize that L current is by no means a noninactivating Ca current. Even with Ba as the charge carrier and with high EGTA levels inside the cell, L current inactivates with multiple time-constants in the range of 100–800 msec. With Ca as the charge carrier and with less internal Ca buffering, inactivation of L current can be very rapid (time-constants of tens of msec); this difference reflects promotion of inactivation by Ca entry (e.g., Kass and Sanguinetti, 1984; Lee et al., 1985; Hadley and Hume, 1987). In fact, at potentials of +10 to +30 mV, inactivation of L current under quasi-physiological ionic conditions is not much slower that of T current. Thus, with Ca as the charge carrier, it is impossible to separate the contributions of T channels and L channels to the macroscopic Ca current simply by inspection of the kinetics of inactivation (except for the smallest depolarizations that elicit current, for which the L current inactivation is very slow). Separation of the two components is much easier when Ba is the charge carrier, when inactivation of L current is far slower.

In cultured pituitary cells, Matteson and Armstrong (1986) distinguished two components of Ca current (which have roughly the characteristics of cardiac T and L currents) by their differing rates of deactivation upon termination of an activating depolarization. The same difference in deactivation kinetics holds for cardiac Ca channels: T channels deactivate relatively slowly and have slow tail currents (time-constant 2–5 msec), while L channels have tail currents that decay many times faster (unpublished observations).

One can confidently speak of the differences in kinetics of T and L type Ca channels only because the distinction between the two current components has been confirmed in many other ways, with differences in ionic selectivity, pharmacology, and single channel behavior that will be discussed. Complex kinetic behavior, by itself, is no evidence for multiple types of channels. In fact, L channels by themselves have fairly complex kinetics: fitting the time-course of inactivation requires at least 2 time-constants (and sometimes a steady, noninactivating component), and tail currents can have multiple time constants.

SINGLE CHANNEL CONDUCTANCE AND SELECTIVITY

L and T channels evidently have different pore structures, since they have different ionic selectivity and different single-channel conductances. In L channels, currents carried by Ba are about twice as large as those carried by the same concentration of Ca. In T channels, currents carried by Ba and Ca are about the same size (Nilius et al., 1985). In 100 mM Ba, the single-channel conductance of T channels (7–9 pS) is about half of that of L channels (15–20 pS), (Nilius et al., 1985; Hagiwara et al., 1988).

Along with these differences in selectivity and single-channel conductance, the two channel types are somewhat different in their sensitivity to inorganic blockers. L channels are more effectively blocked by low concentrations of Cd than are T channels (Nilius et al., 1985; Mitra and Morad, 1986; Bonvallet, 1987; but see Hagiwara et al., 1988). T channels are more effectively blocked by low concentrations of Ni than are L channels (Bonvallet, 1987; Hagiwara, 1988; but see Mitra and Morad, 1986). However, the selectivity of either Ni or Cd is far from perfect; concentrations high enough to completely block either type of current usually inhibit the other component significantly. Both types of channel are also sensitive to block by Co ions, with little difference in sensitivity (Bean, 1985; Hagiwara et al., 1988). Both can also be blocked by La ions, for which differences in sensitivity have apparently not yet been examined.

L channels become very permeable to monovalent cations if external divalents are reduced to submicromolar levels with chelators like EGTA and EDTA (Hess and Tsien, 1984; Matsuda, 1986). This effect has not yet been reported for cardiac T channels, although T-like channels in other preparations do show the phenomenon (Fukushima and Hagiwara, 1985; Suarez-Kurtz et al., 1986; Chen and Hess, 1987). Explorations of monovalent permeation and block by divalents in L channels have led to a model of Ca permeation involving two binding sites for Ca within the pore (Hess and Tsien, 1984; Almers and McCleskey, 1984). It seems possible that the differences in single-channel conductance, ionic selectivity, and divalent block of T channels could all be accounted for by fairly small differences in the hypothetical binding sites or the energy barriers between them. So far, there is no evidence that the mechanism of permeation and selectivity is fundamentally different between the two types of channels (see Tsien et al., 1987).

MODULATION

It is well known (since the first demonstration by Reuter, 1967) that cardiac Ca currents can be modulated by neurotransmitters. Beta-adrenergic stimulation and other transmitters and hormones that increase cyclic AMP levels produce an increase in the Ca current activated by depolarization of the membrane. Such modulation contributes to the positive inotropy and positive chronotropy seen with beta stimulation.

The evidence so far suggests that only L channels, not T channels, are modulated by beta-adrenergic stimulation. In canine atrial cells, beta stimulation clearly did not increase T current, even in cells where large increases in L current were seen (Bean, 1985). The same conclusion was reached by Bonvallet (1987) in experiments on frog atrial cells, and by Hagiwara et al. (1988) on rabbit sinoatrial nodal cells. However, Mitra and Morad (1986), in experiments on guinea pig ventricular cells, concluded that both L current and T current were increased by adrenaline. While it is hard to rule out a species or tissue difference, the apparent discrepancy may arise from the difficulty of separating T and L components when Ca is the charge carrier, as in the experiments by Mitra and Morad. As pointed out by Hagiwara et al., because the L current component is usually so much larger than the T current component, an apparent increase in the T component could easily arise if separation of the two components by holding potential is slightly imperfect. This problem is especially pronounced with Ca as the charge carrier, since inactivation of L current can be so rapid; it is compounded by the fact that the adrenergic increase of L current is voltage-dependent, with larger increases in current for the smallest depolarizations—the region where T current is most easily measured. For these reasons, the evidence for beta-adrenergic modulation of T current is not yet convincing. A clear demonstration of T channel modulation would require single-channel recordings, which so far have yielded negative results (Hagiwara et al., 1988).

An interesting, as yet unexplored, possibility is that T channels could be modulated by other transmitters working through other second messenger systems. T current in neuronal cells can be decreased by adrenergic stimulation (Marchetti et al., 1986), an effect which may be mediated by kinase C, as modulation of high-threshold channels in neurons (Dunlap and Fischbach, 1981) also may be (Rane and Dunlap, 1986). It will be interesting to see whether cardiac T channels can also be regulated by this or other systems. Angiotensin II (Kass and Blair, 1981; Allen et al., 1987), alpha-adrenergic agonists (Alvarez et al., 1987), acetylcholine (Giles and Noble, 1976; Hescheler et al., 1986), adenosine, and ATP modulate cardiac Ca current, and it will be interesting to examine possible selective modulation of L or T channels by these agents.

DISTRIBUTION

All types of cardiac cells so far examined have L channels, but only some have T channels. When present, current from T channels tends to be much smaller than L current. Preliminary experiments suggest that frog ventricular, calf ventricular, calf atrial, and rabbit atrial cells have no T current. T currents in canine ventricular cells are either tiny or nonexistent. In guinea pig ventricular (Nilius et al., 1985; Mitra and Morad, 1986), frog atrial (Bonvallet, 1987), canine atrial (Bean, 1985), and rabbit sinoatrial cells (Hagiwara et al., 1988), peak T current is typically only 5%–20% of peak L current, even under ionic conditions that maximize the relative size of the T component (low external Ca). It therefore seems clear that L channels carry almost all of the classical cardiac Ca current recorded as I_{si} in multi cellular preparations.

FUNCTION

It seems clear that L channels support the functional roles commonly ascribed to Ca channels in working myocardium: helping maintain the plateau of the action potential, and providing an influx of Ca to initiate contraction (mainly by triggering release of more Ca by the sarcoplasmic reticulum). A primary role for T channels in contraction seems very unlikely, since they do not exist in some working myocardial cells. It also seems unlikely that T channels could play much of an electrical role in normal atrial or ventricular tissue, since current through them would be swamped by much larger Na channel currents, which activate in a similar voltage range. However, a role for T channels in abnormal electrical activity in damaged, depolarized atrial or ventricular tissue is a possibility, since Na channels can be inactivated at membrane potentials at which some T channels are still available (Bean, 1985).

An electrical role for T channels in normal cardiac pacemaking is a strong possibility. Both the absolute density of T current and its density relative to L current are greater in rabbit sinoatrial cells than in other types of cells (Hagiwara et al., 1988). Hagiwara et al. found that 40 μM Ni, with a fairly selective blocking action on T current, slows the later phase of diastolic depolarization in sinoatrial cells. The low threshold of T channels is obviously consistent with activity in this voltage range, especially in cells with more negative maximum diastolic potentials, where removal of T channel inactivation would be greatest. T channels have also recently been described in Purkinje fiber cells (Hirano et al., 1988), where they could also play a role in pacemaking. It also seems possible that T channels could be involved in A-V nodal action potentials, although studies of T channels in A-V nodal cells have not yet been reported.

PHARMACOLOGY

Since L channels carry most or all of the current in the multicellular preparations used to characterize cardiac Ca channel pharmacology, the pharmacology of cardiac L channels has been fairly thoroughly explored. L channels can be blocked by various dihydropyridine drugs (nifedipine, nitrendipine, nisoldipine, nimodipine, (+) PN200-110, etc.), verapamil (and its methoxy derivative D600), and diltiazem. Other dihydropyridine molecules (e.g., (−) BAY K 8644, (+)-(S)-202-791) act as *Ca channel agonists,* increasing the current carried through L channels.

Dihydropyridine effects on L channels are quite complicated. Inhibition by dihydropyridine blockers is strongly dependent on holding potential, with more potent block at more depolarized holding potentials (Sanguinetti and Kass, 1984; Uehara and Hume, 1985; Bean, 1984). This effect is quite similar to block of Na channels by lidocaine and other antiarrhythmic agents and it can be understood by the same modulated receptor hypothesis (Hille, 1977; Hondeghem and Katzung, 1977)—that the binding of dihydropyridine blockers to inactivated channels is much tighter than to closed, resting channels.

In cultured pituitary cells, there is convincing evidence that dihydropyridines also bind very tightly to the open state of the channel (Cohen and McCarthy, 1987). It seems likely that this is also true of cardiac L channels, but distinguishing open and inactivated channel block in cardiac cells is much more difficult because it seems impossible to have channels open without rapidly entering the inactivated state. It remains possible to hypothesize that dihydropyridines bind tightly only to open channels, not to inactivated channels. No experiments directly addressing this issue have yet been reported.

Another interesting, related question is: if dihydropyridines do bind tightly to inactivated channels, is there a difference in binding to inactivated states reached by Ca-dependent inactivation and those reached by voltage-dependent inactivation? This question could be approached by comparing the potency of dihydropyridine block at various membrane potentials with and without Ca-dependent inactivation (for example, comparing cells using Ba as the charge carrier and strong internal Ca buffering with cells using Ca as the charge carrier and weak Ca buffering).

Another issue related to dihydropyridine block is the possibility of understanding dihydropyridine interactions by a *guarded receptor* model like that proposed for antiarrhythmic interaction with Na channels (Starmer and Courtney, 1986). There is more experimental data to discriminate between various models in the case of dihydropyridine interaction with Ca channels, since there are ligand binding experiments that directly show changes in binding affinity as a function of holding potential (Kokubun et al., 1987).

Another interesting complication of dihydropyridine effects on Ca channels is that the same molecule can both decrease or increase Ca current, depending on the pulse protocol. It is well-established that, under some circumstances, nitrendipine can increase Ca current (Brown et al., 1984, 1986) and BAY K 8644 can decrease the current (Sanguinetti et al., 1986; Hadley and Hume, 1987). These effects may partially be due to competing effects of the different isomers in these drugs (both of which are racemic mixtures), but experiments by Kokubun et al., (1987) on separated enantiomers of the dihydropyridine Sandoz 202–791 show that even a pure isomer can have both effects. A model for dihydropyridine action has been proposed that can account for both blocking and potentiation as arising from changes in a single kinetic step (slowing of a back reaction from open to closed, nonactivated states of the channel) (Sanguinetti et al., 1986). However, it is not clear that the model can fit all the changes in single-channel behavior seen with the drug (e.g., Hess et al., 1984; Brown et al., 1986). Also, binding data indicate that there are at least two high affinity binding sites on the cardiac L channel (Kokubun et al., 1987).

T channels are much less sensitive than L channels to block by dihydropyridines. For example, nifedipine and nitrendipine at 1–2 μM have no effect on T current (Bean, 1985; Hagiwara et al., 1988). However, T channels are not completely insensitive to dihydropyridine block. At 10 μM, nitrendipine does block T current by about 10%; this is not surprising since at similar concentrations dihydropyridine blockers also have small inhibitory effects on Na (Yatani et al., 1985) and K (Hume, 1985) channels.

A particularly promising area for development of new drugs is identification of selective blockers of T channels. It seems quite possible that T channels could be involved in the generation of some ectopic arrhythmias and that a T channel blocker could be useful therapeutically. The only selective organic T channel blocker described so far is tetramethrin (an insecticide that also acts on Na channels by prolonging channel open time). At 100 nM, tetramethrin completely blocks T current in rabbit sinoatrial cells (Hagiwara et al., 1988), without any effect on L current. The block of cardiac T current is more potent than block of T current in neuroblastoma cells, where T channel block was first described (Tsunoo et al., 1985). Because of its effects on Na channels, tetramethrin itself is unlikely to be a useful therapeutic agent, but it demonstrates the possibility of selective block of T channels.

In neuroblastoma cells and in central neurons, the antiarrhythmic and anticonvulsant agent diphenylhydantoin has been found to be an effective blocker of T current (Twombley and Narahashi, 1986; Yaari et al., 1987). It will be interesting to see whether this (or other antiarrhythmics commonly thought to act mainly on Na channels, like lidocaine and quinidine) might also—or even preferentially—block cardiac T channels.

There may be still another type of Ca channel in heart muscle cells (Lee et al., 1984), which may have a pharmacology of its own.

BIBLIOGRAPHY

Allen IS, Cohen NM, Dhallan RS, Rogers TB. Angiotensin II increases the calcium current in neonatal rat single cardiac myocytes.*Proc Physiol Soc* March 1987.

Almers W, McCleskey EW. Non-selective conductance in calcium channels of frog muscle: calcium selectivity in a single-file pore. *J Physiol (Lond)* 353:585–608, 1984.

Alvarez JL, Mongo KG, Vassort G. Effects of alpha 1-adrenergic stimulation on the Ca current in single ventricular frog cells. *Proc Physiol Soc* March 1987.

Armstrong CM, Matteson DR. Two distinct populations of calcium channels in a clonal line of pituitary cells. *Science* 227:65–66, 1985.

Bean BP. Nitrendipine block of cardiac calcium channels: High-affinity binding to the inactivated state. *Proc Nat Acad Sci USA* 81:6388–6392, 1984.

Bean BP. Two kinds of calcium channels in canine atrial cells. Differences in kinetics, selectivity, and pharmacology. *J Gen Physiol* 86:1–30, 1985.

Bechem M, Pott L. Removal of Ca current inactivation in dialysed guinea-pig atrial cardioballs by Ca chelators. *Pflugers Arch* 404:10–20, 1985.

Bonvallet R. A low threshold calcium current recorded at physiological Ca concentrations in single frog atrial cells. *Pflugers Arch* 408:540–542, 1987.

Brown AM, Kunze DL, Yatani A. Dual effects of dihydropyridines on whole cell and unitary calcium currents in single ventricular cells of guinea pig. *J Physiol (Lond)* 379:495–514, 1986.

Brown AM, Kunze DL, Yatani A. The agonist effect of dihydropyridines on Ca channels. *Nature* 311:570–572, 1984.

Chen C, Hess P. Calcium channels in mouse 3T3 and human fibroblasts. *Biophysical J* 51:226a, 1987. Abstract.

Cohen CJ, McCarthy RT. Nimodipine block of calcium channels in rat anterior pituitary cells. *J Physiol (Lond)* 387:195–225, 1987.

Dunlap K, Fischbach GD. Neurotransmitters decrease the calcium conductance activated by depolarization of embryonic chick sensory neurones. *J Physiol (Lond)* 317:519–535, 1981.

Fukushima Y, Hagiwara S. Currents carried by monovalent cations through calcium channels in mouse neoplastic B lymphocytes. *J Physiol (Lond)* 385:255–284, 1985.

Giles W, Noble SJ. Changes in membrane currents in bullfrog atrium produced by acetylcholine. *J Physiol (Lond)* 261:103–123, 1976.

Hadley RW, Hume JR. An intrinsic potential-dependent inactivation mechanism associated with calcium channels in guinea-pig myocytes. *J Physiol (Lond)* 389:205–222, 1987.

Hagiwara N, Irisawa H, Kameyama M. Contribution of two types of calcium currents to the pacemaker potentials of rabbit sino-atrial node cells. *J Physiol* 395:233–253, 1988.

Hescheler J, Kameyama M, Trautwein W. On the mechanism of muscarinic inhibition of the cardiac Ca current. *Pflugers Arch* 407:182–189, 1986.

Hess P, Tsien RW. Mechanisms of ion permeation through calcium channels. *Nature* 309:453–456, 1984.
Hess P, Lansman JB, Tsien RW. Different modes of Ca channel gating behavior favored by dihydropyridine Ca agonists and antagonists. *Nature* 311:538–544, 1984.
Hille B. Local anesthetics: hydrophilic and hydrophobic pathways for the drug: receptor reaction. *J Gen Physiol* 69:497–515, 1977.
Hirano Y, January CT, Fozzard HA. Inactivation of T type calcium current in cardiac Purkinje cells. *Biophys J* 53:554a, 1988. Abstract.
Hondeghem LM, Katzung BG. Time- and voltage-dependent interactions of antiarrhythmic drugs with cardiac sodium channels. *Biochim Biophys Acta* 472:373–398, 1977.
Hume JR. Comparative interactions of organic Ca^{++} channel antagonists with myocardial Ca^{++} and K channels. *J Pharmacol Exp Ther* 234:134–140, 1985.
Kamp TJ, Miller RJ, Sanguinetti MC. The "agonist" enantiomer of the dihydropyridine (DHP) 202–791 blocks I_{Ca} at depolarized potentials. *Biophys J* 51:429a, 1987.
Kass RS, Sanguinetti MC. Inactivation of calcium channel current in the calf cardiac Purkinje fiber: evidence for voltage- and calcium-mediated mechanisms. *J Gen Physiol* 84:705–726, 1984.
Kass RS, Blair ML. Effects of angiotensin II on membrane current in canine Purkinje fibers. *J Mol Cell Cardiol* 13:797–809, 1981.
Kokubun S, Prod'hom B, Becker C, Porzig H, Reuter H. Studies on Ca channels in intact cardiac cells: voltage-dependent effects and cooperative interactions of dihydropyridine enantiomers. *Mol Pharmacol* 30:571–584, 1987.
Lee KS, Noble D, Lee E, Spindler AJ. A new calcium current underlying the plateau of the cardiac action potential. *Proc R Soc Lond B Biol Sci* B 223:35–48, 1984.
Lee KS, Marban E, Tsien RW. Inactivation of calcium channels in mammalian heart cells: joint dependence on membrane potential and intracellular calcium. *J Physiol (Lond)* 364:395–411, 1985.
Marchetti C, Carbone E, Lux HD. Effects of dopamine and noradrenaline on Ca channels of cultured sensory neurons and sympathetic neurons of chick. *Pflugers Arch* 406:101–111, 1986.
Matsuda H. Sodium conductance in calcium channels of guinea-pig ventricular cells induced by removal of external calcium ions. *Pflugers Arch* 407:465–475, 1986.
Matteson DR, Armstrong CM. Properties of two types of calcium channels in clonal pituitary cells. *J Gen Physiol* 87:161–182, 1986.
Mitra R, Morad M. Two types of calcium channels in guinea-pig ventricular myocytes. *Proc Nat Acad Sci USA* 83: 5340–5344, 1986.
Nilius B, Hess P, Lansman JB, Tsien RW. A novel type of cardiac calcium channel in ventricular cells. *Nature* 316:443–446, 1985.
Rane SG, Dunlap K. Kinase C activator 1,2-oleylacetylglycerol attenuates voltage-dependent calcium current in sensory neurons. *Proc Natl Acad Sci USA* 83:184–188, 1986.

Reuter H. The dependence of the slow inward current on external calcium concentration in Purkinje fibres. *J Physiol (Lond)* 192:479–499, 1967.

Sanguinetti MC, Kass RS. Voltage-dependent block of calcium channel current by dihydropyridine calcium channel antagonists. *Circ Res* 55:336–348, 1984.

Sanguinetti MC, Krafte DS, Kass RS. Voltage-dependent modulation of Ca channel current in heart cells by Bay K 8644. *J Gen Physiol* 88:369–392, 1986.

Starmer CF, Courtney KR. Modeling ion channel blockade at guarded binding sites: application to tertiary drugs. *Amer J Physiol* 251:H848-H856, 1986.

Suarez-Kurtz G, Katz GM, Reuben JP. Currents carried by sodium ions through transient calcium channels in clonal GH3 pituitary cells. *Pflugers Arch* 410:345–347, 1987.

Tsien RW, Hess P, McCleskey EW, Rosenberg RL. Calcium channels: Mechanisms of selectivity, permeation and block. *Annu Rev Biophys Biophys Chem* 16:265–290, 1987.

Tsunoo A, Yoshii M, Narahashi T. Differential block of two calcium channels in neuroblastoma cells. *Biophys J* 47:433a, 1985. Abstract.

Twombley DA, Narahashi T. Phenytoin block of low threshold calcium channels is voltage- and frequency-dependent. *Soc Neurosci Abstr* 12:1193, 1986. Abstract.

Uehara A, Hume JR. Interactions of organic calcium channel antagonists with calcium channels in single frog atrial cells. *J Gen Physiol* 85:621–647, 1985.

Yaari Y, Hamon B, Lux HD. Development of two types of calcium channels in cultured mammalian hippocampal neurons. *Science* 235:680–682, 1987.

Yatani A, Brown AM. The calcium channel blocker nitrendipine blocks sodium channels in neonatal rat cardiac myocytes. *Circ Res* 57:865–875, 1985.

Chapter 7

Properties of Myocardial K^+ Channels and their Pharmacological Modulation

Joseph R. Hume

INTRODUCTION

K^+ currents in heart cells are involved in a number of important aspects of cell function. They are believed to play a critical role in: 1) maintenance of the resting membrane potential, 2) control of the cardiac action potential plateau and duration, 3) initiation and regulation of pacemaker activity, 4) mediation of some of the electrical effects of the autonomic transmitters, 5) determination of the effective refractory period of cardiac cells, and 6) modification of electrical activity that occurs during metabolic inhibition. The fundamental nature of many of these effects translates on a larger macroscopic scale into important factors that regulate the initiation and conduction of electrical impulses throughout the heart. Myocardial K^+ channels, therefore, represent potentially important targets for the interaction of a variety of cardiovascular drugs.

In the treatment of cardiac arrhythmias, it is well recognized that uniform prolongation of refractoriness is an important determinant of the efficacy of an antiarrhythmic agent for terminating re-entry arrhythmias (Singh and Nademanee, 1985). Such a prolongation of refractoriness is thought to be mediated through two

Hondeghem, Luc (ed): Molecular and Cellular Mechanisms of Antiarrhythmic Agents, Futura Publishing Company, Inc., Mount Kisco, NY, © 1989.

potential mechanisms. A so-called time-dependent mechanism, involving a prolongation of the recovery kinetics of myocardial Na^+ channels (class I antiarrhythmic action), or a voltage-dependent mechanism, involving prolongation of the action potential duration (class III antiarrhythmic action). Both mechanisms will result in a prolongation of the effective refractory period of cardiac tissue. Although it is well-established that prolongation of the action potential duration is an effective antiarrhythmic mechanism, most of the available antiarrhythmic agents that exhibit this property are pharmacologically diverse and have additional effects on myocardial Na^+ or Ca^{2+} channels, or have anti-adrenergic properties (e.g., sotolol, amiodarone, etc.).

In this chapter, the different classes of myocardial K^+ channels and some of their properties will be reviewed, especially emphasizing those which are believed to be importantly involved in the control of action potential duration under normal conditions. The delayed rectifier K^+ current, which is activated during the action potential plateau in isolated mammalian cardiac myocytes, is shown to be an important determinant of the ventricular action potential duration. In mammalian heart this current is strongly modulated by β-adrenergic receptor stimulation, which is coupled to the enzyme adenylate cyclase by a GTP-binding protein (Harvey and Hume, 1989).

OVERVIEW OF MYOCARDIAL K^+ CHANNELS

Early voltage clamp experiments in multicellular cardiac preparations provided evidence for the existence of a complex variety of myocardial K^+ currents (for review see Carmeliet and Vereecke, 1979, or Noble, 1984). Recently developed techniques for enzymatic dispersion of single cardiac myocytes and new patch clamp techniques (Hamill et al., 1981) for both whole-cell and single-channel current recording have significantly improved our understanding of the different types and properties of myocardial K^+ channels. Table I summarizes some of the properties of most of the important types of K^+ channels that have been studied using the newer techniques. Not all of these channels are present in every type of cardiac cell and it should be mentioned that significant differences may exist even between different species. A clearer picture of the nature of regional and species' differences with regard to cardiac K^+ channels should emerge as these techniques are applied to a greater variety

Table I
Summary of Cardiac K$^+$ Currents

Current	*Gating Potential*	*γs*	*Selectivity for K$^+$*	*Blockers*
I_{K1}	−100 to 0 mV	27 pS	high	Ba, Cs, Mg, quinidine
I_K	−50 to +30	?	high	Cs, Ba, TEA, 4-AP, quinidine phencyclidine
(In isolated frog atrial cells, a single component of delayed rectification is observed[1,2]. In mammalian cells, two kinetic components of delayed rectification have been observed[3,4]. Reported γs values from mammalian heart include 11 ps[5], 60 ps[5], and 15 ps[7]).				
I_{TO}	−70 to +10	?	?	4-AP, Ba, Cs
(Reported γs values from mammalian heart include 120 pS[8], 20 pS[9], and 27 and 12 pS[10]; P_{Na}/P_K = .25 has been reported[9]).				
$I_{K(Ach)}$	gated by Ach and G proteins[11]	35–40 pS	high	Ba, atropine
$I_{K(ATP)}$	−100 to −50	80 pS	high	ATP, Mg, 4-AP, TEA, tolbutamide, glibenclamide
$I_{K(Na)}$	no voltage dependence	207 pS	high	?

1. Hume, et al., 1986
2. Simmons, et al., 1986
3. Daytner, et al., 1984
4. Walsh, et al., 1987
5. Shibasaki, 1987
6. Clapham, et al., 1984
7. Clapham, et al., 1988
8. Callewaert, et al., 1982
9. Nakayama, et al., 1985
10. Benndorf, et al., 1987
11. Brown, et al., 1988

of different isolated cell preparations. One of the major advantages of the new whole-cell and single-channel recording techniques is a significant improvement in the isolation and separation of the different components of ionic current, thereby removing many of the uncertainties associated with earlier attempts to voltage clamp large syncytial myocardial preparations.

I_{K1}

These are inwardly rectifying K$^+$ channels that contribute significantly to the maintenance of the resting membrane potential in many cardiac cells. Earlier studies failed to provide evidence for time-dependent gating of this current, however, recent single-channel recordings in a number of preparations (Sakmann and Trube, 1984 a,b; Bechem et al., 1985; Payet et al., 1985; Kurachi, 1985; Josephson and Brown, 1986) have provided evidence for time-dependent gating of these channels over the voltage range of -100 to 0 mV. When hyperpolarizing voltage clamp pulses are applied from a holding potential of 0 mV, more channels are open at the beginning of the pulses than in the steady state. This has been interpreted as voltage-dependent inactivation, however, an alternative explanation for the time-dependent decline in inward current is that it arises from rapid depletion of K^+ in extracellular spaces (Cohen, et al., 1986). Such a rapid extracellular depletion of K^+ has been shown in multicellular Purkinje fibers using ion sensitive electrodes (Kline and Cohen, 1984), however, whether a similar rapid depletion occurs in dispersed single cells remains to be determined. It has also recently been suggested that the time-dependent decline in inward current is due to voltage dependent block of the channel by external Na^+, and to a lesser degree by external divalent ions (Biermans et al., 1987).

The inward rectifying properties of I_{K1} are an important factor that allows for the generation of long duration action potentials with prominent plateaus in the heart. As such, I_{K1} is an important determinant of the action potential duration in many types of cardiac cells. For example, an elevation of $(K^+)_o$ is known to shorten the duration of the action potential in many areas of the heart, despite a reduction in driving force for K^+ under these conditions. This is believed to be due to *cross-over* of the current-voltage relationship of I_{K1} when $(K^+)_o$ is elevated (Noble, 1965; Hume and Uehara, 1985). The exact mechanism responsible for inward rectification is not known, however, recent studies have suggested that it is due to unidirectional and voltage-dependent block of the channel by internal magnesium ions (Matsuda et al., 1987; Horie and Irisawa, 1987).

I_K

Over the plateau range of potentials, time-dependent outward current is activated in most types of cardiac cells, which is believed to be important in initiating repolarization of the action potential.

This current, which is often referred to as the delayed rectifier, was first analyzed in sheep Purkinje fibers by Noble and Tsien (1969). They observed that voltage clamp pulses applied to the plateau range of potentials elicited time-dependent outward current with kinetics that were not simple exponentials. However, the kinetics were fit as the sum of two exponentials, which was interpreted as reflecting the simultaneous activation of two population of channels (parallel conductances). Due to their less than perfect selectivity for K^+, they were called I_{X1} and I_{X2}. A similar analysis in a variety of other syncytial cardiac preparations, also generally found two components of delayed rectification, with K^+ selectivity either similar to that observed in sheep Purkinje fibers, or more highly dependent upon K^+ (Rougier et al., 1968; Brown and Noble, 1969a,b; McDonald and Trautwein, 1978; DiFrancesco et al., 1979; Kokubun et al., 1982). The finding that voltage clamp protocols may result in significant accumulation and/or depletion of K^+ in the small restricted spaces associated with multicellular preparations has raised serious questions regarding the actual nature of delayed rectification in the heart (Kline and Morad, 1978; Attwell et al., 1979). For example, in frog atrial trabeculae, the decay of outward tail currents following depolarizing voltage clamp steps can be exceedingly complex, requiring up to three exponentials to fit (Brown et al., 1980).

Single-channel recording or whole-cell recording of delayed rectifier currents in single myocytes offer the obvious advantage of minimal complications due to accumulation/depletion phenomena. In the case of recording single-channel currents associated with the delayed rectifier, it has been difficult to identify such currents, possibly due to the small number of such channels in the membrane, or due to a low single-channel conductance. As shown in Table I, an 11 pS channel ($(K^+)_o = 150$ mM) has been described in cell attached patches in isolated nodal cells of the rabbit heart (Shibasaki, 1987), whereas in chick embryonic ventricular cells, 15 and 60 pS channels ($(K^+)_o = 140$ mM) have been described (Clapham and DeFelice, 1984; Clapham and Logothetis, 1988).

Whole-cell recordings in isolated myocytes from frog atrium (Hume and Giles, 1983; Simmons, et al., 1986; Hume et al., 1986) and sinus venosus (Giles and Shibata, 1985) have provided evidence that the delayed rectifier: 1) can be described as a single Hodgkin-Huxley type conductance, 2) activates in a sigmoidal fashion that can be fit by raising the activation gating variable to the second power, 3) exhibits relatively high K^+ permeability, and 4) has a linear fully-activated current-voltage relation. These experiments, in contrast to earlier results obtained in frog atrial trabeculae, have revealed that a single ohmic conductance mechanism is responsible for delayed rectification in this preparation. In isolated mammalian myocytes, a complete analysis of delayed rectification has not yet been forthcoming. However, preliminary studies indicate that even in single mammalian myocytes, the kinetics of this process cannot be described in a simple exponential fashion (Daytner et al., 1984; Walsh, et al., 1987; Shibasaki, 1987; Matsura et al., 1987; Clapham and Logothetis, 1988). An alternative interpretation of the biexponential kinetics associated with delayed rectification in mammalian preparations is that it arises from a single population of channels with multiple closed states ($C_1 \rightleftharpoons C_2 \rightleftharpoons O$; Daytner et al., 1984; Bennett et al., 1985). Some support for this gating scheme as well evidence for a fast inactivation processs has been obtained from single-channel measurements (Shibasaki, 1987). There is reason to believe, therefore, that there may be fundamental differences between delayed rectifier K^+ channels in amphibian and mammalian heart.

Delayed rectifier K^+ channels may be optimal targets for antiarrythmic drugs with class III action. Activation of I_K is thought to be important in triggering repolarization of the action potential in many areas of the heart. An agent that blocks I_K will be expected to significantly prolong the duration of the cardiac action potential. An example of one such drug is phencyclidine, which has been shown to block K^+ channels in nerve and muscle membrane (Albuquerque et al., 1983; Blaustein and Ickowicz, 1983). When applied to ventricular myocytes isolated from guinea-pig, there is a dose-dependent prolongation of the action potential duration (Fig. 1A). In voltage clamp experiments, this compound has been shown to significantly reduce the amplitude of whole-cell delayed rectifier currents at doses similar to those that prolong the action potential duration (Fig. 1B).

I_{TO}

A transient outward current (I_{TO}) that is activated quickly upon membrane depolarization and inactivates during phase 1 of the action potential was originally described in cardiac Purkinje fibers (Deck and Trautwein, 1964; Peper and Trautwein, 1968; Fozzard

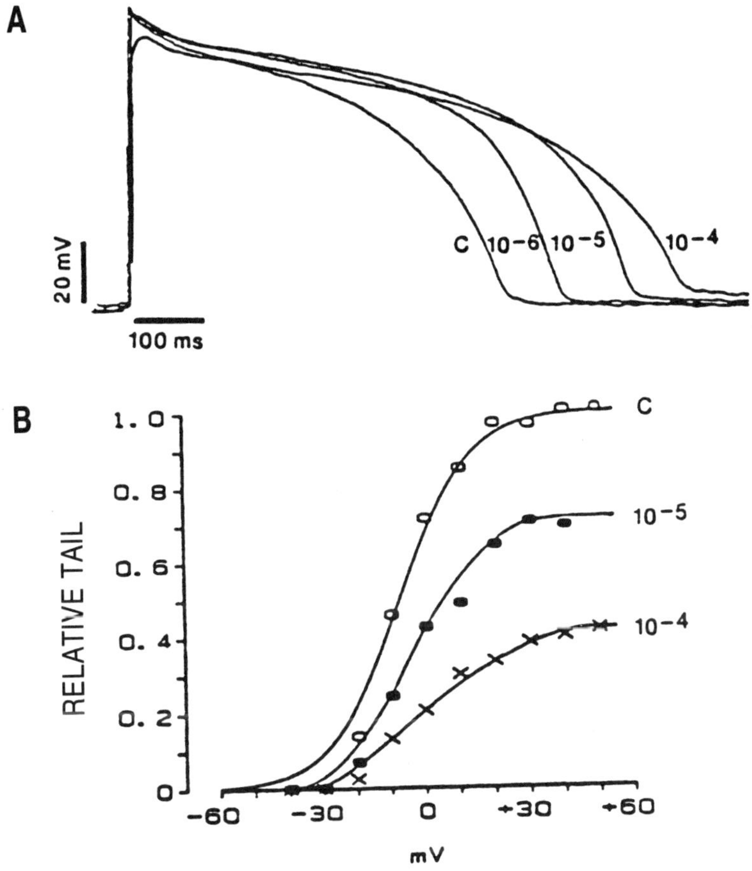

Figure 1. Effect of phencyclidine (PCP) on the action potential and the delayed rectifier K^+ current in isolated guinea-pig ventricular myocytes. A. Action potential under control conditions and after sequential addition of several concentrations of PCP to the bath. Action potentials were elicited by intracellularly applied stimulus of 1 ms duration at a frequency of 0.2 Hz.

Figure 1B. Activation curve of I_K from tail current measurements under control conditions and during exposure to two concentrations of PCP. In these experiments, non-dialyzing pipettes (Hume and Giles, 1983) were used to voltage clamp the cells. Figure adapted from Hadley and Hume (1986).

and Hiraoka, 1973). Since then, this current has been extensively studied in a variety of different cardiac preparations. A major conclusion that emerges in that there is little consenus regarding: 1) the number of components of current, 2) the ionic selectivity of the channels involved, 3) the kinetics of the current(s), 4) whether the current(s) is activated by Ca^{2+}, and 5) the voltage-dependence of the activation and inactivation process. As a result, I_{TO}-like currents have been called at various times *early outward current, initial outward current, positive dynamic current,* I_{Cl}, I_{qr}, I_{bo}, I_{lo} and I_A. Undoubtably, some of this variability may be directly attributable to actual variability in the properties of the channels(s) in different regions of the heart or between various species. This brief review will concentrate on results obtained in isolated single myocytes using the newer voltage clamp techniques.

Recent studies have revealed that I_{TO}-like currents are more prevalent than was originally believed. They have been found in Purkinje fibers, ventricular and atrial tissue, and both the AV and SA node of a variety of different species. In addition to their role in bringing about the early phase of repolarization, they may also play an important role in frequency-dependent changes in the action potential duration and configuration. Transient outward currents have been described in whole-cell voltage clamp experiments in isolated rat ventricular myocytes (Josephson et al., 1984), isolated cells from rabbit AV node (Nakayama and Irisawa, 1985), rabbit crista terminalis (Giles and van Ginneken, 1985), and cells isolated from canine Purkinje fibers (Nakayama and Fozzard, 1988) and ventricular myocardium (Tseng et al., 1987). In most of these studies, I_{TO} appeared to be rather insensitive to Ca^{2+} and exhibited inactivation over the voltage range of -70 to -10 mV. In dog ventricular cells, both Ca^{2+}-dependent and -independent componets of I_{TO} have been described.

A few studies have reported single-channel current measurements that may be associated with I_{TO}. A Ca^{2+}-insensitive 20 pS channel has been reported in cell-attached patches of rabbit AV nodal cells (Nakayama and Irisawa, 1985; see Table I). Inactivation kinetics of the ensemble averaged currents resembling those of I_{TO} from whole-cell recordings, and the relative selectivity of the channels was 0.19 (P_{Na}/P_K). In contrast, Ca^{2+}-sensitive large conductance channels (120 pS) have been recorded in cell-attached patches from bovine Purkinje cells (Callewaert, et al., 1986). In a recent study, cell-attached patches from mouse ventricular cells exhibited two types of single-channel activity, 27 pS and 12 pS channels (Benndorf et al., 1987). Ensemble averages of the activity of these channels exhibited transient kinetics expected for I_{TO}. These channels appeared to be rather highly selective for K^+.

I_{TO} currents may prove to be useful targets for class III antiarrythmic agents, since they appear to be involved in initiating the early phase of repolarization. Such compounds may turn out to be rather selective for particular areas of the heart, since the relative importance of these channels in the overall control of the action potential duration is variable. Drug modulation of action potential duration by interaction with this class of K^+ channels might be more rate-dependent than in the case of compounds that block delayed rectifier channels.

Other Myocardial K^+ Channels

A number of other types of K^+ channels have been demonstrated in the heart, some of which are also listed in Table I. $I_{K[ACh]}$ is present in atrial and nodal cells. These channels are activated by muscarinic stimulation (Sakmann, et al. 1983; Soejima and Noma, 1984). Interestingly, the channels appear active in the absence of agonist binding to the muscarinic receptor, and may be the predominent K^+ channels responsible for the resting membrane potential in nodal as well as atrial cells (Sakmann et al., 1983; Hume and Uehara, 1985). The nature of the coupling of the muscarinic receptor to this channel has been an area of intensive recent investigation and it appears to involve guanine nucleotide-binding proteins (G proteins; see Brown and Birnbaumer, 1988); see also Chapter 4.

In 1983, Noma reported the existence of large (80 pS) K^+ channels in cell-attached and -detached patches from rabbit and guinea-pig atrial and ventricular myocytes that were inhibited by intracellular concentrations of ATP in excess of 1 mM and activated during metabolic inhibition (perfusion with glucose-free Tyrode solution containing cyanide). Similar ATP-sensitive K^+ channels ($I_{K[ATP]}$), since this time, have been described in a number of cardiac cells, skeletal muscle and pancreatic β-cells (see Ashcroft, 1988). These channels are possibly responsible for the severe shortening of the action potential duration that is known to occur during anoxia in the heart. Such action potential duration shortening might favor the development of re-entry type of arrythmias, therefore specific antagonists of this class of K^+ channels may well prove to be effective class III antiarrhythmic agents during anoxic conditions. However, if shortening of the action potential duration during anoxia serves to limit the degree of ATP depletion by reducing contractile activity, blockade of these channels may not be necessarily beneficial.

Another type of K^+ channel, which is activated by $(Na^+)_i$ and has a single-channel conductance of 207 pS, has also been observed in detached membrane patches from guinea-pig ventricular myocytes (Kameyama et al., 1984). The functional significance of this class of channels remains to be determined. Other channels that may exhibit some permeability to K^+ include I_f channels (DiFrancesco, 1986) and nonselective channels activated by intracellular Ca^{2+} (Colquhoun et al., 1981; Hill, Coronado and Strauss, 1988).

AUTONOMIC MODULATION OF DELAYED RECTIFIER K^+ CURRENT

The delayed rectifier K^+ current has been shown to be augmented by catecholamines in multicellular preparations of Purkinje fibers (Tsien, et al. 1972) and frog atrium (Brown and Noble, 1974). Such an effect of catecholamines might be mediated by either a direct effect on the channels, or by one of several indirect mechanisms. These might include: 1) mediation by a second messenger, 2) indirect enhancement by an increase in $(Ca^{2+})_i$ (Ca-activated K^+ conductance), or 3) an indirect enhancement by augmentation of the K^+ gradient due to direct stimulation of the Na^+, K^+ -pump. Recent studies in calf Purkinje fibers as well as isolated cardiac myocytes have provided new information with regard to the underlying mechanism of I_K stimulation by β-adrenergic agonists.

Differences Between Amphibian and Mammalian Cells

In non-dialyzed single cells isolated from frog atrium, doses of catecholamines that produce large increases in the magnitude of the Ca^{2+} current do not significantly alter the magnitude of the delayed

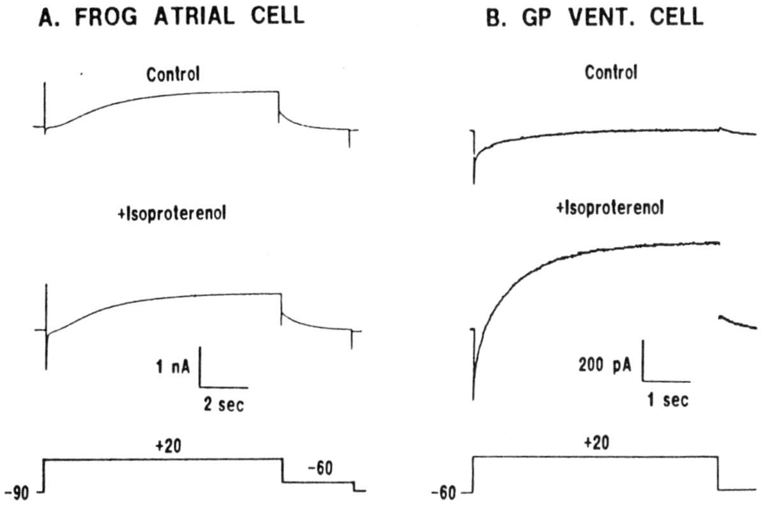

Figure 2. Comparison of the effects of isoproterenol on the delayed rectifier K^+ current in isolated cells from frog atrium (A) and guinea-pig ventricle (B). Panel A is adapted from Hume (1985). In these experiments, non-dialyzing pipettes were used to voltage clamp the cells. In B, dialyzing patch pipettes (Hamill et al., 1981) were used to clamp the cells. The internal pipette solution contained (mM): K-glutamate 130, KCl 10, NaCl 10, $MgCl_2$ 1, ATP-K 2, EGTA 5 and HEPES 5 (pH 7.2).

rectifier K^+ current (Hume, 1985), (Fig. 2A). This surprizing result suggested that part of the effect observed in multicellular preparations of frog atrium might be mediated by changes in local K^+ concentration in restricted extracellular spaces due to stimulation of the Na^+, K^+ -pump. It is now clear that different results are observed in dialyzed myocytes from mammalian heart (Bennett and Begenisich, 1987), (Fig. 2B). In isolated guinea-pig ventricular myocytes, isoproterenol and norepinephrine can greatly augment the amplitude of I_K. One possible reason for the difference observed in isolated cells from frog atrium and mammalian ventricle might be due to differences in temperature. The experiments on amphibian myocytes were carried out at room temperature (19–22° C), whereas many experiments on mammalian myocytes are carried out at 30–35° C. However, the effect of temperature on the response to catecholamines in mammalian myocytes is controversial. The experiment illustrated in Figure 2B shows that isoproterenol enhances I_K in guinea-pig ventricular myocytes at room temperature. A similar effect of isoproterenol also in isolated guinea-pig ventricular myocytes was found by Bennett and Begenisich (1987) to be temperature-independent over the range 20–37° C. However, Walsh, et al., (1988) reported that β-adrenergic stimulation of I_K occurs at 28–32° C, but not at 19–22° C in isolated guinea-pig myocytes. It seems unlikely that differences in temperature can adequately account for the different results observed in amphibian and mammalian myocytes. Another possibility is that there may be fundamental differences between the delayed rectifier K^+ channels in the two types of tissue, or differences in their mode of regulation. It seems clear from whole-cell data that there are certainly important differences in gating properties of the delayed rectifier in the two types of preparations.

Washout of the Delayed Rectifier K^+ Current in Dialyzed Myocytes

In addition to apparent differences in the response of the delayed rectifier to catecholamines in single cells from frog atrium and mammalian heart, there are also apparent differences in their kinetics and magnitude. For example, Figure 2 shows that the peak amplitude of the delayed rectifier K^+ current at positive membrane potentials in frog atrial cells can be in the nanoampere (10^{-9} A) range, whereas in guinea-pig ventricular cells, it is often an order of magnitude smaller under control conditions. Estimates of cell membrane surface areas for the two types of cells can not account for this difference. The difference in current magnitudes might be related to the different type of patch pipettes used to voltage clamp the cells. In the case of frog atrial cells, small-tip diameter pipettes (Hume and Giles, 1983) were used that minimize internal dialysis; in the case of guinea-pig myocytes, standard patch pipettes (Hamill et al., 1981) that allow internal dialysis were used to clamp the cells.

To test whether the smaller amplitude of K^+ currents in the guinea-pig ventricular cells might be attributable to internal dialysis, we compared the stability of K^+ current amplitudes as a function of time using the two types of pipettes in mammalian myocytes. An example of such a comparison is shown in Figure 3. Panel A shows that in a non-dialyzed guinea-pig ventricular cell, K^+ current amplitudes remain relatively stable for several minutes following seal formation and membrane rupture. In contrast, panel B

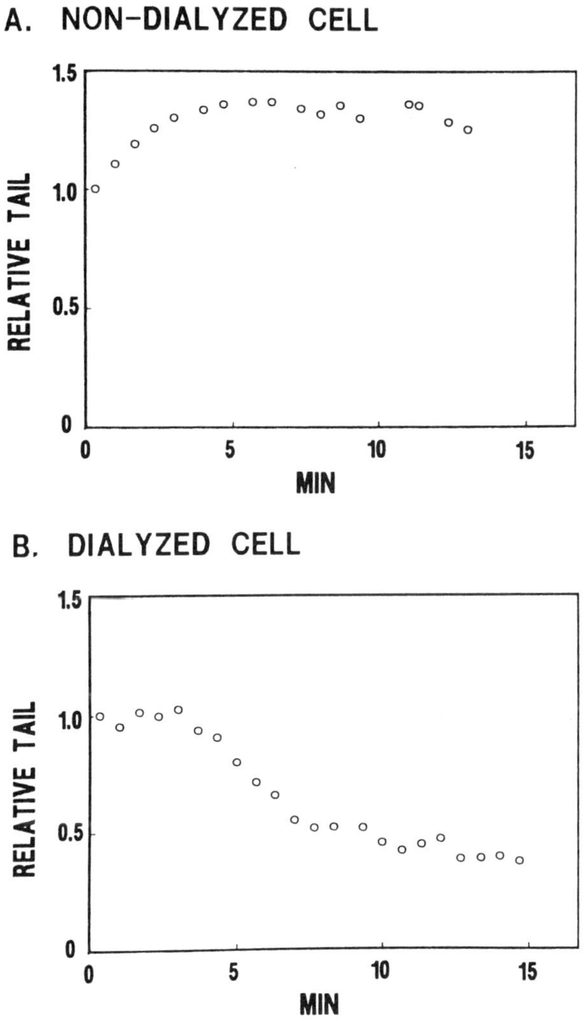

Figure 3. K^+ current stability in non-dialyzed (A) and dialyzed (B) guinea-pig ventricular myoctes. Time 0 represents the occurance of membrane rupture, allowing low resistance access to the interior of the cell. Plotted are the relative amplitudes of the outward tail currents associated with I_K activated by depolarizing voltage clamp steps to +50 mV from a holding potential of −40 mV. Pulses were applied repetitively starting at time 0. Tail current amplitudes were normalized with respect to the first tail current observed. Pipettes and internal solutions the same as described in Fig. 2. External solution contained nisoldipine (0.5 μM).

shows that in a dialyzed cell, K^+ current amplitudes rapidly diminish following membrane rupture. This rundown of I_K resembles that often observed for Ca^{2+} currents in dialyzed cells and implies that some component necessary for channel function is lost due to internal dialysis. It has recently been shown that catecholamines can augment I_K in dialyzed frog atrial cells (Lagrutta et al., 1989). This raises the question of whether β-adrenergic stimulation of I_K represents an important physiological process or reflects reversal of the rundown of I_K in dialyzed myocytes.

Control of the Delayed Rectifier by Adenylate Cyclase

It is believed that β-adrenergic stimulation of myocardial Ca^{2+} currents is due to activation of adenylate cyclase, production of cAMP, activation of cAMP-dependent protein kinase and protein phosphorylation. Furthermore, adenylate cyclase activity is believed to be coupled by guanine nucleotide-binding proteins (G proteins; Gilman, 1987) to β-adrenergic and muscarinic receptors. To test if the delayed rectifier K^+ current is also regulated by adenylate cyclase, the response to forskolin, an activator of adenylate cyclase, was examined. In a dialyzed guinea-pig ventricular cell, in which I_K rundown had stabilized after approximately 10 minutes, the addition of 10^{-6} M forskolin significantly increased the magnitude of I_K (Fig. 4). This result strongly implicates adenylate cyclase and the production of cAMP as important intracellular mediators of the response of I_K to β-adrenergic receptor stimulation.

SUMMARY

Myocardial K^+ channels represent a potentially important site of action for antiarrhythmic agents. Drugs that can selectively cause prolongation of the action potential duration will be especially effective in the treatment of arrhythmias that involve re-entry mechanisms. Of the six known classes of myocardial K^+ channels, those that are probably most important for the control of action potential under normal conditions include I_{K1}, I_K, and I_{TO}. Since cardiac arrhythmias often occur under abnormal conditions, such as local hypoxia or ischemia, agents that selectively act on other types of K^+

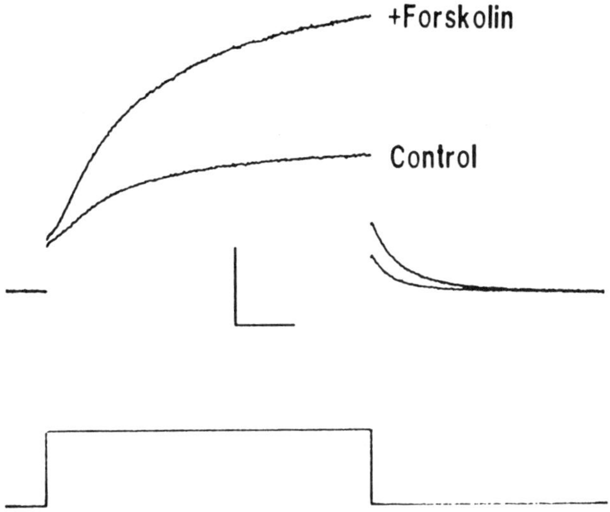

Figure 4. Effect of forskolin (1 μM) on the delayed rectifier K^+ current in dialyzed guinea-pig ventricular myocyte. I_K was elicited by a voltage clamp depolarization to +50 mV from a holding potential of −40 mV before and after exposure to forskolin. Calibrations: 1 second; 1 nA. Same internal solution as in Fig. 2. External solution contained nisoldipine (0.5 μM).

channels (e.g., $I_{K(ATP)}$) may prove to have clinical efficacy in the future.

The delayed rectifier K^+ current is instrumental in initiating phase 3 repolarization of the action potential in many types of cardiac cells. Agents that block this current will significantly prolong the action potential duration. Newer studies are providing important information about the properties of the delayed rectifier K^+ channels and their modulation by intracellular second messengers and enzymes. It is becoming clear that in mammalian heart, delayed rectifier K^+ channel activity is strongly influenced by β-adrenergic receptor occupation, stimulation of adenylate cyclase, production of cAMP, probably resulting in subsequent phosphorylation of K^+ channels: a cascade of events resembling that involved in the regulation of Ca^{2+} currents. The possibility that delayed rectifier K^+ channels may be controlled by G proteins acting on adenylate cyclase should be an active area of future investigation, which may provide new experimental and clinical approaches for altering action potential duration. Recent studies (Tohse, et al., 1987; Walsh and

Kass, 1988) have also implicated protein kinase C in the regulation of the delayed rectifier K^+ current.

Acknowledgments: Most of the experiments described were supported by NIH grant HL 30143 and grants from the American Heart Association. The author wishes to acknowledge the fruitful collaboration of Drs. A. Uehara, R.W. Hadley, and R.D. Harvey in these studies.

BIBLIOGRAPHY

Albuquerque EX, Aguayo LG, Warnich JE, Ickowicz RK, Blaustein MP. Interactions of phencyclidine with ion channels of nerve and muscle: behavioral implications. *Fed Proc* 42:2584–2589, 1983.

Ashcroft FM. Adenosine 5'-triphosphate-sensitive potassium channels. *Annu Rev Neurosci* 11:97–118, 1988.

Attwell D, Cohen I, Eisner D. Membrane potential and ion concentration stability conditions for a cell with a restricted extracellular space. *Proc R Soc Lond* B206:145–161, 1979.

Becham M, Glitsch G, Pott L. Properties of an inward rectifying K channel in the membrane of guinea-pig atrial cardioballs. *Pflugers Arch* 399:186–193, 1983.

Benndorf K, Markwardt F, Nilius B. Two types of transient outward currents in cardiac ventricular cells of mice. *Pflugers Arch* 409:641–643, 1987.

Bennett PB, Mckinney LC, Kass RS, Begenisich T. Delayed rectification in the calf cardiac Purkinje fiber. Evidence for multiple state kinetics. *Biophys J* 48:553–567, 1985.

Biermans G, Vereecke J, Carmeliet E. The mechanism of the inactivation of the inward-rectifying K current during hyperpolarizing steps in guinea-pig ventricular myocytes. *Pflugers Arch* 410:604–613, 1987.

Blaustein MP, Ickowicz RK. Phencyclidine in nanomolar concentrations binds to synaptosomes and blocks certain potassium channels. *Proc Natl Acad Sci (USA)* 80:3855–3859, 1983.

Brown AM, Birnbaumer L. Direct G protein gating of ion channels. *Am J Physiol* 254:H401–410, 1988.

Brown H, DiFrancesco D, Noble D, Noble S. The contribution of potassium accumulation to outward currents in frog atrium. *J Physiol* 306:127–149, 1980.

Brown HF, Noble SJ. A quantitative analysis of the slow component of delayed rectification in frog atrium. *J Physiol* 204:737–747, 1969.

Brown HF, Noble SJ. Membrane currents underlying delayed rectification and pacemaker activity in frog atrial muscle. *J Physiol* 204:717–736, 1969.

Callewaert G, Vereecke J, Carmeliet E. Existence of a calcium-dependent potassium channel in the membrane of cow cardiac Purkinje fibers. *Pflugers Arch* 406:424–426, 1986.

Carmeliet E, Vereecke J. Electrogenesis of the action potential and automaticity. In: Berne R, Sperelakis N, Geiger S, eds.*Handbook of Physiology. The Cardiovascular System. Vol. I: The Heart.* Bethesda, MD: American Physiological Society; 269–334, 1979.

Clapham DE, Defelice LJ. Voltage-activated K^+ channels in embryonic chick heart. *Biophys J* 45:40–42, 1984.

Clapham DE, Logothetis DE. Delayed rectifier K^+ current in embryonic chick heart ventricle. *Am J Physiol* 254:H192–H197, 1988.

Cohen IS, Daytner NB, Gintant GA, Kline RP. Time-dependent outward currents in the heart. In: Fozzard HA, et al. eds. *The Heart and Cardiovascular System* New York, NY: Raven Press; 637–670, 1986.

Colquhoun D, Neher E, Reuter H, Stevens CF. Inward current channels activated by intracellular Ca in cultured cardiac cells. *Nature* 294:752–754, 1981.

Datyner NB, Gintant GA, Cohen IS. Gating of the plateau delayed rectifier in dissociated canine cardiac Purkinje cells. *Circulation* 70 (II,4):74, 1984.

DiFrancesco D. Characterization of single pacemaker channels in cardiac sino-atrial node cells. *Nature* 324:470–473, 1986.

DiFrancesco D, McNaughton PA. The effects of calcium on outward membrane currents in the cardiac Purkinje fiber. *J Physiol* 289:347–373, 1979.

DiFrancesco D, Noma A, Trautwein W. Kinetics and magnitude of the time-dependent potassium current in the rabbit sinoatrial node. *Pflugers Arch* 381:271–279, 1979.

Fozzard HA, Hiraoka M. The positive dynamic current and its inactivation properties in cardiac Purkinje fibers. *J Physiol* 234:569–586, 1973.

Giles WR, Shibata EF. Voltage clamp of bull-frog cardiac pacemaker cells: A quantitative analysis of potassium currents. *J Physiol* 368:265–292, 1985.

Giles WR, Van Ginneken ACG. A transient outward current in isolated cells from the crista terminalis of the rabbit heart. *J Physiol* 368:243–264, 1985.

Giles AG. G Proteins: transducers of receptor-generated signals. *Ann Rev Biochem* 56:615–649, 1987.

Hadley RW, Hume JR. Actions of phencyclidine on the action potential and membrane currents of single guinea pig myocytes. *J Pharmacol Exp Ther* 237:131–136, 1986.

Harvey RD, Hume JR. Autonomic regulation of delayed rectifier K^+ current in mammalian heart involves G proteins. *Am J Physiol* 257:H818–H823, 1989.

Hamill OP, Marty A, Neher E, Sakmann B, Sigworth FJ. Improved patch-clamp techniques for high-resolution current recording from cells and cell-free membrane patches. *Pflugers Arch* 391:85–100, 1981.

Hill JA, Coronado R, Strauss HC. Reconstitution and characterization of a calcium-activated channel from heart. *Circ Res* 62:411–415, 1988.

Horie M, Irisawa H. Rectification of muscarinic K^+ current by magnesium ion in guinea pig atrial cells. *Am J Physiol* 253:H210-H214, 1987.

Hume JR, Giles W. Ionic currents in single isolated bullfrog atrial cells. *J Gen Physiol* 81:153–194, 1983.

Hume JR, Uehara A. Ionic basis of the different action potential configurations of single guinea-pig atrial and ventricular myocytes. *J Physiol Lond* 368:525–544, 1985.

Hume JR. Do catecholamines directly modulate the delay plateau K^+ current in frog atrium? *J Mol Cell Cardiol* 17:813–816, 1985.

Hume JR, Giles W, Robinson K, Shibata EF, Nathan RD. A time and voltage dependent pottassium current in single cardiac cells isolated from bullfrog atrium. *J Gen Physiol* 88:777–798, 1986.

Josephson IR, Brown AM. Inwardly rectifying single-channel and whole cell K^+ currents in rat ventricular myocytes. *J Membrane Biol* 94:19–35, 1986.

Josephson IR, Sanchez-Chapula J, Brown AM. Early outward current in rat single ventricular cells. *Circ Res* 54:157–162, 1984.

Kameyama M, Kakei M, Sato R, Shibasake T, Matsuda H, Irisawa H. Intracellular Na^+ activates a K^+ channel in mammalian cardiac cells. *Nature* 309:354–356, 1984.

Kline RP, Cohen IS. Extracellular $[K^+]$ fluctuations in voltage-clamped canine cardiac Purkinje fibers. *Biophys J* 46:663–668, 1984.

Kline RP, Morad M. Potassium efflux in heart muscle during activity: extracellular accumulation and its implications. *J Physiol* 280:537–558, 1978.

Kokobun SM, Nishimura M, Noma A, Irisawa H. Membrane currents in the rabbit atrioventricular node cell. *Pflugers Arch* 393:15–22, 1982.

Kurachi, Yoshihisa. Voltage-dependent activation of the inward-rectifying potassium channel in the ventricular cell membrane of guinea-pig heart. *J Physiol* 366:365–385, 1985.

Lagrutta AA, Gourdon I, Hartzell HC. β-adrenergic modulation of delayed rectifier K currents in bulfrog atrial cells. *Biophys J* 55:549a, 1989.

Matsuda H, Saigusa A, Irisawa H. Ohmic conductance through the inwardly rectifying K channel and block by internal Mg2+. *Nature* 325:156–159, 1987.

Matsuura H, Ehara T, Imoto Y. An anlysis of the delayed outward current in single ventricular cells of the guinea-pig. *Pflugers Arch* 410:596–603, 1987.

McDonald TF, Trautwein W. The potassium current underlying delayed rectification in cat ventricular muscle. *J Physiol* 274:217–246, 1978.

Nakayama T, Irisawa H. Transient outward current carried by potassium and sodium in quiescent atrioventricular node cells of rabbits. *Circ Res* 57: 65–73, 1985.

Noble D. Electrical properties of cardiac muscle attributable to inward going (anomalous) rectification. *J Cell & Comp Physiol* 66:127–136, 1965.

Noble D. The surprising heart: a review of recent progress in cardiac electrophysiology. *J Physiol* 353:1–50, 1984.

Noble D, Tsien RW. Outward membrane currents activated in the plateau range of potentials in cardiac purkinje fibers. *J Physiol* 200:205–231, 1969.

Noble D, Tsien RW. The kinetics and rectifier properties of the slow potassium current in cardiac purkinje fibers. *J Physiol* 195:185–214, 1968.

Noma A. ATP-regulated K^+ channels in cardiac muscle. *Nature* 305:147–148, 1983.

Payet MD, Rousseau E, Sauve R. Single-channel analysis of a potassium inward rectifier in myocytes of newborn rat heart. *J Membrane Biol* 86:79–88, 1985.
Peper K, Trautwein W. A membrane current related to the plateau of the action potential of Purkinje fibers. *Pflugers Arch* 303:108–123, 1968.
Rougier O, Vassort G, Stampfli R. Voltage clamp experiments on frog atrial heart muscle fibers with the sucrose gap technique. *Pflugers Arch* 301:91–108, 1968.
Sakmann B, Trube G. Conductance properties of single inwardly rectifying potassium channels in ventricular cells from guinea- pig heart. *J Physiol* 347:641–657, 1984.
Sakmann B, Trube G. Voltage-dependent inactivation of inward-rectifying single-channel currents in the guinea-pig heart cell membrane. *J Physiol* 347:659–683, 1984.
Sakmann B, Noma A, Trautwein W. Acetylcholine activation of single muscarinic K^+ channels in isolated pacemaker cells of the mammalian heart. *Nature* 303:250–253, 1983.
Shibasake T. Conductance and kinetics of delayed rectifier potassium channels in nodal cells of the rabbit heart. *J Physiol* 387:227–250, 1987.
Simmons MA, Creazzo T, Hartzell HC. A time-dependent and voltage-sensitive K current in single cells from frog atrium. *J Gen Physiol* 88:739–756, 1986.
Singh BN. Control of cardiac arrhythmias by selective lengthening of repolarization: theoretic considerations and clinical observations. *Am Heart J* 109:421–430, 1985.
Soejima M, Noma A. Mode of regulation of the ACh-sensitive K-channel by the muscarinic receptor in rabbit atrial cells. *Pflugers Arch* 400: 424–431, 1984.
Tohse N, Kameyama M, Irisawa H. Intracellular Ca^{++} and protein kinase C modulate K^+ current in guinea pig heart cells. *Am J Physiol* 253:H1321-H1324, 1987.
Tseng G, Robinson RB, Hoffman BF. Passive properties and membrane currents of canine ventricular myocytes. *J Gen Physiol* 90:671–702, 1987.
Walsh KB, Kass RS. Regulation of a heart potassium channel by protein kinase A and C. *Science* 242:67–69, 1988.

Chapter 8

Modulation of Cardiac Potassium Currents by Antiarrhythmic Drugs: *Present Status and Future Directions*

Focus on the Cardiac Delayed Rectifier

Dan M. Roden
Jeffrey R. Balser
Paul B. Bennett

INTRODUCTION

Prolongation of cardiac repolarization has been associated with both suppression of cardiac arrhythmias and their genesis. Among patients receiving repolarization-delaying agents such as quinidine, paradoxical induction of a morphologically distinctive ventricular tachycardia along with marked prolongation of the QT interval on the surface electrocardiogram (Fig. 1) can occur in 5%–10% of patients, particularly in the presence of hypokalemia and bradycardia (Selzer and Wray, 1964; Roden et al., 1986). Congenital syndromes of marked QT prolongation and similar polymorphic ventricular tachycardias are also well-described. The mechanism(s) underlying the association between marked abnormalities of repolarization and

Hondeghem, Luc (ed): Molecular and Cellular Mechanisms of Antiarrhythmic Agents, Futura Publishing Company, Inc., Mount Kisco, NY, © 1989.

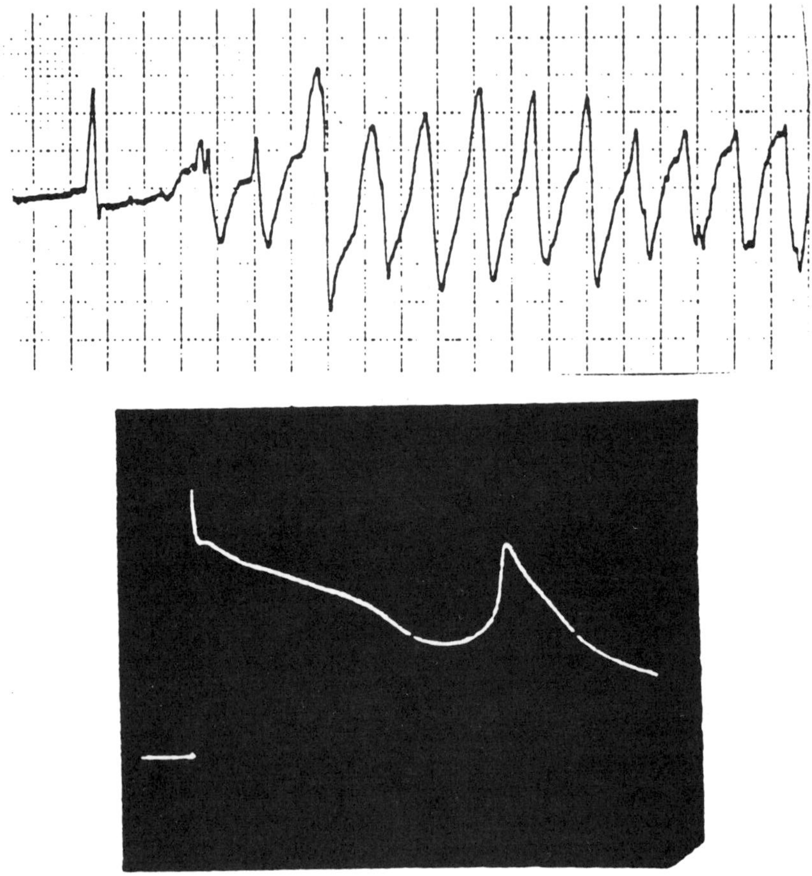

Figure 1. (top) An episode of quinidine-induced polymorphic ventricular tachycardia (Torsades de Pointes). The first beat of the arrhythmia arises at the end of a particularly long QT interval. (bottom) An early afterdepolarization in a canine cardiac Purkinje cell. As with Torsades de Pointes, early after depolarizations are elicited at slow underlying stimulation rates, low K_o, and action potential prolonging agents such as quinidine; moreover, both the initial beat of Torsades de Pointes and triggered activity related to early after-depolarizations arise during terminal repolarization.

the genesis of arrhythmias have not been completely worked out; however, heterogeneity of repolarization times with resultant reentrant arrhythmias (Schwartz and Locati, 1985) and/or early after-depolarizations and triggered activity (Fig. 1) are likely to be involved. The latter have been demonstrated in vitro under experimental conditions mimicking those seen in patients (e.g., quinidine + low K_o + slow rates; Roden and Hoffman, 1985).

Interestingly, prolongation of repolarization in heart also appears to be a major mechanism whereby drugs may suppress arrhythmias (Vaughan Williams, 1985). While certain agents such as amiodarone and quinidine depress maximum action potential upstroke velocity ($\dot{V}_{max}$) and prolong repolarization, agents such as sotalol, its d-isomer, N-acetyl procainamide (NAPA), clofilium, and meobentine are all examples of drugs whose major electrophysiological action is to prolong the cardiac action potential without depressing $\dot{V}_{max}$; these agents often have equivalent or superior arrhythmia-suppressing properties compared to more conventional agents and appear to lack serious adverse hemodynamic actions. Moreover, as a *class*, they appear to raise the electrical energy required to induce ventricular fibrillation (Bacaner et al., 1985) while rendering ventricular defibrillation easier to accomplish (Echt et al., 1989). Because of these pharmacological properties, the determinants of action potential duration and its modification by antiarrhythmic drugs with this so called *class III* action have become a major focus of new drug development (Lumma et al., 1987).

There are at least two possible mechanisms for action potential prolongation: enhancement of inward or inhibition of outward transmembrane ionic current. Enhancement of inward current either through cardiac sodium channels (e.g., DPI-201; Scholtysik and Williams, 1986) or through calcium channels (BAY K 8644, Thomas et al., 1984) may prolong action potential duration and result in this class III antiarrhythmic drug effect. Another mechanism of action potential prolongation is reduction of *outward* current by block of potassium channels.

Modulation of Cardiac Potassium Channels by Antiarrhythmic Agents

The principal voltage-dependent cardiac K^+ channels reported to be blocked by antiarrhythmic agents include the transient outward current (I_{to}), the inward rectifier (I_{K1}), and the delayed rectifier (I_K).

Transient Outward K^+ Current

The importance of the transient outward current varies with tissue and species. In ventricular muscle from guinea pig (Josephson et al., 1984) or cat (TenEick and Robertson, 1983; McDonald et al., 1984), the current is either small or absent. On the other hand, in ventricular muscle from rat (Josephson et al., 1984), rabbit (Kakushkin et al., 1983; Imaizumi and Giles, 1987), and dog (Litovsky and Anzelevitch, 1988; Šimurda et al., 1988), atrial cells from elephant seal (Maylie and Morad, 1984), rabbit AV nodal cells (Nakayama and Irisawa, 1985), rabbit crista terminalis (Giles and van Ginneken, 1985), and sheep Purkinje fibers (Kenyon and Gibbons, 1979), I_{to} is clearly present (for a review, see Cohen et al., 1986). Moreover, I_{to} has been observed in human atrial cells (Shibata et al., 1986; Escande et al., 1987). 4-aminopyridine is a relatively selective blocker of transient outward current and prolongs action potentials in heart (Kenyon and Gibbons, 1979; Giles and van Ginneken, 1985; Šimurda et al., 1988) and other tissue types (Thompson, 1982). However, quinidine blocks I_{to} in rabbit atrial and ventricular cells with 30 times greater potency (Imaizumi and Giles, 1987). Further, quinidine block appeared voltage-dependent (block increased at more positive voltages) and quinidine altered the time course of activation and inactivation (inactivation was more rapid); Imaizumi and Giles speculated that quinidine may act as an open channel blocker.

In some tissues, the early outward K^+ current appears to be Ca^{+2}-activated. Increases in external Ca^{+2} and adrenaline superfusion may increase I_{to} (Maylie and Morad, 1984); both organic Ca^{+2} channel blockers such as D-600 and inorganic blockers such as Mn^{+2} diminished this current in calf Purkinje fibers (Siegelbaum et al., 1977). Maylie and Morad (1984) demonstrated similarities between caffeine-induced suppression of I_{to} activation and caffeine-related attenuation of Ca^{+2} release from the sarcoplasmic reticulum in elephant seal atrial fibers. Further, Kenyon and Sutko (1987) showed that ryanodine, an inhibitor of sarcoplasmic reticulum calcium release, reduced the early outward current in calf Purkinje fibers, providing strong evidence for a Ca^{+2}-sensitive component of transient outward K current in this tissue. Finally, there is some evidence that in isolated canine cardiac Purkinje cells catecholamines enhance I_{to} through the β-adrenergic phosphorylation pathway (Nakayama and Fozzard, 1987).

Inward Rectifier K⁺ Current

Quinidine and a number of other action potential prolonging agents also appear to block the macroscopic steady state outward currents seen at potentials positive to E_K. This current is generally considered to be carried through the inward rectifier potassium channel, although outward current through inward rectifier single channels in this range of potentials has not yet been demonstrated unless internal Mg^{+2} is removed (Vandenberg, 1987; Matsuda et al., 1987). The effects of drugs on the macroscopic outward current attributed to this channel has been studied in a number of laboratories. Salata and Wasserstrom (1988) reported that quinidine blocked this current irreversibly in canine ventricular cells. We have also observed suppression of this current in guinea pig ventricular myocytes by high concentrations of quinidine; however, in guinea pig cells the block was reversible. Action potential prolongation by a binitro analog of clofilium (Arena and Kass, 1987) and several of the benzene sulfonamide analogs described by Follmer et al. (1988) has also been attributed to block of outward I_{K1}. These compounds may provide tools for the pharmacological separation of the delayed rectifier and the inward rectifier.

It has also been possible to study the action of these agents on single inward rectifier K^+ channels conducting in the inward direction. Sato et al. (1987) have reported that externally applied amiodarone (2–5 μM) blocked the inward rectifier irreversibly when assessed by on-cell patches. When these patches were excised to form inside-out patches, block was promptly washed out and could be reestablished by perfusion with amiodarone. Hence, they concluded that an intracellular site may be important for drug-induced block of this channel. The same group reported (Sato et al., 1988) that superfusion with quinidine blocks the channel by reducing both the probability of channel opening and the single channel conductance. We have also found that quinidine blocks single inward rectifier K^+ channels in cell-attached patches using physiological potassium concentrations in the pipette ($[K]_o$ = 4.5 mM; Balser et al., 1988a).

However, under these conditions, quinidine did not appear to reduce unitary conductance; rather, the probability of opening, and especially the probability of opening into a subconductance state (Sakmann and Trube, 1984) was reduced. These findings suggest that quinidine may prevent the channel from entering certain conformational states. Furthermore, in contrast to amiodarone, patch excision was not required to demonstrate reversal of this drug effect.

Delayed Rectifier K^+ Current

Colatsky (1982) attributed action potential prolongation in rabbit Purkinje fibers by quinidine to block of the delayed rectifier. Hiraoka et al. (1986) have more recently demonstrated similar findings in guinea pig ventricular myocytes. We have evaluated the effect of quinidine on time-dependent outward currents in whole-cell voltage-clamped, acutely dissociated guinea pig ventricular myocytes (Roden et al., 1988). As shown in Figure 2, quinidine reduced outward *tail* currents more after short pulses to plateau voltages than after longer ones; conversely, block appeared to be partially relieved by longer pulses. Snyders and Katzung (1985, 1986) have reported that clofilium reduces I_K and I_{Ca} in guinea pig ventricular myocytes. Sotalol and its individual stereoisomers (Carmeliet, 1985) as well as the benzene sulfonamide analogs described by Follmer et al. (1988) have also been reported to reduce the delayed rectifier, but no time- or voltage-dependence was detected. We have examined the effect of amiodarone on I_K elicited by depolarizing steps of varying durations and found that, in contrast to quinidine, amiodarone did not delay I_K activation (Balser et al., 1987a). In fact, block by amiodarone was greatest with long depolarizations, suggesting that

Figure 2. (opposite page) The effect of quinidine on time-dependent outward K current tails in guinea pig ventricular cells. The current was activated by pulses to +20 mV of varying duration (top), and outward tail currents were measured at −30 mV. Quinidine reduced the tail after the 2000 msec pulse from 300 to 125 pA. In contrast, the tail after 100 msec was 46 pA before drug and was completely eliminated by quinidine. Time-dependent reduction in tail currents in eight preparations are shown in the bottom panel. Adapted by permission from Roden DM, Bennett PB, Snyders DJ, Balser JR, and Hondeghem LM. Quinidine delays I_K activation in guinea pig myocytes. *Circ Res* 62:1055–1088, 1988, by permission of American Heart Association.

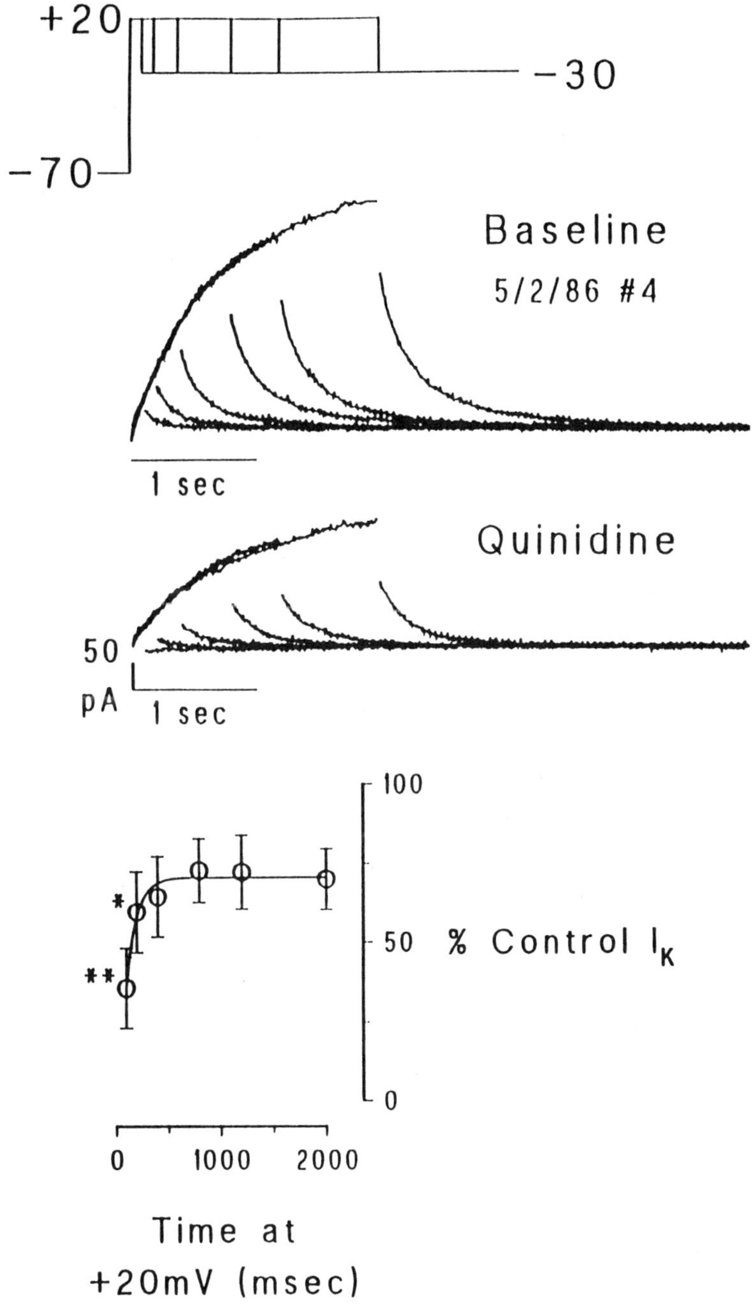
+20
-30
-70
Baseline
5/2/86 #4
1 sec
Quinidine
50
pA
1 sec
100
50
0
% Control I_K
0
1000
2000
Time at
+20mV (msec)

this agent may interact with an open channel state in analogy to block of the delayed rectifier in squid axon by TEA (Armstrong, 1966).

The observation, both in patients (Echt et al., 1986) and in vitro (Roden and Hoffman, 1985), that action potential prolongation by drugs is greatest at slow rates, suggested the hypothesis that quinidine may reduce I_K to a greater extent after long times at negative potentials. We have evidence, using a twin pulse protocol (Balser et al., 1987b), that quinidine block of outward time-dependent current does develop at negative potentials. The time constant for development of block was voltage-dependent: ~140 msec at −100 mV, ~200 msec at −80 mV, and ~350 msec at −40 mV. As discussed further, these time and voltage-dependent effects of quinidine suggest testable model(s) of drug-ion channel interaction.

Ion Channel Modelling

It is now well established that ion channels are intrinsic membrane proteins that permit specific ions to rapidly traverse the lipid bilayer. These channel proteins undergo conformational changes (due to factors such as receptor occupancy or voltage) between conducting and nonconducting states. In heart and other excitable tissue, channels exist in an electric field on the order of 50–100 kV/cm. Changes in this field influence charge distribution and hence the conformation of voltage-activated channels. Transitions between the major conformational states can be represented by voltage-dependent first order rate constants ($k_{ij}[V]$). Development of models that faithfully reproduce macroscopic and unitary gating behavior under a wide range of experimental situations may thus offer insights into the fundamental biological properties of the channel proteins. Furthermore, distinctions among models provide insights into mechanisms of channel behavior while excluding mechanisms that are not important. Similarly, models of drug-induced changes in channel conductance can provide information regarding drug-channel interactions.

Modelling the Delayed Rectifier

The magnitude of a membrane current at any time t and transmembrane voltage V is

$$I(t, V) = N \cdot i \cdot P_{open}(t, V)$$

where $P_{open}(t, V)$ is the probability that the channel is open at time t; N is the number of channels in the cell; and i is the unitary current at voltage V.

The general model most often used to describe delayed rectifier $P_{open}(t, V)$ is a Markovian chain (i.e. voltage-dependent rate constants which are time-independent) that consists of multiple closed (C) states connected in a catenary fashion to an open state:

$$C_n \Longleftrightarrow C_{n-1} \Longleftrightarrow \cdots \Longleftrightarrow C_2 \Longleftrightarrow C_1 \Longleftrightarrow \text{Open}$$

The simplest subset of this general scheme is a two-state model that has the following solution for $P_{open}(t, V)$:

$$\text{Closed} \underset{\beta(V)}{\overset{\alpha(V)}{\Longleftrightarrow}} \text{Open}$$

$$P_{open}(t, V) = A + Be^{-t/\tau}$$

where the time constant τ is a function of the voltage-dependent rate constants α and β. However, this simple probability model cannot reproduce the sigmoidal nature of delayed rectifier activation (Snyders et al., 1986). Hodgkin and Huxley (1952) compensated for this difficulty by assuming there were four identical, independent gating particles each described by the simple model shown above. The channel would only open when all four gating particles were in the open state; under these conditions, the probability of channel opening becomes the above solution raised to the fourth power, $(A + Be^{-t/\tau})^4$, and corresponds to the following state diagram:

$$(\text{Closed} \Longleftrightarrow \text{Open})^4$$

which may also be expressed as the following Markov chain (Young and Moore, 1981):

$$C_4 \underset{\beta}{\overset{4\alpha}{\Longleftrightarrow}} C_3 \underset{2\beta}{\overset{3\alpha}{\Longleftrightarrow}} C_2 \underset{3\beta}{\overset{2\alpha}{\Longleftrightarrow}} C_1 \underset{4\beta}{\overset{\alpha}{\Longleftrightarrow}} \text{Open}$$

$$P_{open}(t, V) = [A + Be^{-t/\tau}]^4$$

The 8 voltage-dependent rate constants, generated by raising the solution to the 2-state model to the fourth power, are integral multiples of each other (α, 2α, 3α, 4α; 4β, 3β, 2β, β). As a result, the system has four time constants that also bear a fixed relationship: τ, $\tau/2$, $\tau/3$, $\tau/4$. Many investigators have used similar variations of the Hodgkin-Huxley formalism to describe the kinetics of the delayed rectifier in various nerve (Young and Moore, 1981; Cole and Moore, 1960) and cardiac cells (Hume et al., 1986; Simmons et al., 1986; Matsuura et al., 1987), although the number of independent gating particles needed to faithfully represent experimental results varies tremendously (exponents ranging from 2 to 25 have been used; Cole and Moore, 1960).

Until recently, studies of the delayed rectifier in mammalian cardiac tissue have been complicated by problems associated with voltage clamping multicellular preparations, including the possibility of accumulation or depletion of K^+ in restricted intra- or extracellular spaces, which causes changes in the concentration of the charge carrier (K^+), thus altering the electrochemical driving force. Since a major aim of the voltage-clamp is measurement of ionic current (current = conductance × $[V - V_{rev}]$), ion accumulation and depletion will confound any interpretation because of changes in transmembrane K gradients and hence V_{rev}. Noble and Tsien first characterized cardiac plateau currents (1969) and described two components of delayed rectifier deactivation kinetics in voltage-clamped Purkinje preparations. Moreover, in their experiments, the two components appeared to have different reversal potentials, which they interpreted as two separate currents, I_{x1} and I_{x2}. Since this work was carried out before problems of ion accumulation were widely recognized, it is unclear to what extent these early recordings of outward potassium currents were influenced by accumulation or depletion of K^+, but the possibility of such experimental problems must be considered when interpreting data from older studies.

Hodgkin-Huxley models with two gating particles have been used to describe I_K kinetics in single frog atrial myocytes (Hume et al., 1986; Simmons et al., 1986) and guinea pig ventricular myocytes (Matsuura et al., 1988), preparations in which ion accumulation should not be a major problem. Bennett et al. (1985), who used shortened calf Purkinje fibers and limited activating pulses to avoid ion accumulation, also detected two exponential components of delayed rectifier deactivation; in these experiments, both components reversed at similar membrane potentials, slightly above E_K. The sim-

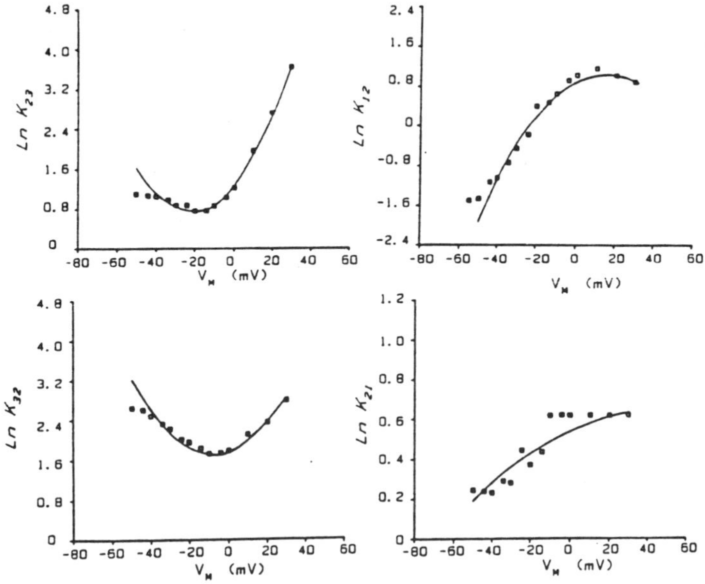

Figure 3. Voltage-dependence of the four rate constants describing the 3-state model for the delayed rectifier in calf Purkinje fibers. The rate constants did not bear a fixed integral relationship to each other, indicating that a conventional Hodgkin-Huxley model is not appropriate for this current. By permission from Bennett PB, McKinney LC, Kass RS, and Begenisich T. Delayed rectification in the calf cardiac Purkinje fiber: evidence for multiple state kinetics. *Biophys J* 48:553–567, 1985, by permission of the Biophysical Society.

plest model consistent with their data was a three state model with two closed states preceding the open state:

$$C_2 \underset{k_{21}}{\overset{k_{12}}{\Longleftrightarrow}} C_1 \underset{k_{10}}{\overset{k_{21}}{\Longleftrightarrow}} \text{Open}$$

$$P_{open}(t, V) = A + Be^{-t/\tau 1} + Ce^{-t/\tau 2}$$

where τ_1 and τ_2 are functions of the voltage-dependent rate constants k_{ij}. However, they found that assumptions regarding fixed integral relationships among rate constants at all voltages were unjustified (Fig. 3); thus, a Hodgkin-Huxley model with multiple independent gating particles was ruled out. Gintant et al. (1985) confirmed that there were two components of delayed rectifier current in acutely dissociated canine Purkinje cells, a preparation in which ion accumulation should be even less likely, and they, too, interpreted their data in the context of a (C-C-Open) model. Further studies in our laboratories have recently suggested a four state non-Hodgkin-Huxley model (C-C-C-Open) may be more appropriate to describe delayed rectifier kinetics.

Establishing a minimal model for the kinetic behavior of I_K will facilitate the process of evaluating models for antiarrhythmic drug action. The finding that quinidine block of I_K develops at negative potentials and is relieved by long pulses to depolarized potentials suggests a state-dependent interaction of drug with the channel. Viewed in the context of the multiple-closed state model for I_K, hypotheses can be proposed and tested. For example, quinidine might alter one or more of the rate constants of the drug-free model. Alternatively, quinidine may create new drug-associated states in analogy to the modulated receptor hypothesis proposed for interaction of drugs and sodium or calcium channels (Hondeghem and Katzung, 1977, 1984; Hille, 1977; Hondeghem and Bennett, 1989). Numerical methods based on a global fitting scheme, which simultaneously evaluates data obtained at multiple transmembrane voltages (Balser et al., 1988b), are now in use in our laboratory to evaluate competing models for I_K and its interactions with drugs.

Obstacles to Further Studies of I_K: Insights into Metabolic Control

Several experimental difficulties must be overcome before a fuller understanding of drug interactions with the delayed rectifier can be developed. These include 1) the possibility that other current(s) contaminate commonly used preparations; and 2) the apparent metabolic regulation of the channel. In our experiments with guinea pig ventricular myocytes, we noted that the time course of activating current during a long depolarizing pulse to +50 mV does not parallel the time course of deactivating tail current tail amplitudes (*envelope test*; Noble and Tsien, 1969). This finding suggests that other current(s) may contaminate these measurements. Extracellular solutions were, therefore, modified (Balser and Roden, 1987) to eliminate nonpotassium currents thereby minimizing any contribution from pumps, ionic exchangers (sodium calcium exchange), and fast and slow inward sodium and calcium currents. Even under these conditions, the *envelope test* was not completely satisfied until 30–100 μM La^{3+} was added to the perfusate (Balser and Roden, 1988). Interestingly, La^{3+} appeared to alter the time course of the tail current amplitudes more than the time course of the activating current measured directly during the longest depolarizing step. The exact nature of the La^{3+}-sensitive current is not yet clear; however, since all known inward currents are eliminated in these experiments through ion substitution and inorganic blocking agents, a smaller time-dependent K^+ current in addition to I_K (such as I_{to}) may be present. An alternate explanation was that K^+ accumulation developed with long depolarizing pulses even in these single cells and thereby distorted the *envelope test*; however, we find that the reversal potential of the current is no different following 200 or 5000 msec prepulses to +50 mV, indicating significant K^+ accumulation does not occur.

Like several other channels, the delayed rectifier in mammalian species is subject to metabolic regulation. We and others frequently observe *run-down* of I_K when using dialyzed cells; we have not found the current to increase over a 10–60 minute period of whole-cell voltage clamp, and often it gradually decreases and eventually vanishes. When a fairly large electrode (1 MΩ) is used with an internal solution (150 mM KCl, Ca^{+2} and pH-buffered) supplemented with 10 mM ATP, I_K ran down rapidly, reaching 10% of its initial value in under 10 min (T = 30°C). When much smaller 5 MΩ electrodes with the same internal solutions were used, I_K retained half its initial value after 20 minutes. When smaller electrodes (with elevated [433 mM] KCl concentrations providing a series resistance of 4–5 MΩ) were used, I_K rundown was virtually eliminated. Using the latter technique, similar to that initially employed by Hume and Giles (1983) in their study of delayed rectifier in frog atrial cells, we have verified that net dialysis of the cell by KCl is minimal over 45 minutes to 1 hour since there is no appreciable change in the reversal potential of I_K during this time.

In contrast to studies in frog cardiac cells (Hume, 1985), it is well-known that catecholamines and cAMP increase the delayed rectifier current in mammalian heart (Tsien et al., 1972; Kass and Weigers, 1982; Bennett et al., 1986a; Bennett and Begenisich, 1987; Fig. 4). In fact, recent experiments on the delayed rectifier in single guinea pig ventricular myocytes (Matsuura et al., 1988) were conducted in 10–20 nM isoproterenol, as this was found to increase the

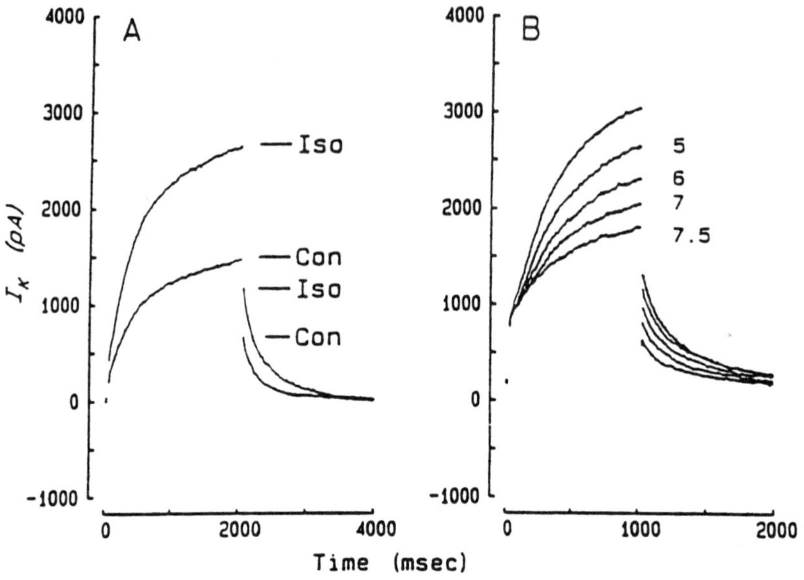

Figure 4. Effect of isoproterenol on I_K and on the inward current elicited immediately after depolarization. As shown in panel A, isoproterenol increases both the time-dependent outward I_K and the current immediately upon depolarization. The fast component of outward current is increased from 200 to 450 pA. As indicated in panel B, I_K returns to its control value 7.5 min after wash out of isoproterenol but the outward current seen at the start of activation remains elevated, indicating that this component may be a different catecholamine-modulated current. From Bennett PB and Begenisich TB. Catecholamines modulate the delayed rectifying potassium current (I_K) in guinea pig ventricular myocytes. *Pflugers Arch* 410:217–219, 1987, by permission.

size of the current sufficiently for study. Catecholamines appear to have multiple effects on the delayed rectifier. Bennett et al. (1986a) attributed the effects of norepinephrine on delayed rectifier kinetics to an alteration in one of the four rate constants in the (C_2-C_1-Open) model, $k_{C2 \rightarrow C1}$. However, these kinetic changes could not account fully for the large (4–6 fold) increase in current magnitude. The mechanism underlying this action of catecholamines has not been established completely. Channel phosphorylation is one possibility raised by the results of Bennett et al. (1989), who analyzed nonstationary current fluctuations before and during norepinephrine and found that the increased macroscopic current did not correspond to a change in unitary current amplitude (i); they concluded that the number of available channels (N) was increased, and speculated that this was probably due to cAMP-dependent phosphorylation of the channel. We have recently demonstrated direct modulation of the channel by using free catalytic subunit of cAMP-dependent protein kinase (cA kinase; Flockhart and Corbin, 1984) in the cell dialysate (also see Kameyama et al., 1985). I_K was increased, when measured either as the time-dependent current activated during depolarization to +30 mV or as the amplitude of the deactivating current tail upon repolarization at −30 mV. Moreover, rundown was often delayed, although not eliminated by addition of cA kinase; this may result from limited diffusion of the cA kinase from the patch electrode to the cell membrane, as described by Belles et al. (1987) for limited intracellular diffusion of ATP in long whole-cell recordings of the ATP-dependent K^+ channel. In addition, Tohse et al., (1987) have recently shown that external application of phorbol esters, which activate protein kinase C, increased I_K in guinea pig ventricular myocytes. Hence, the delayed rectifier may be a substrate for a variety of phosphorylating enzymes.

Interestingly, catecholamines not only increase the delayed outward current, but also increase another outward current component seen immediately upon depolarization, prior to I_K activation (Bennett and Begenisich, 1987; Fig. 4). No information is available on whether this represents metabolic regulation of the inward rectifier or some other outward current such as a *plateau* current, I_{Kp}, recently described in guinea pig ventricle by Yue and Marban (1988), or I_{to} which may be catecholamine-sensitive (Nakayama and Fozzard, 1987). Finally, we have found that preparations treated with isoproterenol or the catalytic subunit of cAMP-dependent protein kinase appear to be more resistant to the actions of quinidine on I_K, raising the interesting possibility that this agent may act at a metabolic step in the channel regulatory pathway. This hypothesis is consistent with earlier studies in canine cardiac Purkinje fibers reported by Mirro et al. (1980) who found that, in the presence of β-adrenergic and muscarinic stimulation by isoproterenol and acetylcholine, quinidine actually shortened action potential duration, suggesting that the electrophysiological effects of quinidine are modulated by autonomic receptor activation.

The most exciting advances in understanding ion channel physiology have resulted from use of the patch clamp method (Hamill et al., 1981), which allows direct measurement of single ion channel activity. While this technique has been successfully used to describe drug effects on cardiac inward rectifier channels as described above, measurement of single channels that constitute the delayed rectifier in mammalian ventricle have not been previously described. This may either result from an extremely low unitary conductance, or from a very low density of channels on the cell membrane. Clapham and DeFelice (1984) found a 62 pS conductance in embryonic chick ventricle that they believed was a delayed rectifier channel with a very low density. Clapham and Logothetis (1988) have more recently described a 15 pS channel in embryonic chick ventricle that may represent a second type of delayed rectifier in that species. However, in mammalian cells the only reported single channel studies of a *delayed rectifier-like* channel were in the nodal pacemaker cells of rabbit heart (Shibasaki, 1987); inward currents were examined using elevated pipette K^+ concentrations due to difficulties in recording outward currents through channels presumed to have a very small unitary conductance. However, the macroscopic current through these channels appears different from the delayed rectifier. First, the nodal current inactivated and second, the steady state activation curve had a mid-point near -25 mV and saturated near 0 mV (DiFrancesco et al., 1979; Shibasaki, 1987). This is unlike I_K in Purkinje and ventricular cells which does not inactivate, and has a steady state activation curve with a midpoint at more positive potentials, and saturates at potentials $\geq +40$ mV (Bennett, et al., 1985; Tohse et al., 1987; Clapham and Logothetis, 1988; Matsuura et al., 1987). These differences suggest that the nodal K^+ channels differ qualitatively from those which underlie I_K in ventricle.

In initial attempts to measure delayed rectifier single channel properties, we have applied nonstationary fluctuation analysis to whole cell I_K measurements. We have found a single channel conductance of 4–7 pS ($K_o = 4.5$) and an estimated channel density of 0.3 channels/μ^2. This agrees with the 6 pS slope conductance reported in avian hepatocytes (Marchetti et al., 1988) and in other cells (see Latorre and Miller, 1983, for review), but differs from the values reported in chick ventricle noted previously (Clapham and Logothetis, 1988). We have also occasionally successfully measured outward unitary K^+ currents using on-cell patches in guinea pig ventricular myocytes. The channels open after a delay, and the ensemble average resembles the time-dependent behavior characteristic of the delayed rectifier. Chord conductance estimated at 140 mV positive to E_K was 6 pS, a value in close agreement to those given for other cell types and predicted from fluctuation analysis in these cells.

Summary and Clinical Implications

Action potential prolongation appears to be an important antiarrhythmic drug action. Marked increases in action potential duration have been associated with paradoxical induction of a specific ventricular arrhythmia; continued research at both the clinical and basic levels into the mechanisms and precipitators of this rhythm disturbance may allow better identification of the patient at risk and improve methods for avoiding this complication. On the other hand, it is now quite clear that selective action potential prolongation is a potent arrhythmia suppressing drug action with a number of associated desirable clinical features including relatively few hemodynamic effects and beneficial effects on ventricular fibrillation and defibrillation. Thus, intensive exploration of the mechanism(s) responsible for action potential modulation by antiarrhythmic drugs has become a major focus of research. Intensive study of drug-sodium channel interactions has yielded insights not only into molecular mechanisms of drug action but also had direct clinical implications in terms of approriate choices of drug combinations, predictions of drug action based on in vitro effects, etc. Potassium channels in heart, like those in many other tissues, are considerably more heterogenous than sodium channels. Nevertheless, critical features of drug block of a range of potassium channels in heart are now becoming evident. Ultimately, delineation of varying drug mechanisms may become important both in the design of new agents as well as the rational use of available agents alone and in combination.

Acknowledgments: We wish to thank Dr. Jackie Corbin for providing the free catalytic subunit of cAMP-dependent protein kinase used in these studies. We also thank Dr. James T. Davis and Holly T. Gray for excellent technical assistance, and Betty Hondeghem and Terri Seale for editorial help. Supported in part by grants from the USPHS (HL32694, HL36020, HL40608, GM07347) and the American Heart Association (Tennessee Affiliate).

BIBLIOGRAPHY

Arena JP, Kass RS. Pharmacological dissection of two heart K channels: the inward rectifier and the delayed rectifier. *Biophys J* 51:367a, 1987.

Armstrong CM. Time course of TEA^+-induced anomalous rectification in squid giant axons. *J Gen Physiol* 50:491–503, 1966.
Bacaner MB, Clay JR, Shrier A, Brochu RM. Potassium channel blockade: a mechanism for suppressing ventricular fibrillation. *Proc Natl Acad Sci* 83:2223–2227, 1985.
Balser JR, Hondeghem LM, Roden DM. Amiodarone reduces time dependent I_K activation. *Circulation* 76:SIV-150, 1987a.
Balser JR, Hondeghem LM, Roden DM. Quinidine block of I_K accumulates at negative potentials. *Circulation* 76:SIV-149, 1987b.
Balser JR, Roden DM, Bennett PB. A method for determining microscopic rate constants from whole cell currents. *Biophys J* 53:543a, 1988b.
Balser JR, Roden DM. Lanthanum-sensitive current contaminates I_K in guinea pig ventricular myocytes. *Biophys J* 53:642a, 1988.
Balser JR, Roden DM, Bennett PB. Quinidine preferentially suppresses a subconductance state of the inward rectifier. *Circulation* 78;SII-411, 1988a.
Belles B, Hescheler J, Trube G. Changes of membrane currents in cardiac cells induced by long whole-cell recordings and tolbutamide. *Pflugers Arch* 409:582–588, 1987.
Bennett PB, Begenisich TB. Catecholamines modulate the delayed rectifying potassium current (I_K) in guinea pig ventricular myocytes. *Pflugers Arch* 410:217–219, 1987.
Bennett PB, Begenisich T, Kass RS. Non-stationary fluctuations of a potassium channel conductance in heart: The effects of catecholamines. *Biophys J* 55:731–738, 1989.
Bennett P, McKinney L, Begenisich T, Kass RS. Adrenergic modulation of the delayed rectifier potassium channel in calf cardiac Purkinje fibers. *Biophys J* 49:839–848, 1986a.
Bennett PB, McKinney LC, Kass RS, Begenisich T. Delayed rectification in the calf cardiac Purkinje fiber: evidence for multiple state kinetics. *Biophys J* 48:553–567, 1985.
Carmeliet E. Electrophysiologic and voltage clamp analysis of the effects of sotalol on isolated cardiac muscle and Purkinje fibers. *J Pharmacol Exp Ther* 232:817–825, 1985.
Clapham DE, DeFelice LJ. Voltage-activated K channels in embryonic chick heart. *Biophys J* 45:40–42, 1984.
Clapham DE, Logothetis DE. Delayed rectifier K^+ current in embryonic chick heart ventricle. *Am J Physiol* 254:H192–H197, 1988.
Cohen JS, Datyner NB, Gintant GA, Kline RP. Time-dependent outward currents in the heart. In: Fozzard HA, Haber E, et al., eds. *The Heart and Cardiovascular System.* New York, NY: Raven Press; 637–669, 1986.
Colatsky TJ. Mechanisms of action of lidocaine and quinidine on action potential duration in rabbit cardiac Purkinje fibers. *Circ Res* 50:17–27, 1982.
Cole KS, Moore JW. Potassium ion current in the squid giant axon: dynamic characteristics. *Biophys J* 1:1–14, 1960.
DiFrancesco D, Noma A, Trautwein W. Kinetics and magnitude of the time-dependent potassium current in the rabbit sinoatrial node. *Pflugers Arch* 381:271–279, 1979.

Echt DS, Black JN, Barbey JT, Coxe DR, Cato E. Evaluation of antiarrhythmic drugs on defibrillation energy requirements in dogs: sodium channel block vs. action potential prolongation. *Circulation* 79:1106–1117, 1989.

Echt DS, Kopelman HA, Lee JT, Crawford D, Woosley RL, Roden DM. Control mechanisms for QT interval in man. *Circulation* 74:SII-401, 1986.

Escande D, Coulombe A, Faivre J, Deroubaix E, Coraboeuf E. Two types of transient outward currents in adult human atrial cells. *Am J Physiol* 252:H142–H148, 1987.

Flockhart DA, Corbin JD. Preparation of the catalytic subunit of cAMP-dependent protein. In: *Brain Receptor Methodologies*. San Diego, CA: Academic Press; 209–215, 1984.

Follmer CH, Buzby GC, Jurkiewicz NK, Stein RP, Colatsky TJ. Selective block of Na^+ and K^+ channels in feline ventricular myocytes. *Biophys J* 53:424a, 1988.

Giles WR, van Ginneken ACG. A transient outward current in isolated cells from the crista terminalis of rabbit heart. *J Physiol* 368:243–264, 1985.

Gintant GA, Datyner NB, Cohen IS. Gating of delayed rectification in acutely isolated canine cardiac Purkinje myocytes: evidence for a single voltage-gated conductance. *Biophys J* 48:1059–1064, 1985.

Hamill OP, Marty A, Neher E, Sakmann S, Sigworth FJ. Improved patch clamp techniques for high resolution current recording from cells and cell-free membrane patches. *Pflugers Arch* 391:85–100, 1981.

Hille B. Local anesthetics: hydrophilic and hydrophobic pathways for the drug-receptor reaction. *J Gen Physiol* 69:497–515, 1977.

Hiraoka M, Sawada K, Kawano S. Effects of quinidine on plateau currents of guinea-pig ventricular myocytes. *J Moll Cell Cardiol* 18:1097–1106, 1986.

Hodgkin AL, Huxley AF. A quantitative description of membrane current and its application to conduction and excitation in nerve. *J Physiol* 117:500–544, 1952.

Hondeghem LM, Bennett PB. Models of Antiarrythmic Drugs. In: Hondeghem LM, ed. *Molecular and Cellular Mechanisms of Antiarrythmic Agents*. Mount Kisco, NY: Futura Publishing Co., Inc., 1989.

Hondeghem LM, Katzung BG. Antiarrhythmic agents: the modulated receptor mechanism of action of sodium and calcium channel-blocking drugs. *Annu Rev Pharmacol Toxicol* 24:387–423, 1984.

Hondeghem LM, Katzung BG. Time and voltage-dependent interactions of antiarrhythmic drugs with cardiac sodium channels. *Biochim Biophys Acta* 472:373–398, 1977.

Hume JR. Do catecholamines directly modulate the delayed plateau potassium current in frog atrium? *J Mol Cell Cardiol* 17:813–816, 1985.

Hume JR, Giles W. Ionic currents in single isolated bullfrog atrial cells. *J Gen Physiol* 81:153–194, 1983.

Hume JR, Giles W, Robinson K, Shibata EF, Nathan RD, Kanai K, et al. A time- and voltage-dependent K^+ current in single cardiac cells from bullfrog atrium. *J Gen Physiol* 88:777–798, 1986.

Imaizumi Y, Giles WR. Qunidine-induced inhibition of transient outward current in cardiac muscle. *Am J Physiol* 253:H704–H708, 1987.

Josephson IR, Sanchez-Chapula J, Brown AM. Early outward current in rat single ventricular cells. *Circ Res* 54:157–162, 1984.

Kakushkin NI, Gainullin RZ, Sosunov EA. Transient outward current and rate dependence of action potential duration in rabbit cardiac ventricular muscle. *Pflugers Arch* 399:87–92, 1883.

Kameyama M, Hoffmann F, Trautwein W. On the mechanism of β-adrenergic regulation of the Ca^{++} channel in the guinea-pig heart. *Pflugers Arch* 405:285–293, 1985.

Kass RS, Weigers S. Ionic basis of concentration-related effects of noradrenaline on the action potential of cardiac Purkinje fibres. *J Physiol* 322:541–558, 1982.

Kenyon JL, Gibbons WR. 4-Aminopyridine and the early outward current of sheep cardiac Purkinje fibers. *J Gen Physiol* 73:139–157, 1979.

Kenyon JL, Sutko JL. Calcium- and voltage-activated plateau current of cardiac Purkinje fibers. *J Gen Physiol* 89:921–958, 1987.

Latorre R, Miller C. Conduction and selectivity in potassium channels. *J Membrane Biol* 71:11–30, 1983.

Litovsky SH, Antzelevitch C. Transient outward current prominent in canine ventricular epicardium but not endocardium. *Circ Res* 62:116–126, 1988.

Lumma WC, Wohl RA, Davey DD, Argentieri TM, DeVita RJ, Gomez RP, et al. Rational design of 4-[(Methylsulfonyl)amino]benzamides as Class III antiarrhythmic agents. *J Med Chem* 30:755–758, 1987.

Marchetti C, Premont RT, Brown AM. A whole-cell and single-channel study of the voltage-dependent outward potassium current in avian hepatocytes. *J Gen Physiol* 91:255–274, 1988.

Matsuda H, Saigusa A, Irisawa H. Ohmic conductance through the inwardly rectifying K channel and blocking by internal Mg^{2+}. *Nature* 325:156–159, 1987.

Matsuura H, Ehara T, Imoto Y. An analysis of the delayed outward current in single ventricular cells of the guinea pig. *Pflugers Arch* 410:596–603, 1987.

Maylie J, Morad M. A transient outward current related to calcium release and development of tension in elephant seal atrial fibres. *J Physiol* 357:267–292, 1984.

McDonald TF, Pelzer D, Trautwein W. Cat ventricular muscle treated with D600: effects on calcium and potassium currents. *J Physiol* 352:203–216, 1984.

Mirro MJ, Watanabe AM, Bailey JC. Electrophysiological effects of disopyramide and quinidine on guinea pig atria and canine cardiac Purkinje fibers. *Circ Res* 46:661–668, 1980.

Nakayama T, Fozzard HA. Adrenergic modulation of the transient outward current in isolated canine cardiac. *Purkiophys J* 51:56a, 1987.

Nakayama T, Irisawa H. Transient outward current carried by potassium and sodium in quiescent atrioventricular node cells of rabbits. *Circ Res* 57:65–73, 1985.

Noble D, Tsien RW. Outward membrane currents activated in the plateau range of potentials in cardiac Purkinje fibres. *J Physiol (Lond)* 200:205–231, 1969.

Roden DM, Bennett PB, Snyders DJ, Balser JR, Hondeghem LM. Quinidine delays I_K activation in guinea pig myocytes. *Circ Res* 62:1055–1058, 1988.

Roden DM, Hoffman BF. Action potential prolongation and induction of abnormal automaticity by low quinidine concentrations in canine Purkinje fibers: relationship to potassium and cycle length. *Circ Res* 56:857–867, 1985.

Roden DM, Thompson KA, Hoffman BF, Woosley RL. Clinical features and basic mechanisms of quinidine-induced arrhythmias. The proceedings of the 4th Annual Joint US-USSR Symposium on Sudden Cardiac Death. *J Am Coll Cardiol* 8:73A–78A, 1986.

Sakmann B, Trube G. Conductance properties of single inwardly rectifying potassium channels in ventricular cells from guinea-pig heart. *J Physiol* 347:641–657, 1984.

Salata JJ, Wasserstrom JA. Effects of quinidine on action potentials and ionic currents in isolated canine ventricular myocytes. *Circ Res* 62:324–337, 1988.

Sato R, Hisatome I, Singer DH. Amiodarone blocks the inward-rectifier K^+ channel in guinea pig ventricular myocytes. *Circulation* 76:SIV-150, 1987.

Sato R, Hisatome I, Wasserstrom JA, Singer DH. Quinidine blocks the inward-rectifier K^+ channel (I_{K1}) from the inside of the membrane in guinea pig ventricular myocytes. *Biophys J* 53:642a, 1988.

Scholtysik G, Williams FM. Antiarrhythmic effects of DPI 201-106. *Br J Pharmacol* 89:287–292, 1986.

Schwartz PJ, Locati E. The idiopathic long QT syndrome: pathogenetic mechanisms and therapy. *Eur Heart J* 6:103–114, 1985.

Selzer A, Wray HW. Qunidine Syncope: paroxysmal ventricular fibrillation occurring during treatment of chronic atrial arrhythmias. *Circulation* 30:17–26, 1964.

Shibasaki T. Conductance and kinetics of delayed rectifier potassium channels in nodal cells of the rabbit heart. *J Physiol* 387:227–250, 1987.

Shibata EF, Refsum H, Aldrete T, Ilnicki T, Giles W. A transient outward current in single cells from human atrial muscle. *Circulation* Suppl. II:II-254, 1986.

Siegelbaum SA, Tsien RW, Kass RS. Role of intracellular calcium in the transient outward current of calf Purkinje fibres. *Nature* 269:611–613, 1977.

Simmons MA, Craeazzo T, Hartzell HC. A time-dependent and voltage-sensitive K^+ curent in single cells from frog atrium. *J Gen Physiol* 88:739–755, 1986.

Šimurda J, Šimurdová M, Cupera P. 4-Aminopyridine sensitive transient outward current in dog ventricular fibres. *Pflugers Arch* 411:442–449, 1988.

Snyders DJ, Hondeghem LM, Katzung BG. Sigmoidal time course of I_K activation in cardiac myocytes. *Circulation* 74:SII-255, 1986.

Snyders DJ, Katzung BG. Clofilium reduces the plateau potassium current in isolated cardiac myocytes. *Ciculation* 72:SIII-233, 1985.

Snyders DJ, Katzung BG. Intracellular clofilium reduces I_K in isolated adult cardiac myocytes. *Biophys J* 49:401a, 1986.

TenEick RR, Robertson L. Cat papillary muscle seems to lack transient outward current. *Fed Proc* 42:730, 1983.

Thomas G, Minn C, Cohen CJ. A dihydropyridine (Bay K8644) that enhances Ca^{++} currents in guinea pig and calf myocardial cells. *Circ Res* 56:87–96, 1984.

Thompson S. Aminopyridine block of transient potassium current. *J Gen Physiol* 80:1–18, 1982.

Tohse N, Kameyama M, Isisawa H. Intracellular Ca^{2+} and protein kinase C modulate K^{+} current in guinea pig heart cells. *Am J Physiol* 253:H1321–H1324, 1987.

Tsien RW, Giles W, Greengard P. cAMP mediates the action of norepinephrine on the action potential plateau of cardiac Purkinje fibres. *Nature* 240:181–183, 1972.

Vandenberg CA. Inward rectification of a potassium channel in cardiac ventricular cells depends on internal magnesium ions. *Proc Natl Acad Sci USA* 84:2560–2564, 1987.

Vaughan Williams EM. Delayed ventricular repolarization as an antiarrhythmic principle. *Eur Heart J* 6:145–149, 1985.

Young SH, Moore JW. Potassium ion currents in the crayfish giant axon: dynamic characteristics. *Biophys J* 36:723–733, 1981.

Yue DT, Marban E. A novel cardiac potassium channel that is active and conductive at depolarized potentials. *Biophys J* 53:641a, 1988.

Chapter 9

Molecular Models for Voltage Activated Channels

H. Robert Guy

INTRODUCTION

Properties of voltage activate channels have been studied with conventional voltage clamping methods for more than three decades. These studies have been directed toward understanding how activation and inactivation of channels occur when the membrane voltage is changed, how channels select for some cations over other cations, and how various drugs and toxins affect these processes. Various kinetic schemes have been developed to explain the gating processes and schematic representations have been made of the general shape and dimensions of the pore; however, until recently no structural data have been available to develop more precise molecular models. Polypeptide sequences have been inferred recently from DNA sequences of sodium channels in the electric eel *Electrophorus electricus* (Noda et al., 1984), rat (Noda et al., 1986a), and *Drosophila* (Salkoff et al., 1987). Voltage activated sodium channels are members of a larger superfamily of voltage activated channels. Sequences of a putative calcium channel from rabbit skeletal muscle (Tanabe et al., 1987) and a type A potassium channel from *Drosophila* (Tempel et al., 1987) are homologous to that of the sodium channel.

Sodium and calcium channels are very large proteins containing about two thousand amino acid residues. Modelling these channels

Hondeghem, Luc (ed): Molecular and Cellular Mechanisms of Antiarrhythmic Agents, Futura Publishing Company, Inc., Mount Kisco, NY, © 1989.

is simplified by the fact that the sequences contain four homologous domains and all of the long hydrophobic segments postulated to span the membrane are located within these domains. The type A potassium channel is about one fourth as large and contains only one domain homologous to those of the sodium and calcium channels. It is likely that four identical subunits aggregate to form a potassium channel since functional channels can be expressed in *xenopus* oocytes from the cDNA of a single subunit (Timpe et al., 1988). Hille (1984) postulated that sodium channels evolved from calcium channels based of presences of these channels in different organisms and similarity of gating mechanisms. The four homologous domains of sodium and calcium channels probably arose from gene duplications. This event appears to have occurred before the branch between sodium channels since sequences of sodium and calcium channels within any of the homologous domains are more similar than the domains are to each other. In contrast the branch between the sodium/calcium channel ancestor and the type A potassium channel appears to have preceded the gene duplication since the potassium channel has only one domain and the four sodium/calcium channel homologous domains are more similar to each other than to the potassium channel.

Our model of the sodium channel was first developed from the eel sodium channel alone (Guy and Seetharamulu, 1986). It has since been modified slightly and expanded to include inactivation on the basis of rat and fly sequences (Guy, 1988). Models of calcium and potassium channels that have the same general folding pattern appear feasible. An effort was made to convert conceptual and kinetic models that have been developed from voltage clamping and other experiments (for reviews see Hille, 1984; Armstrong, 1981; French and Horn, 1983; Catterall, 1984; and Bezanilla, 1985) into structural models in which functions are assigned to specific amino acid residues or polypeptide segments.

TRANSMEMBRANE FOLDING SCHEMES

The first step in developing a model of a membrane protein is to decide which segments cross the membrane and to choose secondary structures for these segments. Figure 1 illustrates transmembrane segments of our current sodium channel model. Sodium

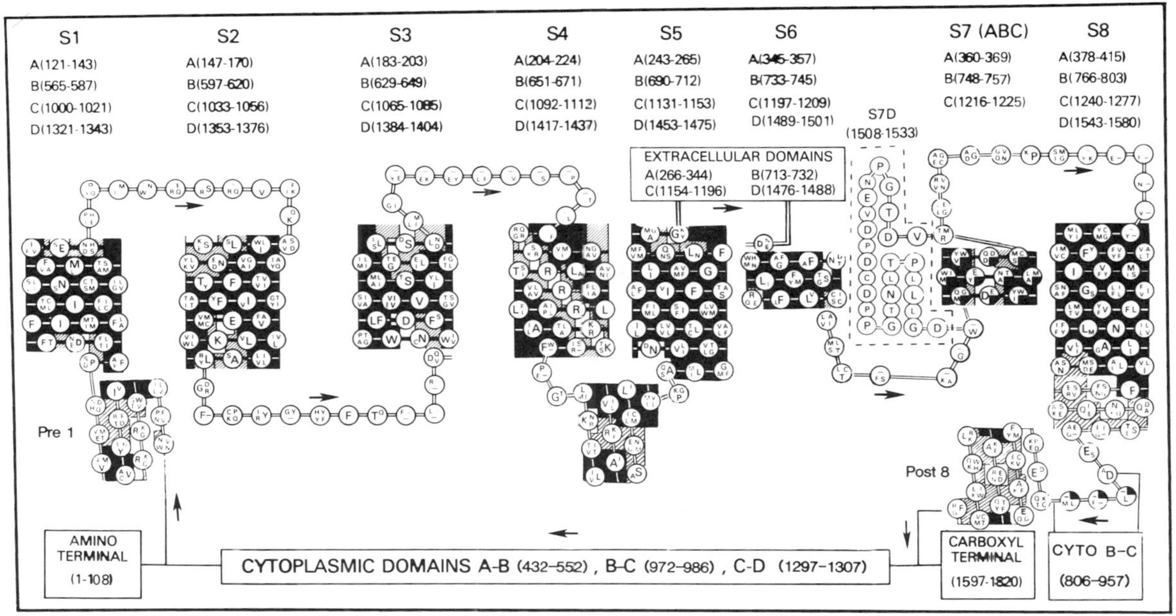

Figure 1. Schematic representation of putative transmembrane segments. Putative transmembrane α helices are represented by a helix net. Sequences for four domains in eel are shown in the single letter code on the same net with residues in the A domain in the upper left of each circle, the B domain in the upper right, the C domain in the lower left, and the D domain in the lower right. If the same amino acid residue is found in adjacent domains (in the circles), a single letter is used for both domains. Positions in which all domains have the same residue have a single letter. Regions of putative α helices with black background are predicted to be buried within the protein or exposed to lipid in all domains; regions with a white background are predicted to be exposed to water in all domains (Guy and Seetharamulu, 1986). Segments are numbered according to the eel sequence.

channel protein sequences contain four homologous domains that are connected by relatively nonhomologous segments of variable length. Noda et al. (1984) identified six segments that are relatively well conserved in each domain: three relatively hydrophobic segments (S1, S2, and S3) that are long enough to span the membrane as α helices and that contain a few charged side chains near their ends; one segment (S4) that has positively charged side chains (usually arginine) at every third position in its sequence and relatively hydrophobic side chains at the other positions; and two very hydrophobic segments (S5 and S8) that have no charged side chains and are long enough to span the membrane as α helices. Noda et al. (1984, 1986a) have suggested that either four or all six of these segments are transmembrane α helices.

Additional segments can also be identified within the homologous domains. S4 and S5 are connected by a segment S(4-5) that may form a short amphipathic α helix in the first three domains (A, B, and C) and is hydrophobic in the last domain (D). S5 is followed by a segment of variable length and that in A and C domain contain five of the ten potential N-glycosylation sites in the eel sequence. These segments have been assigned to the extracellular surface in most models. These extracellular domains are followed by a short hydrophobic segment (S6) that could span about half the membrane as an α helix. The segment connecting S6 to S8 contains a negatively charged segment (S7) that may form a short amphipathic α helix in A, B, and C domains and either a one or three stranded β sheet in the D domain. Guy and Seetharamulu (1986), and Greenblatt et al. (1985) have proposed that S6 and S7 are also in the transmembrane region and that negative charges on S7 are required to balance some of the positive charges on S4. The scheme postulated here differs slightly from that of Guy and Seetharamulu (1986) in that S6D is an α helix (as proposed by Greenblatt et al. (1985) instead of a β strand, S7D has three β strands instead of one, and S7 segments end sooner. Segments that precede S1 (Pre 1) and that follow S8 (Post 8) appear to be distantly homologous and are conserved relatively well among sodium channels. We postulate that these segments form the cytoplasmic entrance to the channel and are involved in inactivation (Guy, 1988). Kosower (1985) proposed a scheme in which each domain has a different folding pattern, S4 segments are 3–10 helices, and very negatively charged segments between domains B and C are also transmembrane 3–10 helices.

SELECTIVITY FILTER

The sodium channel appears to have a negatively charged narrow region near its extracellular entrance that has at least two cation binding sites and a larger funnel shaped cytoplasmic entrance. Based on his studies of the permeability of sodium channels to various organic cation, Hille (1971) postulated that the narrowest portion of the channel that selects for sodium is lined with oxygens and has an rectangular opening of about 3.1 by 5.1 angstroms. Permeability of the sodium channel is affected by internal ions in a manner consistent with a pore that has two cation binding sites, one near the outer entrance and one near the inner entrance of the narrow region of the pore (see Begenisich, 1987 for review). Studies of the voltage dependency of channel blockade by internally perfused drugs suggests that both sodium channels and potassium channels have large funnel-like entrances from the cytoplasmic surface and that most of the voltage drop occurs across a narrow region near the extracellular surface (see Hille, 1984; and Yellen, 1987 for review).

Models that have been proposed for the sodium channel from its sequence differ most by which segments are postulated to form the negatively charged portion of the channel lining that selects for sodium over other ions. In our model S7 segments form the selectivity filter, Greenblatt et al. (1985) chose S3 segments, Noda et al. (1986a) suggested S2, and Kosower (1985) postulated segments between the B and C domains.

Our rationale for selecting S7 segments to form the selectivity filter are listed as follows: (1) Short channel lining segments like S7 are consistent with the hypothesis that the channel is a *funnel shape* with a large entrance on the cytoplasmic surface. (2) Most S7 segments have two negatively charged groups consistent with the hypothesis of two cation binding sites. (3) S4 helices are postulated to fit between the S7 segments but are farther from the center of the channel. Arginine side chains in the central region of S4's can extend between short S7 segments while arginines near the ends of S4 segments can extend over and under S7 segments where they can be exposed to water and form salt bridges with negatively charged side chains from S1, S2, S3, and S6 segments. This arrangement allows the bulky, positively charged side chains that spiral around S4 helices to move during gating activation gating (see Activation Gating). (4) When S7's form the channel lining, charged side chains near the ends of S1, S2, and S3 can be exposed to water and form salt bridges with positively charged side chains near the ends of S4 segments. (6) All side chains on the hydrophilic faces of S7 segments are conserved between eel and rat and most are conserved in fly. One would expect the functionally important selectivity filter to be highly conserved among sodium channels. (7) S7 segments can form a selectivity filter with dimensions consistent with permeability studies and that is consistent with *ridges into grooves* helix packing theory and the postulated activation gating mechanism (Guy, 1988).

S1, S2, and/or S3 are not good candidates for the channel lining because a) by our calculations the central regions of these helices are too hydrophobic (Guy and Seetharamulu, 1986, see Fig. 1); and b) the hydrophobic sides of these helices are not well conserved, suggesting that they are exposed to lipid in some domains (see Homology). We do not consider the very negatively charged segments postulated by Kosower (1985) as good candidates for the selectivity filter because a) they have no hydrophobic residues and thus may be too hydrophilic to be transmembrane segments; and b) there are deletions and several nonconservative substitutions in the rat sequences.

ACTIVATION GATING

Before the sodium channel sequence was determined, Armstrong (1981) postulated that the voltage sensing mechanism of the activation gate could be a string of negative charges associated with a string of positive charges and that one of these strings moves relative to the other when the channel opens. The most conserved feature among the sodium, calcium, and potassium channels is the pattern of positive charges three residues apart on S4 segments. All groups that have modeled the sodium channel from its sequence postulate that movement of positive charges on the S4 segments in the transmembrane region leads to activation of the channel. One can envision several ways that the charges could move in response to the electric field is a way that might open the channel: (1) the arginine and lysine side chains could change conformations while everything else remains static, (2) the S4 segments could move while everything else remains static, (3) each of the four homologous repeats could form a domain that maintains its internal conformation

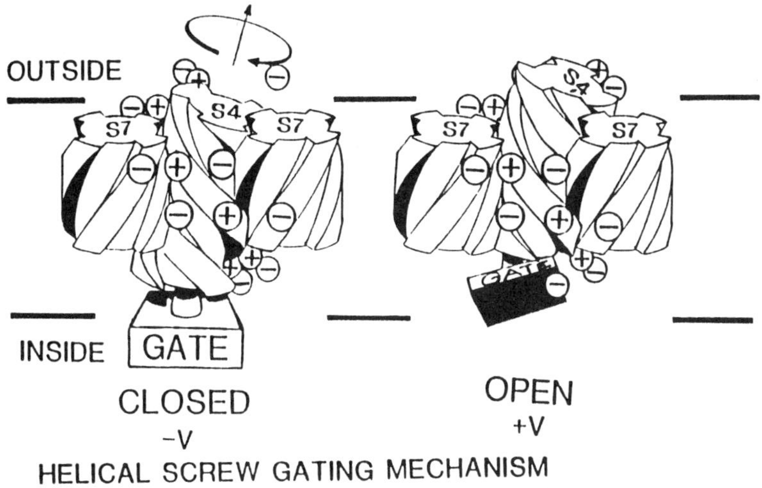

Figure 2. Activation gating mechanisms. (A) Helical screw mechanism. S4 is represented by a cylinder with three ridges spiraling around it in a left handed manner. These ridges, one of which contains all the positively charged side chains on S4, are formed by every third amino acid residue. S4 is positioned between two S7 helices, each of which has four ridges formed by every fourth residue. S4 interacts with S7 helices with 3–4 ridges into grooves packing in which ridges on S4 fit between those on S7's. Positively charged side chains on S4 interact with negatively charged side chains on S7's, S6, S1, S2 and S3 (these latter helices are not shown). When the channel opens, S4 rotates about its axis by 60° and moves along its axis by 4.5 angstroms. Other transmembrane segments do not move. Conformation of the channel lining remains virtually unaltered by this process; however, movement of S4 affects the conformation of the segment linking S4 to S5, represented here by the gate, which may block the channel in the closed conformation.

but moves with respect to the other domains, or (4) the movement could be very complex, involving changes both within and between domains. Any of these mechanisms could produce kinetics complex enough to fit most experimental results.

We tentatively favor the second possibility as illustrated in Figure 2 because it is consistent with postulates on how various agents block the channel and can explain why the charges on S4 segments are three residues apart. Hille (1984) has concluded that positively charged local anesthetics that block the channel from the cytoplasm can enter and exit the channel only when it is in an open conformation but that the channel can close and trap the drug inside. It is difficult to envision how this could occur simply by changing conformations of lysine and arginine side chains. Tetrototoxin and saxitoxin block the channel from the extracellular side. These toxins do not alter gating currents appreciably and bind to both open and closed conformations with only slightly different affinities. If these toxins plug the channel entrance, as postulated by Hille, they should interact with segments from several of the homologous repeats in which case, appreciable movement between domains during gating should disrupt the binding. This argument is weak, however, because the mechanism by which these toxins act has not been proven.

A clue to why every third residue is charged may be given by the *ridges-into-grooves* α helix packing theory. Chothia et al. (1981) noted that side chains four residues apart form four ridges that spiral around the axis of an α helix in a right handed manner and that side chains three residues apart formed three less pronounced ridges that spiral around the axis in a left handed manner. These ridges fit between each other in most helix-helix interactions. If the ridges are formed by side chains four residues apart on both helices, then the axes of the helices will cross at an angle of about −50° and the packing is called *4-4 ridges-into-grooves* packing; if the ridges on one helix is formed by residues four residues apart on one helix and three residues apart on the other helix, then the helices will cross at an angle of about 20° and the packing is called *3-4 ridges-into-grooves* packing. If one assumes that S4 segments are α helices that interact with surrounding helices with *3-4* packing and that charge movement is due to movement of the S4 helices, then the only way this movement can occur and maintain the *3-4* packing is for the helix to rotate about its axis as it moves along its axis. A translation of 4.5 Å and a rotation of 60° results in the movement of each positive charge on the S4 helix to the position occupied by the side chain that preceded it by three residues before the movement. This movement for one S4 helix results in the equivalent movement of one charge and three residues across the membrane. We called this mechanism the *helical screw* because the motion is *screwlike* and ridges formed by every third residue on S4 can be thought of as the threads on a screw, and the ridges on the surrounding α helices can be considered the matrix through which the screw moves.

In the *helical screw* model the portion of the pore formed by the bundle of alternating S4 and S7 segments is virtually identical in the closed and open conformations since S7 segments do not move and arginine side chains near the center of S4's that interact with

S7's in the closed conformations are replaced by other arginine side chains in the open conformation. The main structural differences should be observed for segments connecting S4 to S3 and S4 to S5. The postulated mechanism essentially moves three residues as well as one charge across the membrane when the channel opens. This removes protein from near the cytoplasmic entrance of the channel and adds it to the extracellular side. From studies of drugs that appear to enter and block the open channel from the cytoplasmic side, it has been postulated that the activation gate is near the cytoplasmic entrance (see Armstrong, 1981; and Hille, 1984 for review). It seems reasonable to postulate that protein near the C-terminus of S4 segments form this gate and that they move out of the channel entrance when the channel opens. Negative charges on S1 and S3 that are balanced by positive charges on the C-terminus of S4 in the closed conformation are exposed when the channel opens. It is possible that some of these negative charges interact with some positively charged channel blocking drugs, and drugs such as batrachotoxin (BTX) that favor activation and inhibit inactivation. Helices that surround S4 can be arranged so that each positive charged side chain on S4 can interact with at least one negatively charged side chain on S1, S3, S6, or S7. Note that at most, only two positively charged side chains on S4 interact with negative charges of S7 for a given conformation. S4 helices can be farther from the center of the channel than S7 segments because arginines have long amphiphilic side chains. In soluble proteins of known structure, arginine α carbons tend to be buried within the protein interior while the hydrophilic end guanidinium group is on or near the surface (Guy, 1985). In the helical screw model all positively charged groups on S4, and most charges on S1, S2, and S3 can be partially hydrated either by water inside the channel or on the inner and outer surfaces near the ends of the helices. For this to occur, S7 and S6 must be short so that the arginine side chains on each side of the central residues of S4 can extend above or below these segments (see Fig. 2) and so that charges on S1, S2, and S3 can be partially exposed to water. It is also important for S6 and S7 to be short for the *helical screw* mechanism to work. There would be substantial barriers to moving the very bulky arginine side chains of S4 from one side of an adjacent α helix to the other side, even with *ridges into grooves* packing. This problem is eliminated if these side chains can move above and below S6 and S7 when the channel opens and closes.

INACTIVATION AND CYTOPLASMIC SEGMENTS

When the membrane is depolarized activation is followed by inactivation. Measurements of sodium currents (Bezanilla and Armstrong, 1978; Goldman and Schauf, 1972; Goldman and Kenyon, 1982), gating currents (Armstrong and Bezanilla, 1978), and single channel recordings (Aldrich, 1986; Aldrich, et al., 1983; Horn and Vanderberg, 1986) all indicate that inactivation does not occur independent of activation, as originally proposed by Hodgkin and Huxley (1952). It appears that the probability of inactivation occurring is much greater when the channel is open, but that the channel does not have to be in an open conformation for it to enter or leave the inactivated conformation. Coupling of inactivation to activation is supported by the observation that inactivation immobilizes about two thirds of the activation gating charge. Inactivation can be eliminated by proteolytic cleavage and by various chemical modifying reagents on the cytoplasmic side of the membrane (see Hille, 1984 for review) and can be modulated by binding of sea anemone and α scorpion toxins from the outside (Catterall, 1984).

Armstrong and Bezanilla (1977) postulated that a positively charged inactivation gate plugs the open channel from the inside. Noda et al. (1986a) noted that a positively charged segment following S8C and a negatively charged segment following S8D are well conserved between eel and rat and suggested that these may be involved in activation. These segments are also well conserved in fly (Salkoff et al., 1987). Post 8C has some of the features one might expect for an inactivation gate; it is highly conserved among sodium channels, is very positively charged, it contains sites where cleavage by trypsin can occur, and it contains two tyrosines and an arginine (arginine and tyrosine chains are the most likely sites of action of some reactants that eliminate inactivation, see Hille, 1984). Analyses of amphipathicity and secondary structure predictions (Garnier et al., 1978) suggest that portions of these segments form α helices. One way these segments could form the cytoplasmic entrance to the channel is shown in Figure 3. In this scheme inactivation is caused by movement of the Post 8C segment. In the inactivated conformation a series of salt bridges are formed between positive charges on Post 8C and negative charges on Post 8D.

Figures 3 and 4 illustrate how activation and inactivation may

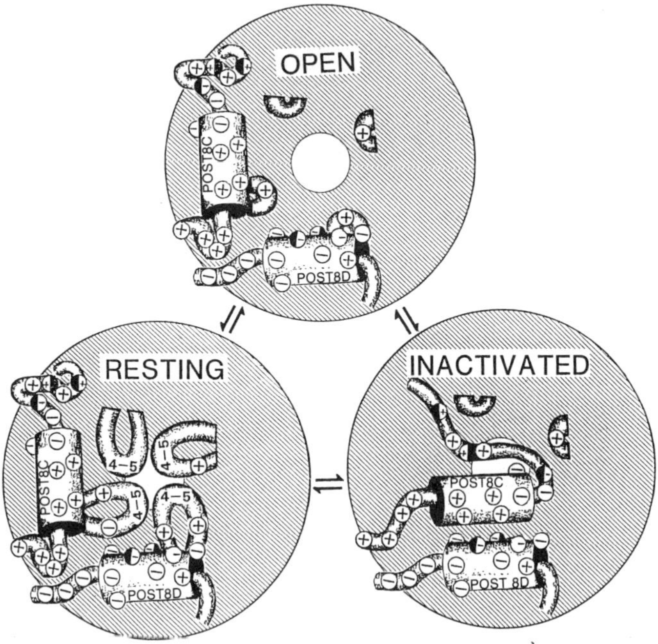

Figure 3. Schematic representation of cytoplasmic entrance to the channel illustrating possible activation and inactivation mechanisms. Segments that follow S8D and S8C are assigned α helical conformations and positioned near the channel entrance. Segments that follow S4 are shown as loops. Circles represent positively and negatively charged side chains; if half of the circle is black, the side chain is not charged in eel (left) or rat (right). The channel is postulated to go from the resting to open conformation when S4's (not shown) of some or all four domains undergo a helical screw conformational change. This removes an occlusion caused by loop segments near the C-termini of S4's. An additional helical screw movement of S4D and possibly S4C then allows the Post 8C segment to move over the channel entrance when the channel inactivates. Note interactions between positive charges on Post 8C and negative charges on Post 8D in the inactivated conformation. The arrows represent a series of conformational changes.

be coupled. In this scheme activation is caused by *helical screw* conformational changes of some or all S4 helices. This removes protein and positive charge from the cytoplasmic entrance of the channel and leaves it open. S4D is postulated to undergo at least one more helical screw conformational change that removes more positive charge and protein from the cytoplasmic entrance. This additional

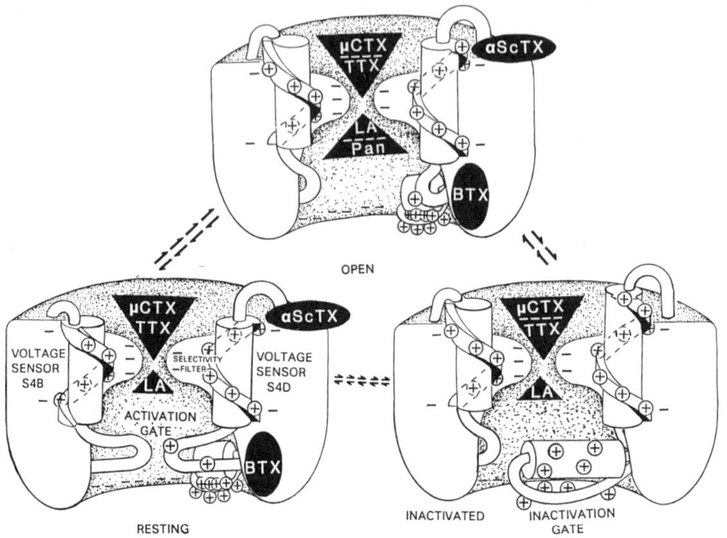

Figure 4. Schematic representation of activation and inactivation mechanisms. The channel is postulated to go from the resting to open conformation when S4's of some or all four domains (only S4B and S4D are shown) undergo a *helical screw* conformational change. This removes an occlusion caused by segments near the C-termini of S4's. Inactivation is caused by an additional *helical screw* conformational change of S4D followed by movement of Post 8C over the channel entrance. Plausible binding sites for TTX, µ conotoxin (µ CTX), local anesthetics (LA), pancuronium (pan), batrachotoxin (BTX) and α scorpion toxin (α SCTX) are shown in black on conformations to which they may bind.

step is possible because the pattern of positive charges repeats more times for the S4D helix, and the segment that connects it on the outside to the S3D helix is longer and better conserved than in the other domains. A transmembrane conformational change associated with inactivation is suggested by modulation of inactivation by α scorpion and sea anemone toxins. The additional movement of S4D in turn, allows the positively charged inactivation gate, Post 8C, to move into the channel entrance. When the channel is inactivated S4D and possibly some of the other S4 segments cannot return to their closed conformations and thus their gating charges are immobilized. The channel could go between the resting and inactivated conformations without passing through the open conformation if some of the S4 helices, say S4A and S4B, can be in closed conformations when the channel is inactivated.

PHARMACOLOGY

Sodium channels are affected by a variety of drugs and toxins (see Hille, 1984; and Catterall, 1984 for review). Tetrodotoxin (TTX) and saxitoxin (STX) inhibit the channel from the outside. These toxins bind to all conformations of the protein. The voltage dependency of binding is the same for TTX and STX even though STX has two charges and TTX has only one charge. This indicates that they do not transverse a substantial portion of the membrane before binding. One hypothesis is that they block the outer entrance of the channel. Figure 4 illustrates that a binding site at the outer entrance would be negatively charged and would not change conformations greatly during activation and inactivation. This region involves segments near the C-termini of S7 segments. The μ conotoxin from cone snails is a very positively charged peptide that competes with TTX and STX binding in some sodium channels (Moczydlowski et al., 1986). It is substantially larger than TTX and STX and would probably bind to additional segments not involved in TTX and STX binding. Segments connecting S7D to S8D and S7C to S8C are more negatively charged in eel, which is blocked by μ conotoxin, than in rat brain, which is not affected.

Sodium channels can be blocked from the inside by a variety of positively charged local anesthetics. Analyses of the effects of these drugs suggests that they can enter and leave the channel only when it is open but can be trapped in resting and inactivated channels (Hille, 1984, Starmer et al., 1986). A variety of larger positively charged toxins such as pancuronium and strychnine also block sodium channels from these inside; however, once the channel is blocked it cannot go to a resting or inactivated conformation, and all gating charge is immobilized. Mimicry of inactivation by these drugs was part of Armstrong and Bezanilla's (1978) rationale for postulating the positively charged inactivation plug. Figure 4 illustrates how in this model, local anesthetics may bind near the N-termini of S7 segments and the larger drugs may interact with this region and also with the activation and inactivation gates.

Sea anemone toxins and α scorpion toxins slow or block inactivation and enhance activation of sodium channels by batrachotoxin (BTX) and similar toxins (Catterall, 1984). Their binding on the extracellular side of the membrane is reduced by depolarization in a way that indicates the binding site undergoes a conformational change during channel activation (Catterall, 1982). These effects can be explained by the model if the presence of either BTX or α scorpion toxin inhibits the final conformational change of S4D and likewise, if the last conformational change of S4D inhibits binding of the toxins. BTX prevents inactivation and also affects activation kinetics and channel ion selectivity. It is difficult to determine from which side of the membrane BTX binds because it is so lipophilic. The model suggests that all these properties could be affected by binding of BTX near the C-terminus of S4D where it could affect the N-termini of S7's that form the selectivity filter, S4D movement, and movement of the inactivation gate, Post 8C.

USING HOMOLOGY IN DEVELOPING MODELS

Having sequences that vary greatly in the extent of homology allows us to determine which features are conserved for all members of the superfamily, which features are conserved within a family (e.g., among sodium channels) but differ among families, and which features can vary within a family.

We use two criteria to select which portions of α helices form the outer surface of the channel that is exposed to the hydrophobic lipid chains: the residues should be hydrophobic and they should be comprised of the least well conserved residues in the transmembrane region when comparing sequences of channels that have the same functional properties. Statistical studies of homologous proteins for which the structure is known indicate that residues on the surface that are not part of a functional site tend to be conserved less well than those buried in the interior of the protein (Go and Miyazawa, 1980). These residues tend to be hydrophilic and are exposed to water surrounding the protein. This pattern is reasonable, since changing the volume or shape of these surface side chains may have little effect on the way the protein packs to form the three-dimensional structure. Likewise, for membrane proteins changing the volume and shape of hydrophobic side chains that extend into the *lipid solvent* may have little effect on the protein's structure. In studying many putative transmembrane α helices we have often observed a pattern, which we call unilateral conservation, in which one face of the helix is conserved better that the opposite face. When the poorly conserved face is hydrophobic we interpret this pattern to indicate that the poorly conserved face is exposed to lipid.

The unilateral conservation pattern is especially apparent when comparing sequences of S1, S2, and S3 segments from eel, rat, and fly sodium channels. More hydrophobic faces of these putative α helices are poorly conserved with many substitutions; whereas, more hydrophilic faces of these helices are conserved extremely well, with most of the residues being the same among the four homologous domains of the sodium and calcium channels and most of the charges on these faces being conserved in the potassium channel. In contrast, most residues of S5 and S6 are the same among the sodium channels but are poorly conserved among the four domains. S5 and S6 exhibit no clear pattern of unilateral conservation.

The most conserved features among the four homologous domains are the positive charges on the S4 segments and the more hydrophilic faces of S1, S2, and S3. The S4 positive charges are conserved in the potassium channel and the hydrophilic faces of S1, S2, and S3 are partially conserved: a glutamate and isoleucine on S1; a glutamate, positive charge (arginine substitutes for lysine), and phenylalanine on S2; and an aspartate, asparagine, and leucine on S3 are conserved. Except for their general hydrophobic properties, S5–S8 segments are poorly conserved among the repeats and are difficult to align with homologous segments in the potassium channel. Many substitutions occur in these segments when comparing sodium and calcium channels. In contrast, these segments are conserved well among the sodium channels. These patterns are consistent with a model in which S1–S4 form a domain involved primarily with a voltage activation mechanism that is on the exterior of the structure where S1, S2, and S3 are exposed to lipid and S5–S8 form a domain involved primarily with ion selectivity that is nearer the center of the channel with few residues exposed to lipid. Many buried and charged residues of the S1–S4 domains may be conserved to preserve a gating mechanism common to these domains in sodium, calcium, and potassium channels whereas buried and charged residues of S5–S8 domain may vary for channels with different ion selectivities but are conserved for channels with the same ion selectivities.

EXPERIMENTAL TESTS

Using the classic definition of the scientific method one examines the available information, formulates alternative hypotheses, and performs experiments to test these hypotheses. Structures of large membrane proteins cannot be predicted confidently using present methods. The major advantage of models is that they may suggest experiments that otherwise would not be performed.

Site Directed Mutagenesis

Site directed mutagenesis combined with single channel recording methods now make it possible to observe how altering the sequence affects the conductance properties, gating kinetics, and pharmacology of a single channel protein (Imoto et al., 1986). Models are very important to this approach because they suggest which of a virtually infinite number of possible mutants should be made, which experiments should be done to test these mutants, and how results of these experiments should be interpreted.

Care must be taken in designing and interpreting mutagenesis experiments. Substantial changes such as deletions are informative only when they have no effect on a particular function; e.g., the fact that deletions through the putative cytoplasmic region of the nicotinic acetylcholine receptor have no detectable effect on the channel or receptor means that these segments are not important for these functions (Mishina et al., 1985). Effects of changes on functional properties can be determined only if the changes do not destroy the ability of the protein to function. Changes that affect functional properties should be very conservative to avoid affecting the general structure of the protein. The ideal type change should alter only one functional property; e.g., a change that alters ion selectivity but does not affect channel gating kinetics or drug binding properties is not likely to be caused by unpredictable changes in the overall structure of the protein. Hydrophobic residues should not be changed since they are usually buried, and changes are likely to alter the three-dimensional structure of the protein. Aspartates and glutamates may be good candidates for mutagenesis experiments since these residues are likely to be on the protein's surface and very conservative changes can be made. Changing an aspartate or glutamate to an aspargine or glutamine removes a negative charge without affecting the geometry or hydrophobicity of the side chain and, changing an aspartate to a glutamate, or visa versa, changes the geometry and volume only slightly without changing the charge. These substitutions occur frequently for nonfunctional surface residues in homologous soluble proteins.

Mutagenesis experiments may be better for analyzing some functions than others. For example, effects of substitutions on channel conductance properties may be easier to interpret than effects on gating mechanisms in voltage activated channels because: (1) substitutions can be more conservative for glutamates and aspartates postulated to control ion selectivity than for arginines and lysines postulated to be involved in gating; (2) if segments involved in gating are more buried than those involved in ion selectivity (as we postulate), changes in gating segments are more likely to affect the protein structure in unpredictable ways; (3) fewer groups are postulated to control ion selectivity than gating; thus, fewer experiments may be required to test selectivity filter models than gating models, and effects of changing residues involved with ion selectivity may be more detectable and interpretable; and (4) we are more likely to be able to predict how a change will affect channel conductance properties than how it will affect a complex series of conformational changes like those involved in gating.

Some proteins may be better suited for specific mutagensis experiments than others. If type A potassium channels are comprised of four identical subunits then effects of a mutation on channel conductance and/or gating properties may be more detectable than in a sodium or calcium channel comprised of one subunit. On the other hand the effects of changing four charges in the selectivity filter region may be so drastic that properties of the modified channel cannot be measured. In these cases it may be better to study sodium and/or calcium channels in which only one residue is altered.

Mutagenesis experiments may be valuable for simplifying the analysis of some processes. Inactivation of sodium channels greatly complicates studies of its activation kinetics. If modifications of Post 8C and/or Post 8D segments eliminated inactivation without affecting activation it would not confirm our model of inactivation; however, it could greatly simplify studies of activation kinetics and channel conductance properties.

It is important to remember that nature has performed millions of mutagenesis experiments. Comparison of homologous protein sequences can be extremely useful in designing mutagenesis experiments as well as in designing models. When different proteins have indistinguishable functional properties one can assume that sites that differ are not crucial for the function. When their functional properties differ then mutagenesis can be used to identify which sequence changes cause the differences. Models may prove useful in identifying which sequence changes are likely to be responsible for the functional change. Model independent approaches may also be used. For example, Imoto et al., (1986) identified which segment made conductance properties of torpedo and bovine nicotinic acetylcholine receptor differ by demonstrating that *bovine* nAChR's that had a torpedo M2 segment of the δ subunit had conductance properties like those of the torpedo, and that *torpedo* nAChR's that had a δ subunit M2 segment had conductance properties of a bovine nAChR.

Other Experimental Tests

Mutagenesis experiments by themselves are unlikely to prove a model of a complex protein structure. Experiments such as determination of the shape and size of channel proteins by electron microscopy or X-ray diffraction, measurement of protein secondary structure, identification of drug and toxin binding sites, locations of disulfide bridges, and identification of which segments are on the extracellular and intercellular surfaces, line the channel and are in contact with the lipid are also important in testing models. These experiments have not been emphasized because their design is usually model independent; however, many of these experiments are intended to test models or aid in their design.

CAN PRECISE MODELS OF VOLTAGE ACTIVATED CHANNELS BE CONSTRUCTED AND TESTED THEORETICALLY?

Models such as the one presented here would be much more convincing and valuable if 1) they could be used to make quantitative predictions about conductance and ion selectivity properties of the channel, the kinetics and rate constants of channel gating, and binding constants of drugs and toxins and 2) if it could be shown that the postulated structure is the most energetically favorable structure. Unfortunately, there are several reasons why the kind of precise energy calculations required to accomplish these goals are not yet possible.

The first step required to do this is to develop a three dimensional model that includes the positions of all the functionally important atoms. We have used computer graphics to generate models to do this. These models help demonstrate that a postulated model is feasible, and they provide an attractive means of illustrating the primary features of the model. However, the computer graphic models we have developed thus far should be considered a rather crude approximation. The spatial arrangement and even secondary structure of putative transmembrane segments are still uncertain; no segments connecting helices have been modeled, putative transmembrane α helices were constructed with 'standard' backbone and side chain conformations commonly observed in known structures or by manually adjusting them using computer graphics to eliminate overlaps, most transmembrane α helices were positioned so that the perpendicular distance between their axes is 10.2 angstroms and so they cross each other at an angle of 20° as predicted by optimal values for '3–4 ridges into grooves' packing; however, in known structures these values range from 8.9° to 11.3 angstroms and 7° to 39°. These methods were used because the sodium channel structure is far too complex to generate structural models on the basis of energy calculations alone. We have been developing models of membrane channels formed by small peptides and have used the program CHARMM to obtain more energetically favorable models. Unfortunately, it does not appear energies calculated by the program CHARMM can be used to distinguish between a protein that has been folded correctly and one with the same sequence that has been folded incorrectly into a completely different structure (Novotny, et al., 1984). If the postulated model is basically correct, it may be possible however to use energy calculations to refine computer graphic representation of models and to develop models that include connecting segments. The important point is that the initial model, including all transmembrane segments, must be basically correct in order for the refined model to be meaningful.

At the present time it is unlikely that an energy refined model—one that includes all the transmembrane segments in basically the correct positions—can be used to evaluate potential drug binding sites, energy barriers encountered by alternative gating mechanisms, energy barriers encountered by ions passing through the channel, and/or effects of mutations on these processes. A major difficulty is that even small errors in the structure could drastically alter results of these calculations. The prospect of calculating the structure of a protein this size without any errors is remote. It is also not clear that all energetic parameters have been defined well enough to accurately calculate these energies even if the model is correct.

FUTURE OF MEMBRANE CHANNEL MODEL BUILDING

The need to develop reliable methods to model membrane channel protein structures and functional mechanisms should be obvious given 1) the present rate at which membrane channel sequences are being determined, 2) the prospect that this rate will increase sharply in the next few years as efforts to clone the human genome begin, 3) the number of groups interested in using site directed mutagenesis and patch clamping methods to study membrane channel proteins, 4) the difficulty in determining membrane channel structure experimentally, and 5) the importance of these proteins, especially in pharmacology. Present efforts to model membrane proteins are still in the embryonic stages. Although existing methods have produced some promising models, these models have not been proven and the methods usually have subjective elements that are often very time consuming. These methods need to be verified, quantified, and automated to make the modelling objective and rapid. Also, predictions of the models are not usually quantitative. We would like to explain the molecular basis for relative ion permeabilities and conductance of a channel, why it opens and closes at a particular rate, why drugs and toxins bind with a particular binding constant, and how modifying the protein sequence or drug structure in a particular way will affect these values. If we could do this then mutagenesis experiments would be much better tests of models.

There are several reasons to be optimistic that at least some of these goals can be accomplished. (1) Massive efforts are currently underway to understand how proteins fold, and to quantify energies involved in these processes. Many methods developed for proteins and macromolecules in general should be applicable to membrane proteins. (2) Computer technology is rapidly improving. Computer graphic systems coupled with powerful computers to perform extensive energy calculations will soon be available at reasonable prices. Model building processes described require that numerous factors be considered. Computer methods such as those used in artificial intelligence continue in their development toward solving these kinds of problems. (3) Experimental determination of the photosynthetic reaction center structure (Deisenhofer et al., 1985) has stimulated much interest in determining structures of other membrane proteins. The paucity of known membrane channel protein structure makes theoretical efforts to understand their structures difficult. As more structures are determined, we should be able to determine which methods are valid and improve the methods. Having known structures will also encourage more groups with experience in modelling proteins to work on membrane proteins. This will be especially true if transmembrane regions prove easier to model than soluble proteins.

BIBLIOGRAPHY

Aldrich RW. Voltage-dependent gating of sodium channels: towards an integrated approach. *Trends in Neurosci.* 9:82–85, 1986.

Armstrong CM. Sodium channels and gating currents. *Physiol Rev* 61:644–683, 1981.

Armstrong CM, Bezanilla F. Inactivation of the sodium channel II: Gating current experiments. *J Gen Physiol* 70:567–590, 1977.

Bezanilla F. Gating of sodium and potassium channels. *J Membr Biol* 88:97–112, 1985.

Begenisich T. Molecular properties of ion permeation through sodium channels. *Ann Rev Biophys Biophys Chem* 16:247–263, 1987.

Catterall WA. Voltage-dependent gating of sodium channels: correlating structure and function. *Trends in Neurosci* 9:7–10, 1986.

Catterall WA. The molecular basis of neuronal excitability. *Science* 223:653–661, 1984.

Chothia C, Levitt M, Richardson D. Helix to helix packing in proteins. *J Mol Biol* 145:215–250, 1981.

Deisenhofer J, Epp O, Mike K, Huber R, Michel H. Structure of the protein subunits in the photosynthetic reaction centre of *Rhodopseudomonas viridis* at 3 angstroms resolution. *Nature* 318:618–623, 1985.

French RJ, Horn R. Sodium channel gating: models, mimics, and modifiers. *Annu Rev Biophys Bioeng* 12:319–356, 1983.

Garnier J, Osguthorpe DJ, Robson B. Analysis of the accuracy and implications of simple methods for predicting the secondary structure of globular proteins. *J Mol Biol* 120:97–120, 178.

Go M, Miyazawa S. Relationship between mutability, polarity and exteriority of amino acid residues in protein evolution. *Int J Peptide Protein Res* 15:211–224, 1980.

Greenblatt RE, Blatt Y, Montal M. The structure of the voltage-sensitive sodium channel: Inferences derived from computer-aided analysis of the *Electrophorus electricus* channel primary structure. *FEBS Letters* 193:125–134, 1985.

Guy HR. Amino acid side-chain partition energies and distribution of residues in soluble proteins. *Biophy J* 47:61–70, 1985.

Guy HR. A model relating the sodium channel's structure to its function. In: Agnew W, Claudio T, et al., eds. *Molecular Biology of Ion Channels: Current Topics in Membrane Transport.* San Diego, CA: Academic Press; 289–308, 1988.

Guy HR, Seetharamulu P. Molecular model of the action potential sodium channel. *Proc Natl Acad Sci (USA)* 83:508–512, 1986.

Hille B. The permeability of the sodium channel to organic cations in myelinated nerve. *J Gen Physiol* 58:599–619, 1971.

Hille B. *Ionic Channels of Excitable Membranes.* Sunderland, Mass: Sinauer Assoc., Inc.

Hodgkins AL, Huxley AF. A quantitative description of membrane current and its application to conduction and excitation in nerve. *J Physiol (Lond)* 117:500–544, 1952.

Horn R, Vandenberg CA. Inactivation of single sodium channels. In: Ritchie JM, Keynes RD, et al., eds. *Ion Channels in Neural Membranes.* New York, NY: Alan R. Liss; 71–84, 1986.

Imoto K, Methfessel C, Sakmann B, Mishina M, Mori Y, Konno T, et al. Location of a δ-subunit region determining ion transport through the acetylcholine receptor channel. *Nature* 324:670–674, 1986.

Kosower EM. A structural and dynamic molecular model for the sodium channel of *Electrophorus electricus. FEBS Lett* 182:234–242, 1985.

Mishina M, Tobimatsu T, Imoto K, Tanaka K, Fujita Y, Fukuda K, et al. Location of functional regions of the acetylcholine receptor α-subunit by site-directed mutagenesis. *Nature* 313:364–369, 1985.

Moczydlowski E, Olivera BM, Gray WR, Strichartz GR. Discrimination of muscle and neuronal Na-channel subtypes by binding competition between [^{3}H]saxitoxin and μ-conotoxins. *Proc Natl Acad Sci (USA)* 83:5321–5325, 1986.

Noda M, Ikeda T, Kayano T, Suzuki H, Takeshima H, Kurasaki M, et al. Existence of distinct sodium channel messenger RNAs in rat brain. *Nature (Lond)* 320:188–192, 1986a.

Noda M, Ikeda T, Kayano T, Suzuki H, Takeshima H, Takahashi T, et al. Expression of functional sodium channels from cloned cDNA. *Nature (Lond)* 322:826–828, 1986b.

Noda M, Shimizu S, Tanabe T, Takai T, Kayano T, Ikeda T, et al. Primary structure of *Electrophorus electricus* sodium channel deduced from cDNA sequence. *Nature* 312:121–127, 1984.

Novotny J, Bruccoleri R, Karplus M. An analysis of incorrectly folded protein models. *J Mol Biol* 177:787–818, 1984.

Salkoff L, Butler A, Wei A, Scavarda N, Giffen K, Ifune C, et al. Genomic organization and deduced amino acid sequence of a putative sodium channel gene in *Drosophila. Science* 237:744–748, 1987.

Starmer CF, Yeh JZ, Tanguy J. A quantitative description of QX222 blockade of sodium channels in squid axons. *Biophys J* 49:913–920, 1986.

Tanabe T, Takeshima H, Mikami A, Flockerzi V, Takahashi H, Kangawa K, et al. Primary structure of the receptor for calcium channel blockers from skeletal muscle. *Nature* 328:313–318, 1987.

Tempel BL, Papazian DM, Schwarz TL, Jan YN, Jan LY. Sequence of a probable potassium channel component encoded at *Shaker* locus of *Drosophila*. *Science* 237:770–774, 1987.

Timpe, LC, Schwarz TL, Tempel BL, Papazian DM, Jan YN, Jan LY. Expression of functional potassium channels from *Shaker* cDNA in *Xenopus* oocytes. *Nature* 331:143–145, 1988.

Yellen G. Permeation in potassium channels: implications for channel structure. *Ann Rev Biophys Chem* 16:227–246, 1987.

Chapter 10

Characterizing Ion Channel Blockade with the Guarded Receptor Hypothesis

C. F. Starmer
V. V. Nesterenko
A. I. Undrovinas
D. L. Packer
F. R. Gilliam
A. O. Grant
L. V. Rosenshtraukh
H. C. Strauss

INTRODUCTION

How much complexity must a model of ion channel blockade exhibit in order to account for observations made under experimental conditions? Further, can an unambiguous estimation procedure be developed from such a minimal model? These questions are central to developing a framework for quantitatively studying the modulation of cellular communication with pharmacological agents.

In contrast to ligands that bind to continuously accessible binding sites, many ion channel antagonists appear able to bind only to certain conformations of the ion channel (Armstrong, 1966; Strichartz, 1973; Courtney, 1975; Khodorov et al., 1976). With repetitive

Hondeghem, Luc (ed): Molecular and Cellular Mechanisms of Antiarrhythmic Agents, Futura Publishing Company, Inc., Mount Kisco, NY, © 1989.

excitation of an excitable membrane, availability of or access to the binding site appears to be periodic, i.e., limited to a short interval of time during each stimulation pulse. Total access time accumulates with each additional stimulus and thus binding becomes dependent on the frequency of excitation. Such systems exhibit frequency-dependence induced either by periodic changes in membrane potential (for voltage-gated channels; Strichartz, 1973) or by periodic changes in agonist concentration (for agonist activated channels; McDonald et al.,1987). Starting with the standard first order model of ligand binding to continuously accessible sites, are additional features required to account for frequency-dependent patterns of ligand-channel binding?

Our work in this area started almost 8 years ago with a review of the work of Armstrong (1966), Strichartz (1973), Courtney (1975), Khodorov et al., (1976), Hille (1977), Hondeghem and Katzung (1977), and Yeh (1979). Our goal was to quantitatively characterize antiarrhythmic agents in order to study the effects of membrane potential, pH, and stimulation frequency. We focused on the Modulated Receptor Hypothesis (Hille, 1977; Hondeghem and Katzung, 1977) since it was by far the most cited idea in the literature and sought to evolve a procedure for assessing rate constants. This scheme postulated a single binding site whose affinity for an agent changed with the state of the channel. One of us (Starmer) had the responsibility for developing the appropriate estimation procedures. Developing the modulated receptor simulation and estimation programs was not difficult but due to the inherent complexity of this model, debugging and validating them was beyond our capability. Thus we took a step back and asked whether there were simpler frameworks that would be easier to manipulate. In particular, we began to explore what would happen with an Armstrong-like model (fixed affinity, limited access) applied to sodium channels.

Questions about applicability of the Armstrong model were based on the role of the inactivation process in antagonist bound sodium channels. When using the Hodgkin-Huxley (1952) two pulse protocol, a number of investigators (Hille, 1977; Sanchez-Chapula et al., 1983; Courtney, 1975) had observed shifts in apparent inactivation measured in the presence of drug. Observations of this shift in apparent inactivation coupled with thermodynamic considerations led Hille (1978) to state that "gating continues to occur in blocked channels, (and) at least one of the rate constants α_h^* or β_h^* must be different from the normal, stabilizing the blocked inactivated state as is seen in the inactivation experiments. Such considerations must be included in any quantitative model of inactivation in the presence of drugs." This statement can be viewed as a direct result of a mass balance around the reaction loop: open → inactivated → inactivated blocked → open blocked → open.

Early investigations reported by Hille (1977) and Hondeghem and Katzung (1977) were based on studies of tertiary agents such as lidocaine. One can view these agents as comprised of two active moieties that compete for the same binding site: the hydrophilic, charged moiety, and the hydrophobic, neutral moiety. If we postulate that the charged moiety binds to the open channel and the neutral moiety binds to the inactivated channel, then the reaction loop utilized by these investigators requires modification. While their view of transitions between blocked states was limited to a single step:

$$\mathrm{OD} \rightleftharpoons \mathrm{ID}$$

it did not explicitly accommodate the protonation process. We have viewed transitions between inactivated blocked (ID°) and open blocked (OD^{+}) states as requiring a change in channel conformation as well as movement of a proton (two steps):

$$\mathrm{OD}^{+} \rightleftharpoons \mathrm{H}^{+} + \mathrm{OD}^{0} \rightleftharpoons \mathrm{ID}^{0}$$

The addition of the protonation/deprotonation step adds an additional state for the tertiary binding model and makes it possible to maintain a detailed balance in the reaction loop: open → inactivated → neutral blocked inactivated → neutral blocked open → charged blocked open → open, and have different binding affinities for the open-channel charged-drug interaction and the inactivated-channel neutral-drug interaction. In view of this modification, the Armstrong scheme appeared to be a good candidate for consideration as a general model of channel blockade.

For us, the detailed balance requirement and its implied requirement for modified channel gating transition rates as asserted by Hille (1977) and Hondeghem and Katzung (1977) presented a paradox. On one side of the puzzle is the thermodynamic requirement for the mass balance. On the other side of the puzzle is the missing proton exchange step in blockade by tertiary agents. Were modified gating kinetics essential for drug induced shifts in apparent inactivation? Apparently not in the light of the following argument. There is general agreement that blockade by most channel antagonists exhibits a dependence on voltage, i.e., $b = b(V_m)$ where b is the fraction of blocked channels and V_m is the membrane potential, although the source of the voltage dependence is unresolved. The source of voltage dependence could be that of a voltage- or state-dependent affinity or it could result from a voltage dependent mixture of bindable and unbindable sites. If blockade were voltage independent, its effect would be a reduction in the maximum conductance and inactivation and activation curves measured in the presence of drug would appear as scaled versions of their control representation. On the other hand, if blockade exhibited voltage dependence, a shift is required. Apparent inactivation, h^*, as measured by the H-H two pulse protocol in the presence of drug is described by the currents measured in the remaining conducting channels: $h^* = h(1-b)$ where 1-b represents the remaining fraction of conducting channels. Since b is always greater than 0 and increases with membrane potential, the apparent inactivation will always be less than control inactivation and therefore obligated to shift away from true inactivation in the hyperpolarizing direction. Thus the paradox is readily resolved. To support the idea of modified gating kinetics, one would need evidence that the shift in observed apparent inactivation exceeds that derived from the mixture effect. Thus to meet the thermodynamic requirements as specified in Hille's mass balance required either a variable affinity receptor and modified gating kinetics, as suggested by Hille (1977) and Hondeghem and Katzung (1977), or a fixed affinity receptor and a different sequence of state transitions (perhaps including the protonation/deprotonation of drug-complexed channels). The lack of evidence of a shift different from that expected by mixture dependent binding suggested that simple extensions of the Armstrong scheme might be adequate for a general description of ion channel blockade. Here we show that frequency-dependent responses and concentration-dependent shifts in apparent activation and/or inactivation are consistent with transient access to (or availability of) a binding site and that the postulated modified gating kinetics of drug-complexed channels may, in many cases, be unnecessary for meeting thermodynamic requirements.

CHARACTERIZING LIGAND BINDING TO TRANSIENTLY ACCESSIBLE SITES

We consider a simple voltage- or agonist- sensitive mixture of bindable and unbindable channels. We consider two processes of blockade, the untrapped scheme of Armstrong:

$$C \underset{\beta}{\overset{\alpha}{\rightleftharpoons}} O \underset{l}{\overset{kD}{\rightleftharpoons}} B$$

and a trapped scheme:

$$C \underset{\beta}{\overset{\alpha}{\rightleftharpoons}} O \underset{l}{\overset{kD}{\rightleftharpoons}} B \underset{\alpha}{\overset{\beta}{\rightleftharpoons}} B^t$$

where C represents the unbindable conformation, O represents the bindable conformation, D represents the antagonist, B and B^t represent blocked and trapped conformations, α and β represent the conformation transition rates and kD and l represent the rates of drug binding and unbinding. Although we use the same symbols for the trapped and untrapped models, we do not mean to suggest that the unbindable or bindable conformations associated with the untrapped and trapped schemes are the same. For instance, the bindable conformation for the trapped model might be the open, conducting conformation while the bindable conformation for the untrapped model might be the inactivated conformation. Let b represent the fraction of blocked channels. Then the macroscopic current is represented by:

$$I = g_c(1 - b)(V - V_{rev}) \qquad [1]$$

where g_c is the macroscopic conductance.

When the conformation equilibration time $(\alpha+\beta)^{-1}$ is short when compared with the blockade equilibration time $(kD+l)^{-1}$ then both schemes can be represented as special cases derived from a framework of models specified by:

$$U + D \underset{gl}{\overset{fk}{\rightleftharpoons}} B$$

and where the time dependent properites of the fraction of blocked channels is described by the solution to

$$\frac{db}{dt} = fkD(1 - b) - glb$$

where U represents the concentration of unbound sites, b is the fraction of bound sites (B/(U+B)), f represents the fraction of unbound sites with an exposed binding site and g represents the fraction of bound sites where drug is able to unbind. The apparent equilibrium dissociation constant, $K_d^* = gl/fk$, demonstrating the dependence on the voltage- or agonist- induced mixture of channel conformations. There is the possibility of an additional modification to k or l in order to describe the interaction between the dipole moment of a drug and the membrane electric field. This is typically represented by including a term like $\exp(-z\delta VF/RT)$ as part of the binding or unbinding rates. Here δ reflects the fraction of the membrane potential, V, through which a charge moves to the binding site. For convenience we will not include this term for the remainder of the discussion.

EQUILIBRIUM ANALYSIS

Under conditions where both the channel conformation transitions and channel blockade are at equilibrium, a number of useful relationships can be derived. The equilibrium fraction of blocked channels is:

$$b_\infty = \left(1 + \frac{gl}{fkD}\right)^{-1} = \left(1 + \frac{K_d^*}{D}\right)^{-1} \qquad [2]$$

clearly demonstrating the sensitivity of the dose-response relationship to the voltage- or agonist- controlled mixture of channels (Fig. 1). Here, the ratio of the trap to guard functions acts to modify the true equilibrium dissociation constant, creating an apparent dissociation constant that reflects both the true value and the mixture of bindable and unbindable sites. Using this relationship, one can predict apparent activation and inactivation when measured under equilibrium conditions. Thus:

$$h^* = h(1 - b_\infty) = h\left(1 + \frac{fkD}{gl}\right)^{-1} = h\left(1 + \frac{D}{K_d^*}\right)^{-1} \qquad [3]$$

indicating that since $fkD/gl > 0$ then $h^* < h$, consistent with a shift in the hyperpolarizing direction (Fig. 2). Furthermore for neutral

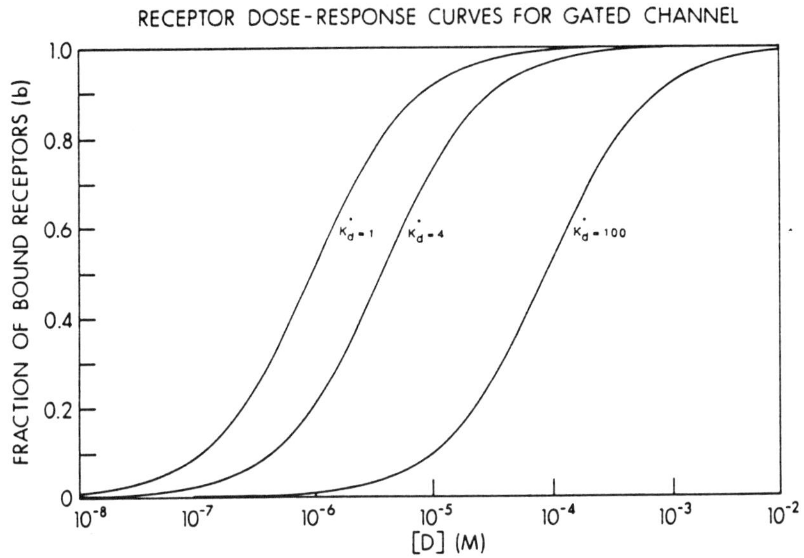

Figure 1. Dose-response curves for transiently accessible binding sites. Here the membrane potential is held constant for each binding curve. The left most curve reflects the true equilibrium dissociation curve where the membrane potential is at a depolarized potential (0 mV). As the membrane potential is progressively polarized, the dose-response relationship shifts to the right, indicating an apparent decrease in the binding affinity.

agents binding to inactivated channels, the apparent inactivation is described by:

$$h^* = 1\Big/\left[1 + \left(1 + \frac{D}{K_d}\right) e^{(V - V_h)/s}\right] \quad [4]$$

and the amount of shift in the midpoint of h and h^* is defined by:

$$\Delta V = V_h - V_h{}^* = s \ln\left(1 + \frac{D}{K_d}\right) \quad [5]$$

where s is the slope factor of the Boltzmann function describing the inactivation factor, h:

$$h = \left(1 + \exp\left(\frac{(V - V_h)}{s}\right)\right)^{-1} \quad [6]$$

Similarly, for drug binding to activated channels, the induced

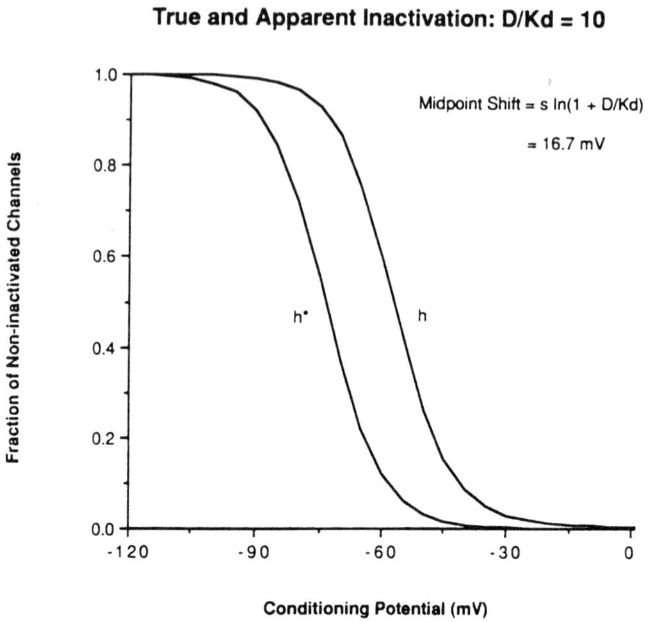

Figure 2. Inactivation curves under control and drug conditions. For a drug concentration 10-fold greater than the true equilibrium dissociation constant, the midpoint of the apparent inactivation curve is shifted approximately 17 mV in the hyperpolarizing direction. The slope factor of the control curve, s, is 7.0 yielding a predicted shift of 16.7 mV.

shift in activation is approximated by the same function where s is now the slope of the activation Boltzmann function.

Under continuous activation, blockade follows a typical exponential response (Fig. 3A) described by:

$$b(t) = b_\infty + (b_0 - b_\infty)\exp(-\lambda t) \qquad [7]$$

where b_o is the initial fraction of blocked channels, b_∞ is the equilibrium block and λ is the blocking event rate, as:

$$\lambda = fkD + gl; \; b_\infty = \left(1 + \frac{gl}{fkD}\right)^{-1} \qquad [8]$$

NON-EQUILIBRIUM ANALYSIS

Pulse train stimulation reflects a slightly more complex pattern of excitation. Consider a stimulus protocol consisting of repeated

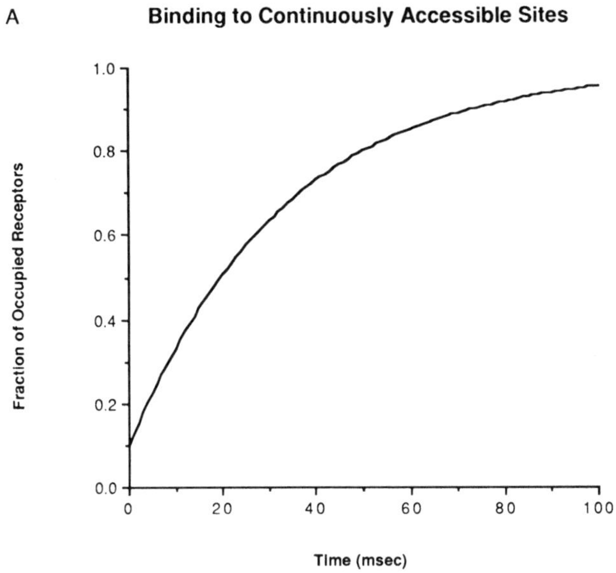

Figure 3A. Panel A illustrates the expoential binding curve associated with continuously accessible binding sites.

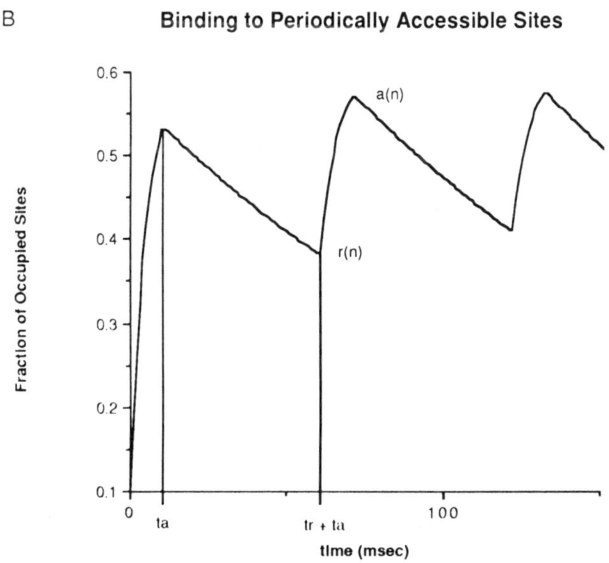

Figure 3B. Panel B illustrates the piecewise expoential binding curve associated with periodically activated binding sites. The peak of each segment is denoted a_n and the valley is denoted by r_n.

instances of a pulse defined by an activation phase of duration, t_a, and a recovery phase of duration, t_r. Initially, we (Starmer et al., 1984) evaluated blockade acquired with pulse train stimulation by using functions of the H-H gating equations to represent guard and trap functions and by numerically solving the differential equation that characterizes time-dependent blockade. In response to criticism of the gating model we utilized, we investigated computed block associated with several other gating models. Remarkably, the results were almost identical—with the pattern of blockade exhibiting little sensitivity to the underlying gating model. If this lack of sensitivity could be theoretically demonstrated, then it would be possible to obtain a very general closed-form analytic solution to the blockade equation since we could substitute a constant amplitude pulse function for the variable amplitude gating parameter. Taking advantage of single-channel observations, we reasoned that if we considered block in all channels to take place during an interval equal to the mean conformation dwell time then we could substitute a pulse with equivalent duration for the H-H like time-dependent gating behavior. We (Starmer and Grant, 1985) used a statistical argument to show that the amount of block expected with a constant dwell time that is equal to the mean dwell time of an exponentially distributed process was a first order approximation of that associated with stochastic dwell times generated by the same exponential probability distribution. Using a fixed access interval and under conditions of periodic activation, we then showed that blockade followed a piecewise exponential pattern (Starmer et al., 1987; Starmer, 1988). When the activation interval and recovery interval are such that blockade equilibrium is not achieved, then the response pattern reflects the cumulative response from prior stimuli (Fig. 3B). For the case of periodic (in contrast to random) stimulation, a number of useful relationships between stimulus parameters, steady state blockade and the time course of blockade can be developed. From these relationships, procedures can be derived for use in comparing drugs and evaluating interventions.

Let a_n and r_n represent, respectively the fraction of blocked channels at the end of the activation interval, t_a, and at the end of the recovery interval, t_r. Also let k_a, l_a, k_r, l_r represent the apparent binding and unbinding rates associated with the activation and recovery intervals. These rates reflect the product of the drug binding or unbinding rate and the associated guard or trap function. The fraction of blocked channels associated with each transition in the stimulus function can be related to the block associated with the previous transition by:

$$a_n = a_\infty + (r_n - a_\infty)e^{-\lambda_a t_a} \qquad [9]$$

$$r_n = r_\infty + (a_{n-1} - r_\infty)e^{-\lambda_r t_r} \qquad [10]$$

where

$$\lambda_a = k_a D + l_a; \qquad \lambda_r = k_r D + l_r;$$

and

$$a_\infty = \left(1 + \frac{l_a}{k_a D}\right)^{-1}; \qquad r_\infty = \left(1 + \frac{l_r}{k_r D}\right)^{-1}.$$

Combining the equations defining a_n and r_n results in an equation that describes the fraction of blocked channels at the end of two successive stimulation intervals.

$$r_n = r_{n-1}\, e^{-(\lambda_a t_a + \lambda_r t_r)} + a_\infty(1 - e^{-\lambda_a t_a})e^{-\lambda_r t_r} + r_\infty(1 - e^{-\lambda_r t_r}) \qquad [11]$$

Let

$$\lambda^* = \lambda_a t_a + \lambda_r t_r \qquad [12]$$

then at steady state when $r_n = r_{n-1}$ the steady state fraction of blocked channels is

$$r_{ss} = a_\infty + \gamma(r_\infty - a_\infty) \qquad [13]$$

where

$$\gamma = \frac{1 - e^{-\lambda_r t_r}}{1 - e^{-\lambda^*}} \qquad [14]$$

The description of frequency-dependent blockade is expressed by the solution to equation (11):

$$r_n = r_{ss} + (r_0 - r_{ss})e^{-n\lambda^*} \qquad [15]$$

which demonstrates that the theoretical pattern of frequency-dependent blockade follows an exponential pattern (similar to the exponential time course observed with binding to continuously accessible sites) but where the pulse constant, λ^*, reflects the weighted sum of binding that takes place with the activated and recovery mixtures of channel conformations.

The linear relationship between the apparent rate, λ^*, the mixture dependent rates, λ_a and λ_r, the stimulus intervals, t_a and t_r, and the antagonist concentration, D, provides a number of potential experimental protocols for estimating apparent rates. A frequently used protocol is to evaluate blockade using different frequencies of stimulation where t_a remains fixed and the recovery interval, t_r, is varied from one train of stimuli to the next. Another strategy is to hold t_r constant and to vary the activation interval, t_a. Both of these protocols will provide data that allow estimation of the mixture dependent rates, λ_a and λ_r. Since r_{ss} as expressed in equation 13 is a linear function of the mixture-specific equilibria, then a_∞ and r_∞ are easily estimated. The two rates and two equilibrium values allow direct estimation of the apparent binding and unbinding rates.

Sometimes, the stability of the membrane preparation is such that steady-state block cannot be compared from one pulse train to the next (e.g., calcium channel rundown). When rundown is negligible during a short pulse train but significant over the duration of a study, an alternative strategy is available for estimating rate constants. Above, we showed that the apparent pulse rate, λ^*, is a linear function of the stimulus intervals and drug concentration. It can be rewritten in the form:

$$\lambda^* = \lambda_a t_a + \lambda_r t_r = l_a t_a + l_r(t_r) + k_a t_a(D) + k_r(t_r D) \qquad [16]$$

When t_a is held constant and t_r and D are varied, then each apparent rate constant can be estimated using a multiple regression procedure. In this case, one would use several (>2) pulse trains at several (>2) concentrations of the antagonist in order to obtain the diversity of frequency-dependent rates required for the analysis. These results provide the basis for estimating apparent rate constants from frequency-dependent data.

TERTIARY AGENT BLOCKADE

Though the guarded receptor concepts have been developed for single agents, it has also been useful in characterizing tertiary amines where both the neutral and charged moiety may be active. Extending the model to describe two agents competing for a single binding site (Starmer and Courtney, 1986; Starmer, 1987) showed that one would expect the frequency-dependent uptake and recovery to reflect the sum of two exponentials. That this is not frequently seen suggests that one of the moieties dominates the blockade process during the activated interval and one moiety (not necessarily the same) dominates (un)binding during the recovery interval. In other words, for quinidine, one might consider the charged moiety dominating the binding during the activated interval but trapped by the channel during recovery. Unblocking then might be due to deprotonation of the drug-complexed channel and escape of the neutral moiety via the hydrophobic path. Analysis of frequency-dependent data in this case would yield results that would characterize the hydrophilic binding path and the hydrophobic unbinding path. Extraction of the remaining rates would require modification of the pH in order to influence the protonation/deprotonation of drug-complexed channels.

Currently, we have simplified our characterization of tertiary agents in order to avoid the problems associated with analyzing sums of exponentials. Therefore, instead of viewing blockade by both moieties as taking place in parallel, we have tentatively viewed the process as a sequence, with open conformation block preceding inactivated conformation block. In other words, we are currently ignoring the effects during the interval where there are significant fractions of both open and inactivated conformations. Thus for tertiary agents we make the following assumptions:

1. the bindable conformations controlling access to a common binding site for the charged and neutral moieties are not necessarily identical;
2. the binding affinities of the charged and neutral moieties for a common binding site are not necessarily identical;
3. for the sodium channel, the hydrophilic moiety dominates the binding to open or activated channels while the hydrophobic moiety dominates the binding to inactivated channels. Schematically this is represented by:

$$U + D^+ \underset{g_+ l_+}{\overset{f_+ k_+}{\rightleftharpoons}} B^+$$

$$l_p \downarrow\uparrow k_p$$

$$H^+$$

$$+$$

$$U + D^0 \underset{g_n l_n}{\overset{f_n k_n}{\rightleftharpoons}} B^0$$

This scheme seems consistent with much of the data relating to the sensitivity of recovery to pH (Grant et al., 1980; Grant et al., 1982).

A candidate model of quinidine blockade would include the following assumptions:

1. dominant binding via the hydrophilic path for D^+ ($f^+ = m^3h$), with negligible hydrophobic binding for D^o ($f_n = 1\text{-}h$);
2. trapping of the charged moiety in resting channels ($g_+ = m^3h$);
3. no trapping of the neutral moiety in resting channels ($g_n = 1$);
4. drug pK_a in free solution $\neq$ pK_a of drug-complexed channels.

Reduction of extracellular pH thus would result in an increase in the number of charged drug-complexed channels. Since these are trapped, the recovery time constant would increase with reduction in the pH. The difference in the pK_a for the drug in free solution and the pK_a for drug-complexed channels would reflect the requirements for a microscopic balance (assuming different affinities of the neutral and charged moieties). In fact, one would expect a difference in the pK_a since proton access to the drug in free solution is unrestricted while proton access to a drug-complexed channel is probably constrained.

A similar model can be constructed for lidocaine. Here, though, instead of assuming dominant binding via the hydrophilic path, we would assume binding to be dominated by the neutral moiety via the hydrophobic path. Here, the guard function for the neutral moiety is best characterized by (1-h), while the trap is 1 indicating that drug can unbind at any time. We assume the changed moiety binds to activated channels [guardism] and unbinding is accelerated by hyperpolarization [trap is exp (f(V)]. Thus the effect of pH on extending the recovery time constant would be similar to that proposed for quinidine.

EXAMPLE

These ideas can be illustrated by considering an example. Cibenzoline, a sodium channel antagonist, has been studied by Arena and colleagues (Arena, et al., 1987). Using the maximum first derivative of the upstroke of the action potential as a measure of sodium channel conductance (now currently out of favor), frequency-dependent uptake curves were obtained from 16 μM concentration as shown in panel A of Fig. 4. Stimulus intervals of .5, 1.0, 1.5, 2.0, and 2.5 seconds were utilized. For each curve, an exponential of the form

$$\left.\frac{dV_n}{dt}\right|_{max} = V_{ss} + (V_0 - V_{ss})e^{-n\lambda^*} \qquad [17]$$

was fit using a non-linear least squares procedure. Steady state block, b_{ss}, was estimated from

$$b_{ss} = \frac{(V_{control} - V_{ss})}{V_{control}}. \qquad [18]$$

The results of the fitting procedures are as shown in Table I.

Table I

Uptake Rates and Steady State Estimates

isi (sec)	λ^*	b_{ss}	γ
0.5	.230	.482	.429
1.0	.277	.388	.610
1.5	.308	.335	.710
2.0	.437	.261	.773
2.5	.554	.241	.816

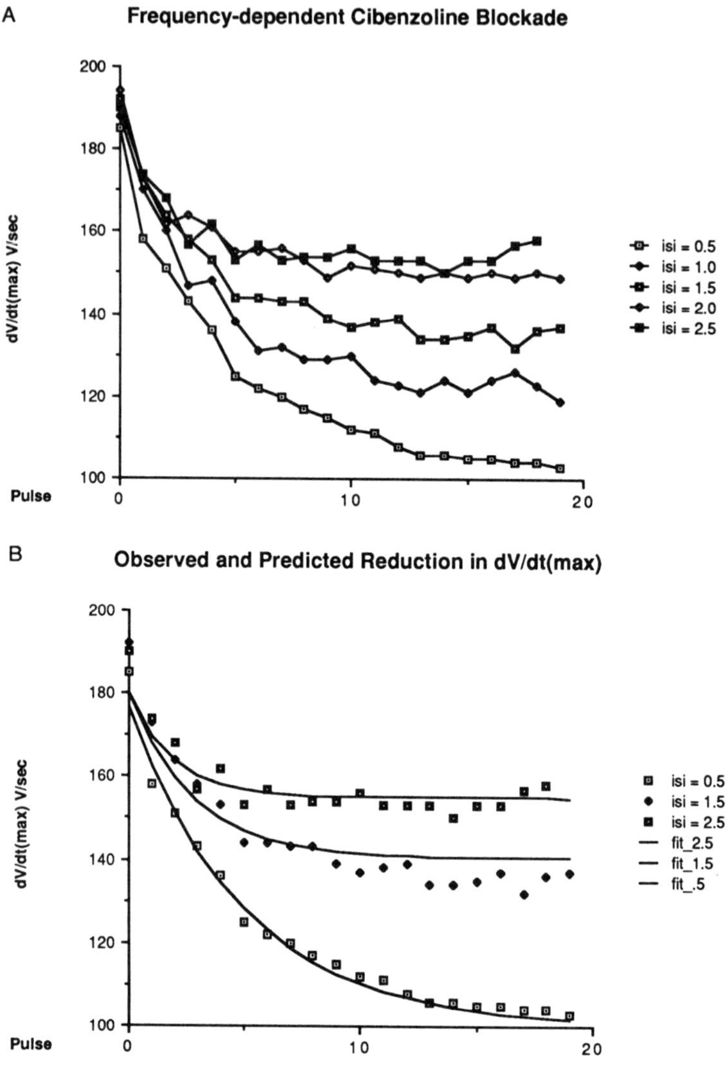

Figure 4. Panel A illustrates the frequency-dependent uptake of cibenzoline by sodium channels in guinea pig papillary muscle. Stimulus rates were varied from 2/sec to .4/sec. The uptake rate as monitored by reduction in dV/dt (max) was greatest for the longer intervals and progressively decreased with increasing frequency of stimulation. The resultant steady state also was frequency-dependent with the greatest blockade associated with the fastest stimulation rate. Panel B illustrates the observed and predicted patterns of reduction in dV/dt (max) utilizing rate constants derived from the uptake rates, λ^*, and the values of steady state block, b_{ss}.

The apparent uptake rates, λ^*, were plotted as a function of the stimulus interval in order to estimate λ_r from the slope (.162 sec^{-1}) and $\lambda_a t_a$ from the intercept (.119) as shown in Fig. 5A. With these values, γ was estimated (equation 14) for each stimulus interval and a plot of b_{ss} against γ was made (Fig. 5B) yielding the activated mixture equilibrium (a_∞) from the intercept (.761) and the recovery mixture equilibrium, r_∞ = .132, from the slope (−.629), ($r_\infty - a_\infty$). Once a value of t_a is selected, e.g., 1 msec, the mixture-specific apparent rate constants can be directly estimated since $k_xD = \lambda_x \chi_\infty$, $l_x = \lambda_x(1 - \chi_\infty)$ where χ indicates the channel mixture (a or r) under consideration. Results of these computations yield values of k_a = 5.66×10^6 M^{-1} sec^{-1}, l_a = 28.4 sec^{-1}, k_r = 1.33×10^3 M^{-1} sec^{-1}, and l_r = .141 sec^{-1}. With the activated and rest rates estimated above, we predicted the pattern of frequency-dependent reduction in dV/dt (max) for stimulus intervals of 0.5, 1.5, and 2.5 seconds. The predicted curves as well as the observed values are shown in panel B of Fig. 4 and are in close agreement.

It is worth noting that the estimation of the apparent rate constants here has not required specification of access paths. The apparent rates we have estimated represent the product of the true rates and the access function (guard or trap). Only when the true rate constants are desired is it necessary to define the guard and trap functions. In other words, the estimation of frequency-independent apparent rate constants is independent of the detailed mechanism of blockade. Only when one seeks to refine the interpretation of these values is it necessary to postulate guard and trap functions. Thus one can investigate the voltage dependence of apparent binding and unbinding rates and then compare these results with a model of the access control. For instance, one might compare the voltage dependence of the activated mixture binding rate, k_a, with the voltage dependence of the activation process and with the voltage dependence of the inactivation process to try to discern what controls drug access for the particular agent under study. Similarly, one can study the voltage dependence of the unbinding rate. These values, combined with measures of drug solubility, charge, pKa, and size will provide a rich arena for investigation of structure-activity relationships.

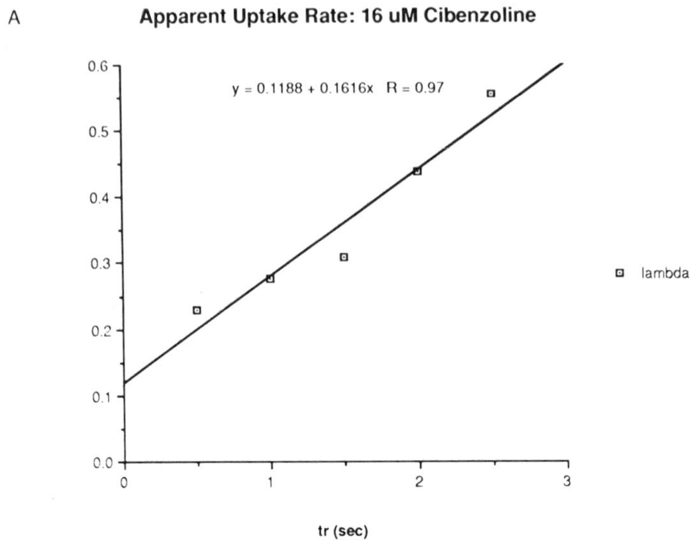

Figure 5A. Panel A depicts the relationship between the uptake rate (pulse^{-1}) and recovery interval. The agreement between the observed data and the predicted (equation 12) relationship is evident from the good correlation (r = .97).

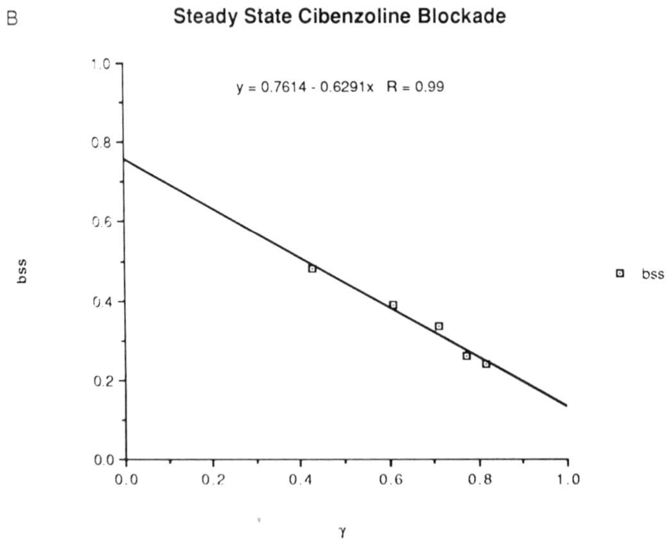

Figure 5B. Panel B (similar to panel A) depicts the expected linear relationship between steady state block and the stimulus parameter, γ. Equation 13 predicts this linear relationship and the high correlation (r = .99) supports the simple binding scheme that lead to the theoretical prediction.

CONCLUSIONS

We have presented a minimal model of ion channel antagonism that describes most of the patterns of blockade observed in studies of frequency-dependent blockade. The assumption underlying our characterization is that the ion channel binding site is either accessible or inaccessible as determined by the conformation of the channel protein. Here we have assumed resting channels represent a mixture of conformations dominated by inaccessible sites while the depolarized mixture is dominated by accessible sites. Furthermore, we assume that agents bind to an accessible site with an affinity that does not vary with channel conformation. The binding site affinities of charged and neutral moieties of a tertiary amine are assumed not necessarily equal. By utilizing constant dwell times for the lifetime of the accessible conformation and the rest conformation, it is possible to solve the equations that describe blockade. These solutions provide a method for directly estimating apparent binding rates for each mixture of channel conformations induced by a pulse train stimulus protocol. Interpretation of these apparent rates can be further refined by considering the detailed properties of candidate models of access control to the binding sites.

No doubt, this minimal scheme will be found inadequate in characterizing all drug-channel interactions. However, it has been found adequate to describe antagonism for sodium, calcium, and potassium channels by several drugs (Starmer, 1986). It has also been found to predict paradoxical agonism (Starmer, 1987). Since very few assumptions are present in the current model, it should be easy to add additional features as dictated by new experimental results.

Does this work offer anything to the practicing clinician? Perhaps the major utility of this model is that of providing a foundation for predicting the effect of antiarrhythmic drugs on myocardial conduction as reflected by intracardiac and surface electrocardiograms. To a first approximation, the squared conduction velocity, θ^2, is proportional to the sodium conductance. Thus one can approximate frequency-dependent changes in conduction velocity in terms of the exponential reduction in conducting channels as described in equation 15 where

$$\Theta^2 = \Theta^2_{control} (1 - r_n)$$

This predicted effect on conduction is not only reflected in measures of conduction between two points but also in measures of average conduction as reflected by the surface EKG. Thus, one would expect the QRS and QT intervals to exhibit frequency-dependent changes due to sodium channel blockade while the PR interval would reflect changes due to calcium channel blockade. Further, these intervals may provide direct measures of drug effects and allow the clinician to monitor drug effects through measures of myocardial conduction. Because channel blocking agents slow myocardial conduction, they can potentially exhibit proarrhythmic effects by increasing the likelihood of creating a reentry path. Since blockade is voltage-, concentration- and frequency-dependent, the critical concentration associated with proarrhythmic effects may be difficult to ascertain. However, if one could quantitatively predict drug effects on conduction, then perhaps it is possible to develop a strategy to anticipate the conditions surrounding proarrhythmic effects. Use of frequency-dependent conduction delay data allows direct estimation of binding and unbinding rates in man. Thus it may be possible to estimate the concentration and frequency range where a particular channel blocking agent exhibits antiarrhythmic effects and thus avoid situations where proarrhythmic effects are anticipated.

In summary, the guarded receptor hypothesis provides a minimal physical model for characterizing the effects of ion channel blocking agents. More important, it is the only model of antiarrhythmic drug action that includes both the *tonic* as well as *phasic* components of block and that admits to unique estimates of binding and unbinding rates. Thus for the first time, the kinetic properties of these agents can be readily estimated using standard pulse protocols and therapeutic effects predicted.

Acknowledgements: This research was supported in part by grants HL11307, HL17670, and HL32994 from the National Institutes of Health, by contract 4414804 from the Office of Naval Research, and by the joint US-USSR scientific exchange in problem area 5, sudden death.

BIBLIOGRAPHY

Arena JP, McArdle JJ, Laxminarayan S. Characterization of the class 1 antiarrhythmic activity of cibenzoline succinate in guinea-pig papillary muscle. *J Pharmacol Exp Ther* 240:441–450, 1987.

Armstrong CM. Time course of TEA^+ induced anomalous rectification in squid giant axons. *J Gen Physiol* 50:491–503, 1966.

Courtney KR. Mechanism of frequency-dependent inhibition of sodium currents in frog myelinated nerve by the lidocaine derivative GEA 968. *J Pharmacol Exp Ther* 195:225–236, 1975.

Grant AO, Strauss LJ, Wallace AG, Strauss HC. The influence of pH on the electrophysiological effects of lidocaine in Guinea pig ventricular myocardium. *Circ Res* 47:542–550, 1980.

Grant AO, Trantham JL, Brown KK, Strauss HC. pH-dependent effects of quinidine on the kinetics of dv/dt max in Guinea pig ventricular myocardium. *Circ Res* 50:210–217, 1982.

Hille B. Local anesthetics: hydrophilic and hydrophobic pathways for the drug-receptor reaction. *J Gen Physiol* 69:497–515, 1977.

Hille B. Local anesthetic action on inactivation of the Na Channel in nerve and skeletal muscle: possible mechanisms for antiarrhythmic agents. In: Morad M, ed. *Biophysical Aspects of Cardiac Muscle*. New York, NY: Academic Press; 55–74, 1978.

Hodgkin AL, Huxley AF. A quantitative description of membrane current and its application to conduction and excitation in nerve. *J Physiol (Lond)* 117:500–544, 1952.

Hondeghem LM, Katzung BG. Time and voltage-dependent interactions of antiarrhythmic drugs with cardiac sodium channels. *Biochim Biophys Acta* 472:373–398, 1977.

Khodorov BI, Shishkova LD, Peganov EM, Revenko SV. Inhibition of sodium currents in frog Ranvier node treated with local anesthetics: role of slow sodium inactivation. *Biochim Biophys Acta* 433:409–435, 1976.

McDonald JF, Miljkovic Z, Pennefather P. Use-dependent block of excitatory amino acid currents in cultured neurons by Ketamine. *J Neurophysiol* 58:251–266, 1987.

Sanchez-Chapula J, Tsuda Y, Josephson IR. Voltage and use-dependent effects of lidocaine on sodium current rat single ventricular cells. *Circ Res* 52:557–565, 1983.

Starmer CF. Characterizing activity-dependent processes with a piecewise exponential model. *Biometrics* 44:549–559, 1988.

Starmer CF. Theoretical characterization of ion channel blockade: competitive binding to periodically accessible receptors. *Biophys J* 52:405–412, 1987.

Starmer CF. Theoretical characterization of ion channel blockade: ligand binding to periodically accessible receptors. *J Ther Biol* 119:235–249, 1986.

Starmer CF, Courtney KR. Modeling ion channel blockade at guarded binding sites: application to tertiary drugs. *Am J Physiol* 251:H848-H856, 1986.

Starmer CF, Grant AO. Phasic ion channel blockade: a kinetic model and parameter estimation procedure. *Mol Pharmacol* 28:348–356, 1985.

Starmer CF, Grant AO, Strauss HC. Mechanisms of use-dependent block of sodium channels in excitable membranes by local anesthetics. *Biophys J* 46:15–27, 1984.

Starmer CF, Packer DL, Grant AO. Ligand binding to transiently accessible sites: mechanisms for varying apparent binding rates. *J Ther Biol* 124:335–341, 1987.

Strichartz GR. The inhibition of sodium currents in myelinated nerve by quaternary derivatives of lidocaine. *J Gen Physiol* 62:37–57, 1973.

Yeh JZ. Dynamics of 4-aminoacridine block of sodium channels in squid axons. *J Gen Physiol* 73:1–21, 1979.

Chapter 11

Models of Antiarrhythmic Drug Action

Luc M. Hondeghem
Paul B. Bennett

Antiarrhythmic drugs suppress arrhythmias primarily by alteration of transmembrane ionic current flow. Many of the drugs act by blocking sodium channels, thus reducing the sodium current, slowing the upstroke velocity of the cardiac action potential, slowing conduction, and widening the QRS complex. Block of sodium channels is a function of voltage and time. Useful antiarrhythmic agents have a voltage-time profile such that at normal heart rates and membrane potentials they have relatively little effect, while severely interfering with abnormal rates or rhythms especially in depolarized tissues. The transmembrane potential alters the conformation of sodium channels, and although there exist numerous conformations, they can be grouped into three primary states: rested (**R**), activated (**A**) and inactivated (**I**). **R** exists primarily at potentials negative to −70 mV, **I** prevails at potentials positive to −50 mV, while **A** occurs transiently upon depolarization. Most antiarrhythmic agents have a low affinity for **R** channels (K_{dR} in the mM to M range) and have slow interaction kinetics with this state (τ = 0.1 to 30 sec). They frequently have a much higher affinity for activated or inactivated sodium channels (K_{dA} and K_{dI} in μM range). Moreover, whereas the rate of interaction with the **I** state is also slow (frequently slightly slower than for the **R** state), interactions

Hondeghem, Luc (ed): Molecular and Cellular Mechanisms of Antiarrhythmic Agents, Futura Publishing Company, Inc., Mount Kisco, NY, © 1989.

with the **A** state are very fast (μsec range). Thus, the affinity for and rate of interaction with the sodium channel are modulated by channel conformation. Various mathematical models simulating the time- and voltage-dependence of sodium channel block have been proposed, their individual strengths and weaknesses are summarized: the κ model is computationally convenient, but is valid at only one membrane potential and for one action potential duration. The guarded receptor, although simpler than the modulated receptor, is incompatible with numerous experimental observations. The modulated receptor can simulate drug effects over a wide range of potentials and pulse patterns. However, since the time- and voltage-dependence of the drug-free channel has substantially changed, we have constructed a drug-free model that incorporates this new information.

INTRODUCTION

Antiarrhythmic agents were first introduced to medicine by de Senac (1749), who observed that rebellious arrhythmias succumbed to the action of quinine. It was, however, not until Wenckebach (1914) had a patient who consistently could suppress his arrhythmias with quinine that the value of antiarrhythmic agents were recognized by the medical community. Lewis (1925) observed that quinidine slowed cardiac conduction, which is reflected in a widening of the QRS complex of patients on quinidine.

Understanding of the electrophysiological basis for the slowing of conduction by antiarrhythmic agents at the cellular level started with the classic work of Silvio Weidmann (1955). He concluded that quinidine reduced the rate of rise of the upstroke of the action potential while having little effect upon the resting potential. Furthermore, hyperpolarization of the membrane could restore the rate of rise of the action potential, despite the presence of quinidine. He concluded that quinidine shifts the availability of sodium carriers to more negative potentials.

A few years later (1957), Johnson and McKinnon demonstrated that the reduction of the rate of rise of the action potential was minimal when the preparation was rested, but increased on a beat by beat basis during stimulation until a steady level of block was reached. Following stimulation, the effect of quinidine slowly dissipated. Chen, Gettes and Katzung (1975) observed that for lidocaine the recovery rate from block was faster the more negative the membrane potential.

Strichartz (1973), showed that like in heart (Johnson and McKinnon, 1957), in nerve sodium channel block is also use-dependent. More importantly, he proposed that the drugs block and unblock the sodium channel primarily while the channel is open. Courtney (1975), confirmed that like in heart (Weidmann, 1955), in nerve inactivation is shifted to more negative potentials by local anesthetics. He made the very important proposal that the shift only occurs in channels that are occupied by the drug.

MODULATED RECEPTOR

Brief Review

Hondeghem and Katzung (1977) deemed it necessary in order to account for the diastolic recovery from block (Chen et al., 1975), i.e., unblocking while the channel is closed, that sodium channels can also interact with the channel receptor while the channel is closed (**R** and **I**). Thus, the drug interacts not only with activated state of the channels (**A** ⇔ **AD**) as proposed by Strichartz (1973) and Courtney (1975), it can also interact with the inactivated (**I** ⇔ **ID**) and the rested (**R** ⇔ **RD**) states (Fig. 1). Indeed, recovery from block could develop at depolarized membrane potentials when drug-associated channels were in the **ID** state, as well as at negative potentials when drug-associated channels were in the **RD** state.

Moreover, as the channels assume different conformations, the rate constants and affinities for the drug interactions with the sodium channel receptor change, i.e., they are modulated by channel conformation. As proposed by Weidmann (1955) and Courtney (1975) the voltage-dependence of gating of drug-associated channels is modified such that drug-associated channels become inactivated at more negative membrane potentials. Consequently, at certain potentials drug-associated channels will remain trapped in the **ID** state, while drug-free channels become rested (**R**). As a result with each depolarization new block accumulates.

Since it was not clear whether the *open* channel block occurred just prior to opening, during opening proper, or just following opening, Hondeghem and Katzung (1977) preferred to refer to this block as activated state interactions.

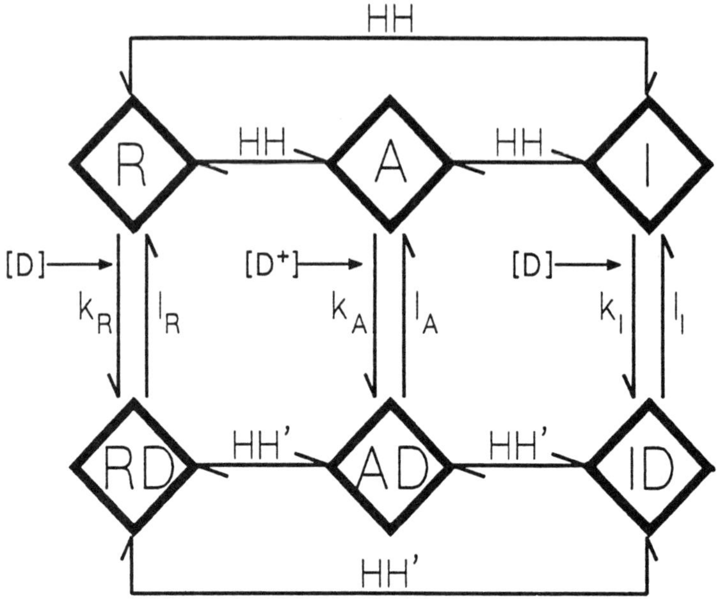

Figure 1. Modulated receptor. R: rested, A: activated, I: inactivated, D: drug.

While studying the interactions of neutral and cationic local anesthetics in nerve, Hille (1977) also concluded that the drug had to have access to the channel receptor while the channel was closed (**R** and **I**). Furthermore, charged drug had access to the receptor through a hydrophilic route, only while the channel was open (indicated by $\mathbf{D}^+$ in Fig. 1), while neutral drug (indicated by **D**) could interact with the sodium channel receptor through a lipophilic pathway (the lipid of the membrane), even when the channel was closed (**R** and **I**). So far no convincing evidence is available to indicate that neutral drugs also interact significantly with activated sodium channels.

Since antiarrhythmic agents are weak bases, having a pK_a ranging from 7.5 to 10, they exist in both the neutral and cationic form at body pH. More importantly, the ratio of charged/uncharged changes with pH, so that it is not surprising that in heart, too, the kinetics of block/unblock are markedly altered by pH (Grant et al., 1982).

Hondeghem and Katzung (1977) formulated the modulated receptor in differential equations. They also estimated rate constants for lidocaine and quinidine based upon limited experimental data. Nevertheless, these rate constants could relatively accurately describe the actions of antiarrhythmic agents over a wide range of cycle lengths and voltages.

To date, the modulated receptor scheme has been extensively tested and used by numerous laboratories as a basis for the explanation of experimental results (for reviews see Hondeghem and Katzung, 1984; Bennett et al., 1989).

Predictions by the Modulated Receptor

The computer model predicted several unexpected features: (1) the use-dependent block by lidocaine would reach steady state in just a few depolarizations; (2) the availability of sodium channels could exhibit a two-slope appearance or exhibit bumps. More importantly, availability of drug-associated channels continues to increase at potentials where drug-free channels are fully available, (3) combinations of drugs, with dissimilar kinetics of interaction with the sodium channel for any given level of block at the basic cycle length can achieve more block throughout diastole than either drug alone, (4) blockers with fast kinetics at appropriate cycle lengths can competitively displace a slower agent, (5) agents with extremely fast kinetics could have virtually no effect of their own upon the sodium conductance, while inhibiting the block of other agents (Hondeghem, 1987). All but the last of these predictions have been verified by experimental tests (Hondeghem and Katzung, 1980; Clarkson and Hondeghem, 1985) and some have found clinical applications (Duff et al., 1983).

OTHER MODELS

Although the modulated receptor model can accurately reproduce the essential aspects of antiarrhythmic agents upon sodium conductance, this does not prove the correctness of this model. Actually, since recent information about single sodium channels conclusively indicates that the drug-free channel behavior is quite different from that described by Hodgkin and Huxley (1952), it is mandatory that this new information be incorporated in any state of the art model. It is also necessary to test whether the modulated receptor assumptions still can adequately account for drug action when attached to a more realistic description of the drug-free sodium channel. Before doing this, we will briefly discuss models that have been proposed as alternates to the modulated receptor.

Indeed, the modulated receptor model is computationally quite intensive so that it is very time consuming to fit experimental results. For these reasons, other models have been proposed. The three most prevalent ones are: 1) Kappa (κ) model, 2) Guarded receptor, and 3) Analytical modulated receptor.

Kappa (κ) Model

In order to obtain a quantitative description of block and unblock, Courtney (1978) lumped the closed state interactions and combined them with a term for open channel block, resulting in a 4 state approximation of the modulated receptor. Unfortunately, since the interactions of drugs with rested and inactivated channels is quite different, such scheme is not very satisfactory. In a later version Courtney (1983) therefore lumped block development during depolarization (open and inactivated channel block) into a single process (κ). The block accumulated during depolarization declined exponentially during diastole, resulting in a 3 state approximation of the modulated receptor (see Fig. 2). The major advantage of such a description is that it results in simple equations that can be used to estimate numeric values for amount and rate of block development and recovery from block. These values provide not only a handy summary of experimental results, but they can be used successfully to make comparisons between drugs (Courtney, 1987).

Unfortunately, because block development appears to contain at least 2 components (one in association with the upstroke of the action potential and one associated with the plateau), the estimates are only valid for a limited range of cycle lengths. Indeed, action potential duration and consequently the relative contributions of upstroke and plateau block are a function of cycle length and membrane potential. Therefore, the parameters of this simplified scheme can not be used to describe block at other driving rates or potentials.

Guarded Receptor

A simplified version of the modulated receptor can be made by assuming that (1) the voltage-dependence of inactivation gating of

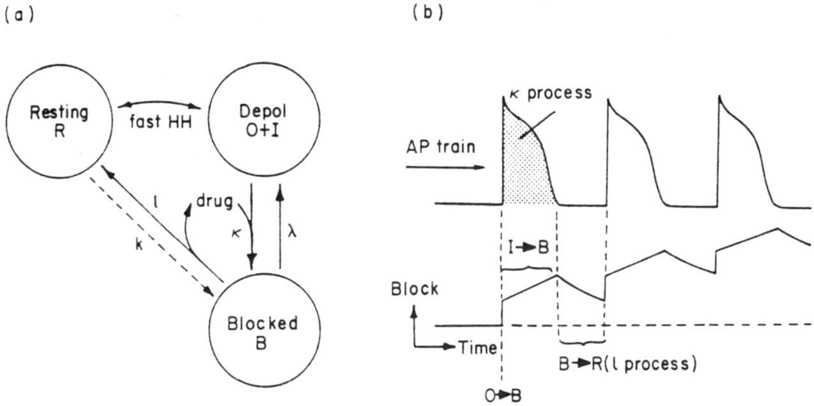

Figure 2. A simplified 3–state model for the frequency-dependent action of antiarrhythmic drugs. R: rested, O: open, I: inactivated, B: blocked. κ: net blocking of open and inactivated channels, λ net unblocking. Reproduced from Courtney (1983) with permission of the *Journal of Molecular and Cellular Cardiology.*

drug-associated channels is not modified; and (2) the sodium channel receptor has a fixed affinity for the drug. Instead, the receptor is guarded from occupancy by the gates (Starmer et al., 1984). Such simpler scheme must *a priori* be considered the preferred model, until it is ruled out by experimental tests.

The lack of alteration of the voltage-dependence of inactivation in drug-associated channels (assumption I) creates a serious deviation from experimental observations. Indeed, although the guarded receptor hypothesis can simulate some shift of the sodium channel availability curve (see for example Fig. 3 in Starmer et al., 1984), this shift is substantially different from that observed experimentally in at least four ways. First, the slope of the availability curve for a cationic activated channel blocker ($z = +1$; Starmer et al., 1984; Fig. 3) does not become steeper than that of control. To the contrary, it is substantially shallower (Fig. 3, Chapter 11). For neutral drugs that block inactivated channels, the sodium channel availability curve can, of course, be steeper, because as inactivation becomes available the block progressively increases (see Chen et al., 1975). Second, in the presence of drug the availability of channels increases, even at potentials where the drug-free channels are *fully* available (see −120 to −160 mV in Fig. 3). Third, under conditions where both drug-free and drug-associated channels are present, the

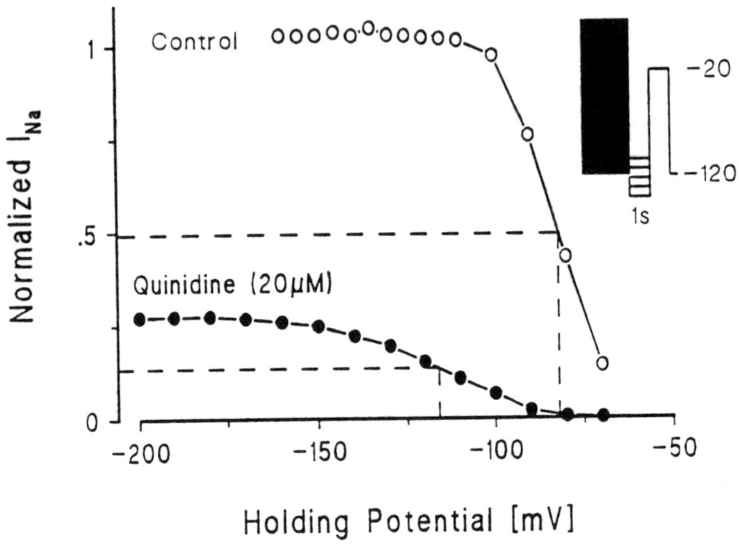

Figure 3. Voltage-dependence of use-dependent unblock from quinidine. Following induction of nearly complete block by a burst, the membrane was clamped for 1 second to various potentials. Dashed lines represent half maximal availability. (Data from Snyders and Hondeghem 1988).

availability curve can exhibit a *bump*: at potentials positive to the bump the increase in availability is dominated by drug-free channels, at potentials more negative than the bump (where all drug-free channels are available) the increase in availability is dominated by the drug-associated channels. Fourth,

> *For a drug with slow recovery kinetics, the modulated-receptor hypothesis suggests that with increasingly negative potentials, the block recovery time constant should stabilize at the potential where h^* (the apparent fraction of non-inactivated drug-complexed channels) becomes 1. The guarded receptor hypothesis suggests that for cationic drugs, accelerated recovery from block should continue for potentials beyond the point where $h^* = 1$.* (Starmer et al., 1984).

At 16°C quinidine has slow diastolic recovery kinetics: $\tau \sim 90$ sec at -120 mV, $\tau \sim 30$ sec at -160 mV. In addition, quinidine has a $pK_a = 8.3$, so that most of the drug is cationic at a pH of 7.4. Hence, according to the guarded receptor for increasing hyperpolarization, a constant recovery interval of 1 sec should yield increasing channel availability. Figure 3 clearly shows that over the potential of -160

to −200 mV availability of sodium channel did not increase. In contrast, the modulated receptor predicts that once inactivation of drug-associated channels is completely removed, further hyperpolarization may not yield further increases in availability, so that the observed plateau in Figure 3 is not unexpected.

Dr. Starmer argued that hyperpolarization might alter the ionization of the drug receptor complex, and result in faster recovery at more negative potentials. We do not agree with this argument, because hyperpolarization would attract hydrogen ions into the channel (receptor is more controlled by external pH than internal pH; Grant et al., 1982), thus promoting the cationic form of the drug and slowing recovery from block. This is contrary to experimental observation. Furthermore, quinidine is already so extensively cationic, that there is little room for further protonation. Thus, once hyperpolarization drives all drug-associated channels into the RD state, further hyperpolarization yields no further recovery.

The fixed affinity of the receptor for the drug (assumption II) creates another serious deviation from experimental observations. Indeed, in the absence of a voltage shift, block induced by frequent activations should approach the same steady state as that for a single long depolarization at the same potential. Instead for lidocaine, a long pulse clearly results in more block than many short pulses (see Fig. 3 of Matsubara et al., 1987). Similarly, for bupivacaine, no open channel block could be measured at a concentration that elicited marked inactivation block (Clarkson and Hondeghem, 1985). Amiodarone was similarly found to only block inactivated channels (Mason et al., 1984). Although the previous examples could possibly be explained away by assuming very fast diastolic recovery from block and infinitely slow open channel block, this reasoning cannot hold for quinidine; block induced by frequent depolarization declines during prolonged depolarization at potentials where all the channels are inactivated (Snyders and Hondeghem, 1989). Of course, one could argue that the receptor has a higher affinity for cationic quinidine during activation than for neutral quinidine during inactivation, but that exact mechanism for state-dependent differences in affinity was proposed in the modulated receptor (see Hille 1977; Hondeghem and Katzung, 1977).

Perhaps the strongest evidence against the guarded receptor scheme results from a series of experiments on quinidine (Snyders and Hondeghem, 1989). Following induction of block, use-dependent unblocking can be induced. For quinidine, at 16° C use-dependent

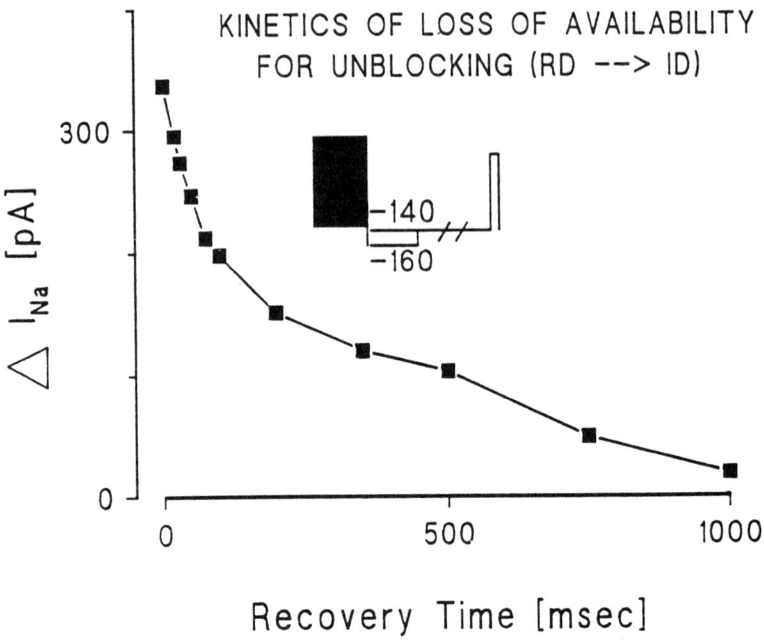

Figure 4. Decline upon stepping to −140 mV of availability for unblocking established by clamping to −160 mV. With a τ in the 100 msec range the sodium channels lose the availability for unblocking induced by a 1 second hyperpolarization to −160 mV. As a result, following a 1 second period at −140 mV, there is no memory of the 1 second period at −160 mV. Thus, hyperpolarization induces a state (**ID** ⇒ **RD**) from which unblocking can occur (**RD** ⇒ **AD** ⇒ **A**), provided an activation is triggered. Upon a less strong depolarization (e.g., to −140 mV), this availability dissipates (**RD** ⇒ **ID**). (Data from Snyders and Hondeghem, 1988).

unblocking reaches a maximum near a holding potential of −160 mV (Fig. 3). However, this maximum unblock is only achieved if an activation is contiguous with the hyperpolarization (Gintant and Hoffman, 1984). If instead, one steps from −160 mV to −140 mV, then the amplitude of the unblock declines with a time constant of about 100 msec (see Fig. 4). We interpret this result to indicate that for drug-associated channels, hyperpolarizations create a state (**RD**) from which unblocking can occur during activation (**RD** ⇒ **AD** ⇒ **A**). However, subthreshold depolarization removes this potential for unblocking (**RD** ⇒ **ID**). Thus, not only is removal of inactivation (**ID** ⇒ **RD**) shifted to more negative potentials in drug-associated channels, inactivation (**RD** ⇒ **ID**) is too. Indeed, no inactivation develops in drug-free channels upon depolarization from −160 to −140 mV. Thus, in contrast to Starmer and Courtney (1986) who "*believe there is no structural analog of resting drug-complexed channels,*" we have demonstrated the existence of a rested drug-associated state. Moreover, since upon activation of **RD** channels drug must first dissociate from the channel receptor before the channel can conduct, it is not unexpected that activation from **RD** takes slightly more time than activation from **R** (Snyders and Hondeghem, 1987).

Analytical Modulated Receptor

Although the modulated receptor is conceptually uncomplicated, the equations, as originally implemented by Hondeghem and Katzung (1977), are computationally very intense. So we, like others, have therefore tried to make computationally simpler approximations. One such version is described in the Ph.D. thesis of Moyer (1985).

Basically, at potentials more positive than −40 mV (during the plateau of the action potential), all channels are inactivated (**I** or **ID**). As a result, the modulated receptor simplifies to a first order linear differential equation, which has a very simple analytical solution.

Activation (during the upstroke of the action potential) can be approximated by a difference equation, such that a fraction (related to the K_{dA}) of the channels in the **R** state become blocked, and a fraction of the **RD** channels unblock.

Finally, since diastolic recovery from block is relatively little voltage-dependent (most of the hyperpolarization induced reduction in block appears to result from use-dependent unblocking), **RD** and **ID** can be lumped until just before activation. This 3 state diastolic modulated receptor (**R**, **I**, Blocked = **RD** + **ID**) is similar to the κ model of Courtney (1983), and can be solved analytically. However, in contrast to the κ model, the contributions of activated and inactivated channel block are actually computed. Thus, the model will simulate changes in action potential duration and resting potential. Just prior to activation the blocked channels can then be distributed between **RD** and **ID**. On an IBM AT this procedure computes so fast (msec range) that one can repeat it with pixel resolution throughout

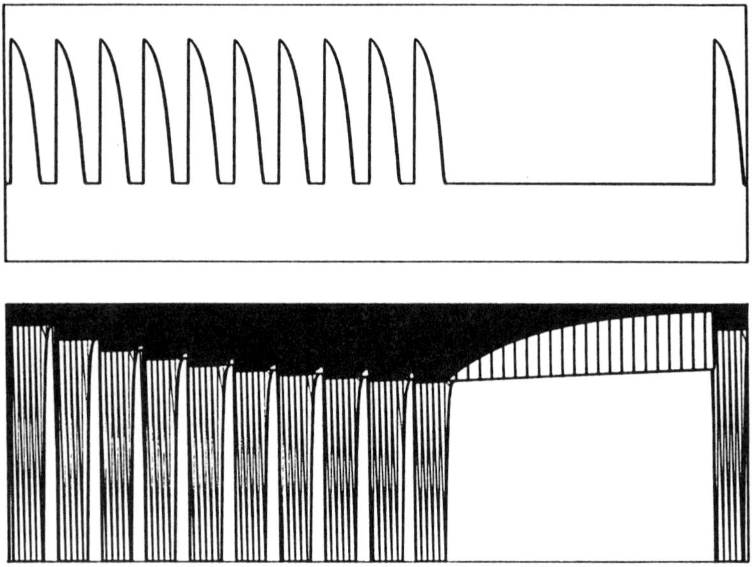

Figure 5. Output of analytical modulated receptor model. For details see text.

any phase of the action potential and still visualize the time course of block/unblock in about *real* time (1–2 action potentials per second).

A copy of this analytical approximation of the modulated receptor enriched with extensive graphical illustrations (see Fig. 6) can be obtained from the authors. The program requires a computer capable of running DOS (preferably an AT or 386 machine, since the program runs rather slowly on a PC) and having an EGA (16 color 640 × 350 capability, i.e., the 64K version will not work) or VGA graphics card. Although a math coprocessor is desirable, it is not mandatory.

In Figure 5, 10 action potentials were generated from a resting potential of −90 mV at a cycle length of 300 msec in the presence of quinidine (8 μM). In this figure white represents **R**, narrow striation **ID**, wide parallel striation **RD**, black **ID**. The available sodium current during the upstroke of the action potential would be equal or larger than the white **(R)**, but less than the white plus wide striation **(R + RD)**. Thus, the analytical version of the modulate receptor will be best defined under conditions where **RD** is small.

Caution: The analytical version of the modulated receptor is intended as an educational tool. **Although the program can be used to find initial estimates for the modulated receptor, it must be realized that it is only an approximation.** There exist two conditions under which the analytical modulated receptor may make serious deviations from the full implementation: (i) when equilibrium between **RD** and **ID** is not reached (fast heart rates at intermediary potentials, where **ID-RD** transitions exist but may be slow). At potentials where **RD** does not exist, or where **ID-RD** is very fast (at very negative potentials) this error should be minimal. (ii) When **RD** is present at the time of activation, full equilibrium between **A** and **AD** is assumed. Although this may be somewhat reasonable for fast drugs as mexiletine and lidocaine, it certainly is not for slower drugs like quinidine, encainide or flecainide (we have not yet examined other drugs). Until the kinetics of activated unblock are determined experimentally, I have therefore opted to generate a beeping warning message when activations are triggered with more than 7% of the channels in **RD**. Under the latter condition, in its present form the analytical modulated receptor will compute an erroneous level of block. Once more is known about activation block/unblock in the presence of **RD** it may be trivial to incorporate this feature. For the time being, these conditions can only be appropriately simulated with the full modulated receptor model.

TEMPERATURE- AND VOLTAGE-DEPENDENCE OF ACTIVATION UNBLOCKING

The shift of the voltage-dependence of inactivation in quinidine-associated channels is much larger than anticipated from $\dot{V}_{max}$ at 37°C. However, as we warmed the preparation to 25°C the shift became progressively less (Snyders and Hondeghem, 1987). In another series of experiments on ODE (O-demethylencanide, a potent metabolite of encainide) we found the shift was so marked that at 15°C there was nearly no activation-associated unblocking at potentials where drug-free channels exhibit no inactivation (−100 to −140 mV), and even when hyperpolarizing to −160 mV, the activation-associated unblocking was less than 2% (Fig. 6). However,

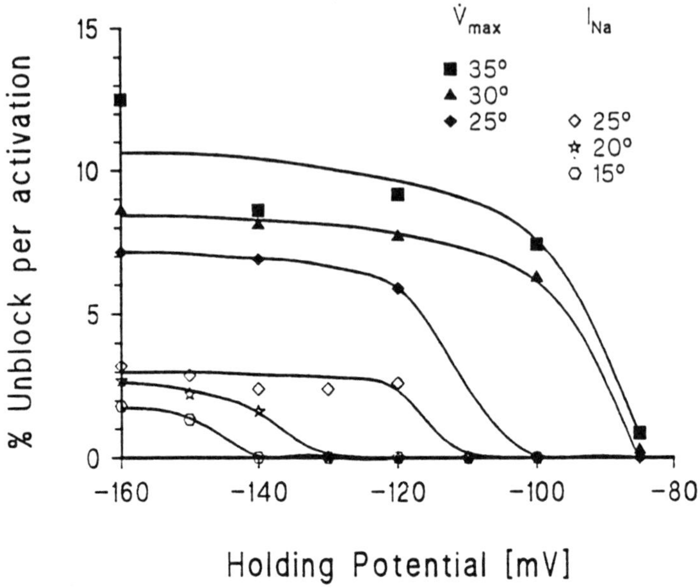

Figure 6. Temperature dependence of availability for activation associated unblocking. 15–25°C using I_{Na}, 25–37°C $\dot{V}_{max}$. (Data adapted from Johns et al., 1989).

as the temperature was increased, the availability for unblocking at each potential became progressively larger (Johns et al., 1989).

At 15°C, upon breaking into the cell the inactivation curve usually drifts to more negative potentials. This negative shift is partially overcome by warming. At 35°C the inactivation curve usually does not drift to more negative potentials; actually it sometimes drifts to more positive potentials. Thus, removal of inactivation requires less negative potentials at warm temperatures than at cold temperatures. Drug occupation of the sodium channel receptor further stabilizes the inactivated state so that even more negative potentials are required to remove inactivation. We have interpreted these results to indicate that drug occupation makes the rested state energetically less likely and increases the energy barriers that separate the **RD** and **ID** states (Johns et al., 1989).

UNBLOCKING

Following development of block, unblocking occurs both during diastole and during activation. Diastolic unblock can occur via two pathways: **RD** ⇒ **R** and **ID** ⇒ **I**. Originally, Hondeghem and Katzung (1977) assumed that lack of use-dependent unblocking at negative potentials resulted from fast diastolic recovery from block. However, more recent experimental results (Snyders and Hondeghem, 1989) indicate that even upon hyperpolarization to −160 mV diastolic recovery becomes only moderately faster. Instead, most of the hyperpolarization induced block appears to result from activation-associated unblocking. The question thus arises whether closed channel unblocking requires two rate constants, i.e., are l_R and l_I different?

When restraining l_R and l_I to be equal in the modulated receptor, the computer appears to have little problem simulating the experimental results. Actually, as one hyperpolarizes, net unblocking becomes independent of membrane potential. The only difference is that as the membrane is made more negative, more of the blocked channels accumulate in the **RD** pool (see Fig. 5), i.e., become available for unblocking. This suggests that the faster diastolic recovery from block at more negative potentials (Chen et al., 1975; Hondeghem and Katzung, 1984) may actually result from activation unblocking during the test pulse. This interpretation predicts that the faster recovery at −160 mV should become similar to the recovery at −120 mV, if the test pulse is preceded by a brief depolarization to a subthreshold potential. The latter brief depolarization before the test pulse provides an opportunity for the **RD** channels to become **ID** channels again, and thus loose their availability for activation-associated unblocking (Fig. 4). Thus diastolic unblocking would only appear voltage-dependent because of the voltage-dependence of availability for activation unblocking.

If the above observation becomes a general feature for antiarrhythmic drug action, then l_R and l_I can be replaced by a single closed state unblocking rate constant. This would suggest that closed channel state unblocking, presumably most relevant to neutral drug (Hille, 1977), is little voltage-dependent.

CRUCIAL PROPERTIES OF A SODIUM CHANNEL

Single channel experiments have greatly enhanced our understanding of the voltage and time-dependent behavior of sodium channels (Bennett 1987, 1988; Aldrich and Stevens, 1983; Grant et al., 1983, 1987; Vandenberg and Horn, 1984; Horn and Vandenberg,

1984; Kunze et al., 1985). In contrast to the original assumptions made by Hodgkin and Huxley (1952), it now appears that the rise and fall of macroscopic sodium conductance (activation and inactivation) are governed by both the activation process and the rate constants of leaving the open state (the latency of channel opening and the open time autocorrelation function; Vandenberg and Horn, 1984). At some membrane potentials delayed openings are quickly followed by channel inactivation. Thus, sodium channels usually open for only a brief period (0.5 to 1.5 msec at 20°C; maybe much shorter at 37°C).

Any model describing the time- and voltage-dependence of drug action on sodium channels should satisfactorily describe the following:

1. *Accurate duplication of macroscopic currents*
   - Standard IV relationship (membrane potential versus peak I_{Na}; Fig. 7) should have a threshold near −60 mV, the peak sodium current should smoothly increase to have a maximum peak near −20 mV, while for larger depolarizations it should linearly (approximately) decline and reverse at the sodium equilibrium potential.
   - Macroscopic inactivation (Fig. 8) must appear faster as the depolarization is increased (e-fold per 26 mV; Vandenberg and Horn, 1984). A double exponential is required to approximate macropscopic inactivation at intermediate potentials, while requiring only one faster exponential at more positive potentials, or one slower one at more negative potentials (Grant et al., 1987).
   - Available sodium current should decline upon depolarization (h-curve; (Fig. 9), with a slope factor of about 6.
   - The rate of recovery from inactivation should increase as the membrane is made more negative (Fig. 10).
2. *Accurate description of single channels currrents*
   - At threshold (small depolarizations near −60 mV), first openings can be delayed for a long time (Fig. 11); many "null" sweeps occur (Fig. 12) and sodium channels reopen frequently (Fig. 13; Grant et al., 1987).
   - For stronger depolarizations first openings occur earlier (Fig. 11), nulls become relatively rare (Fig.

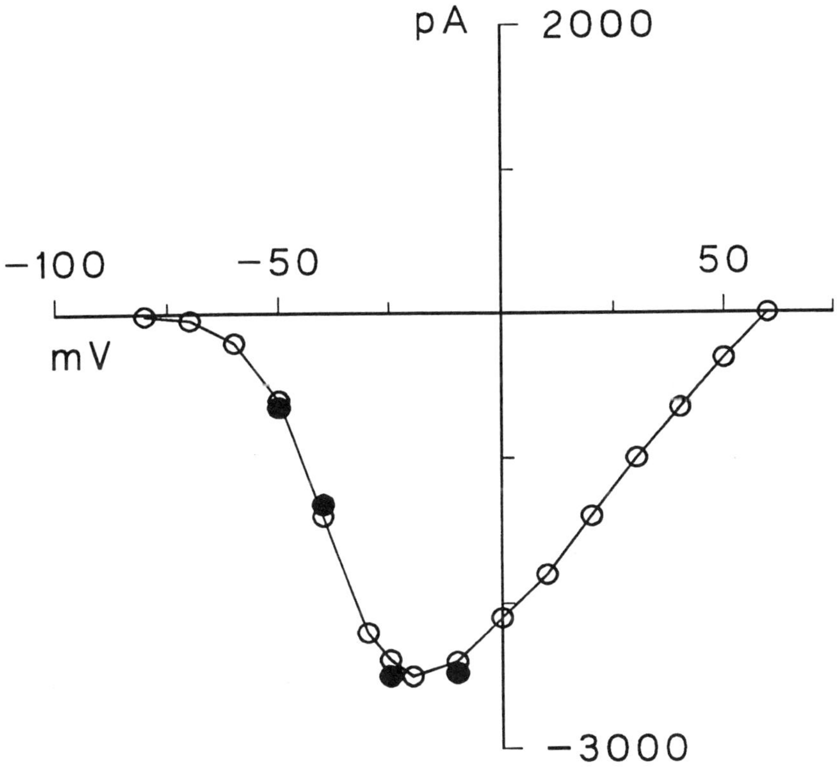

Figure 7. IV relation.

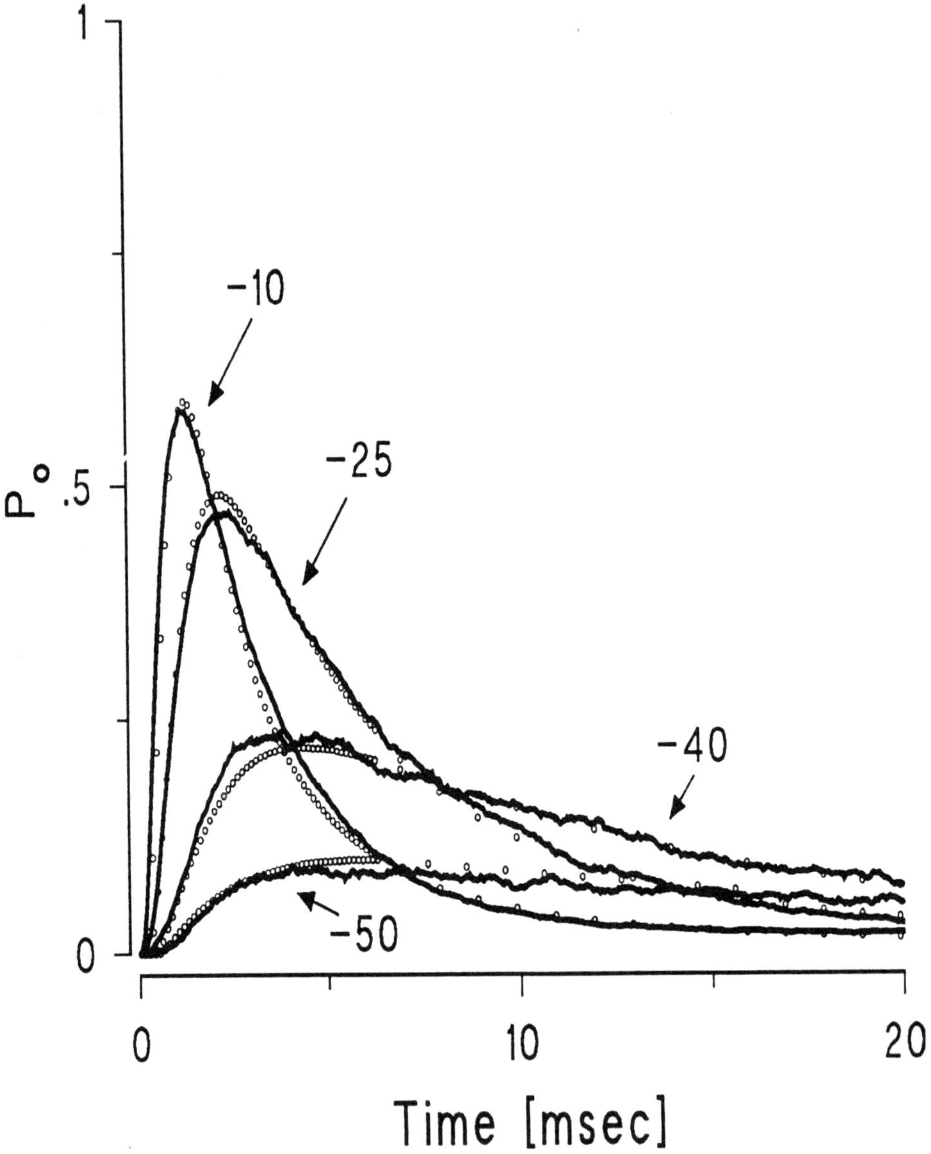

Figure 8. Probability of opening.

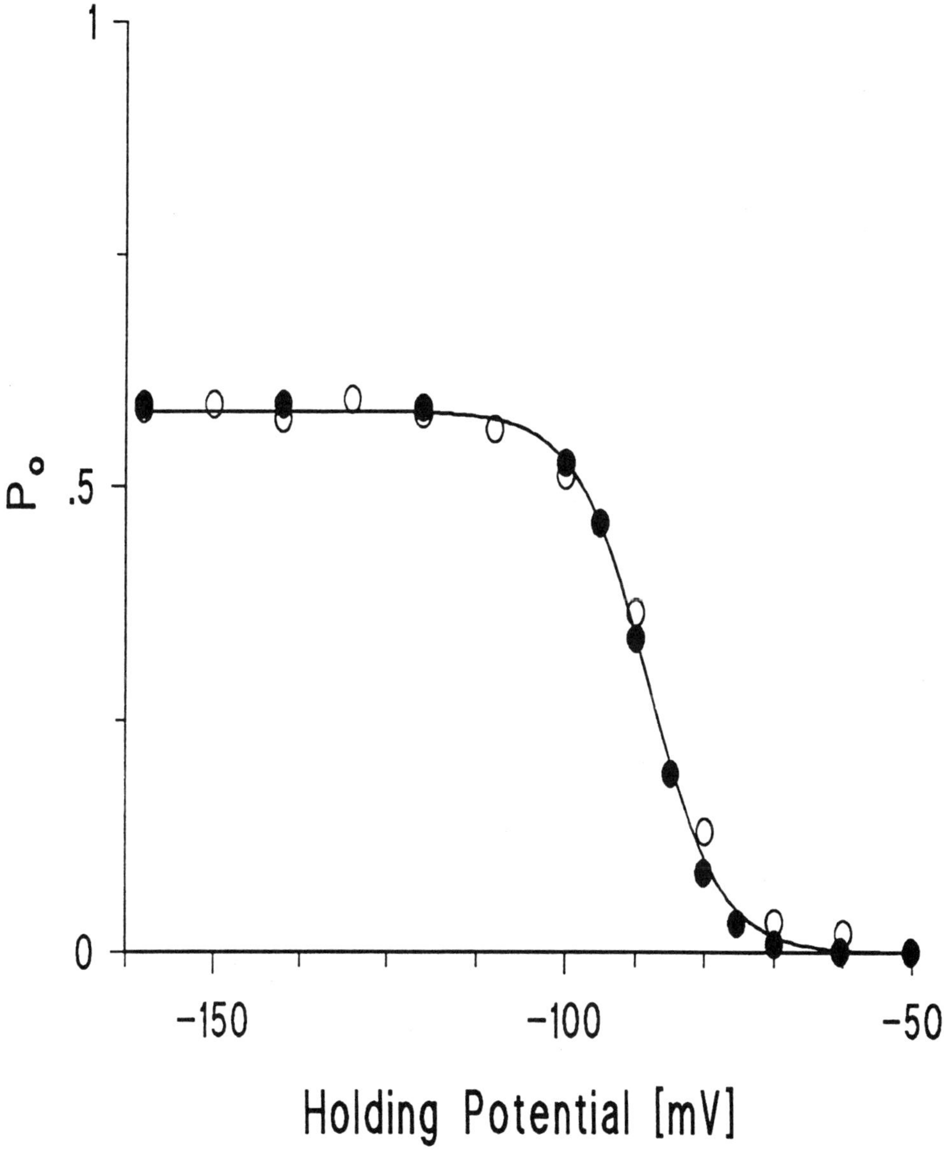

Figure 9. h-curve.

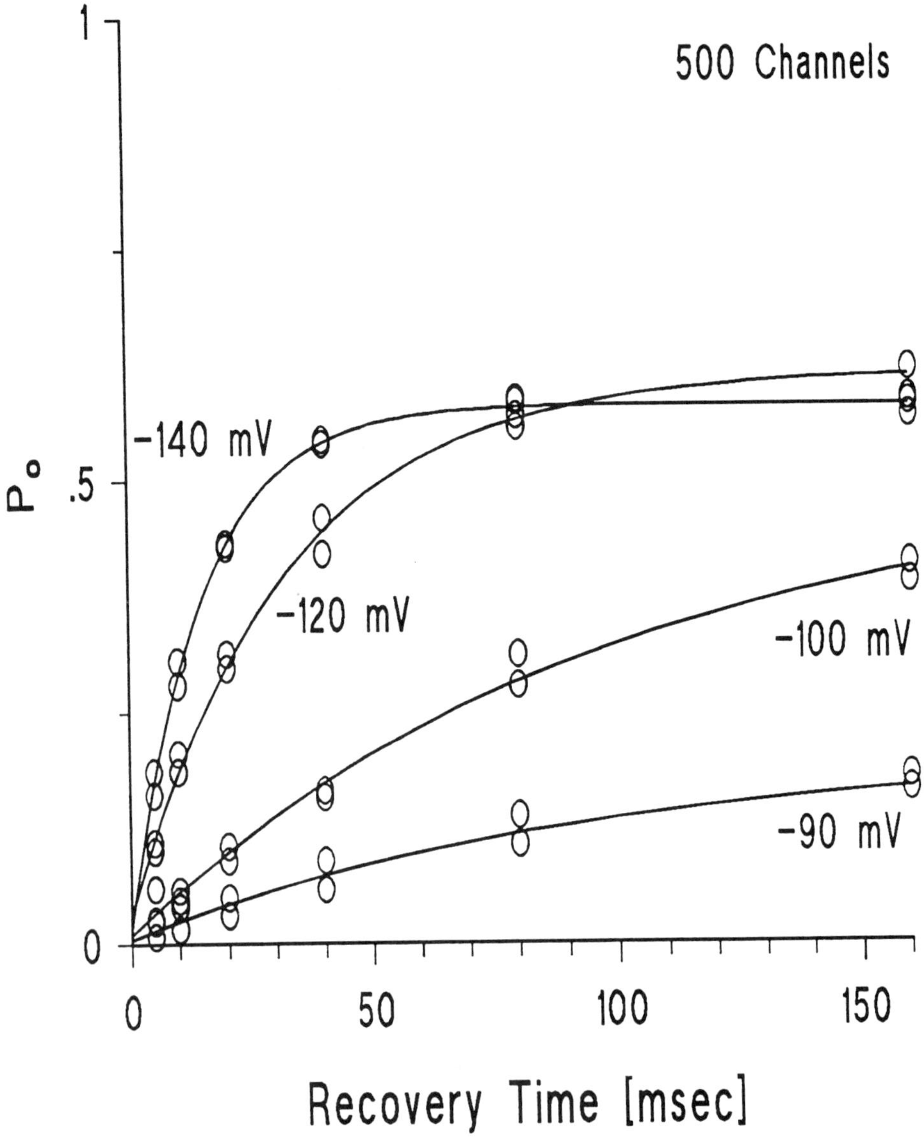

Figure 10. Recovery from inactivation.

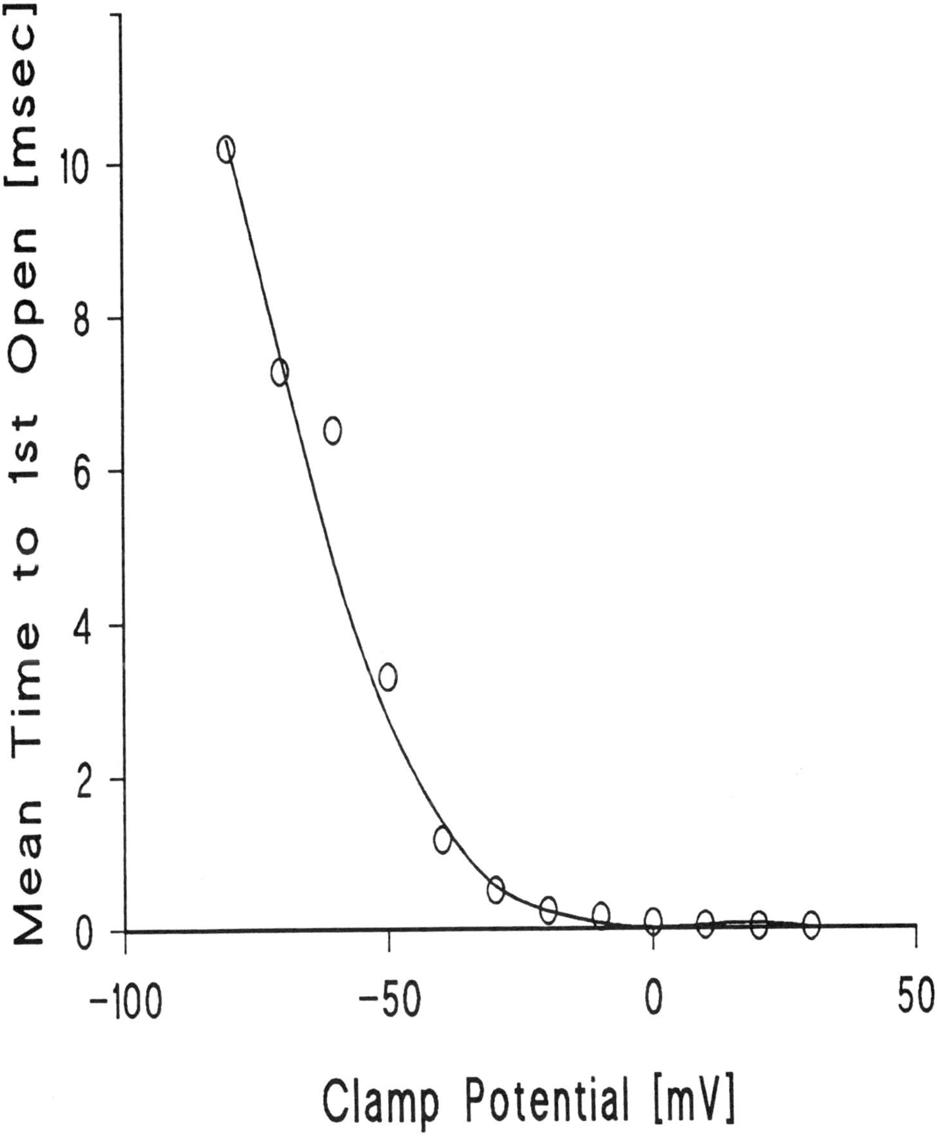

Figure 11. Time to 1st opening.

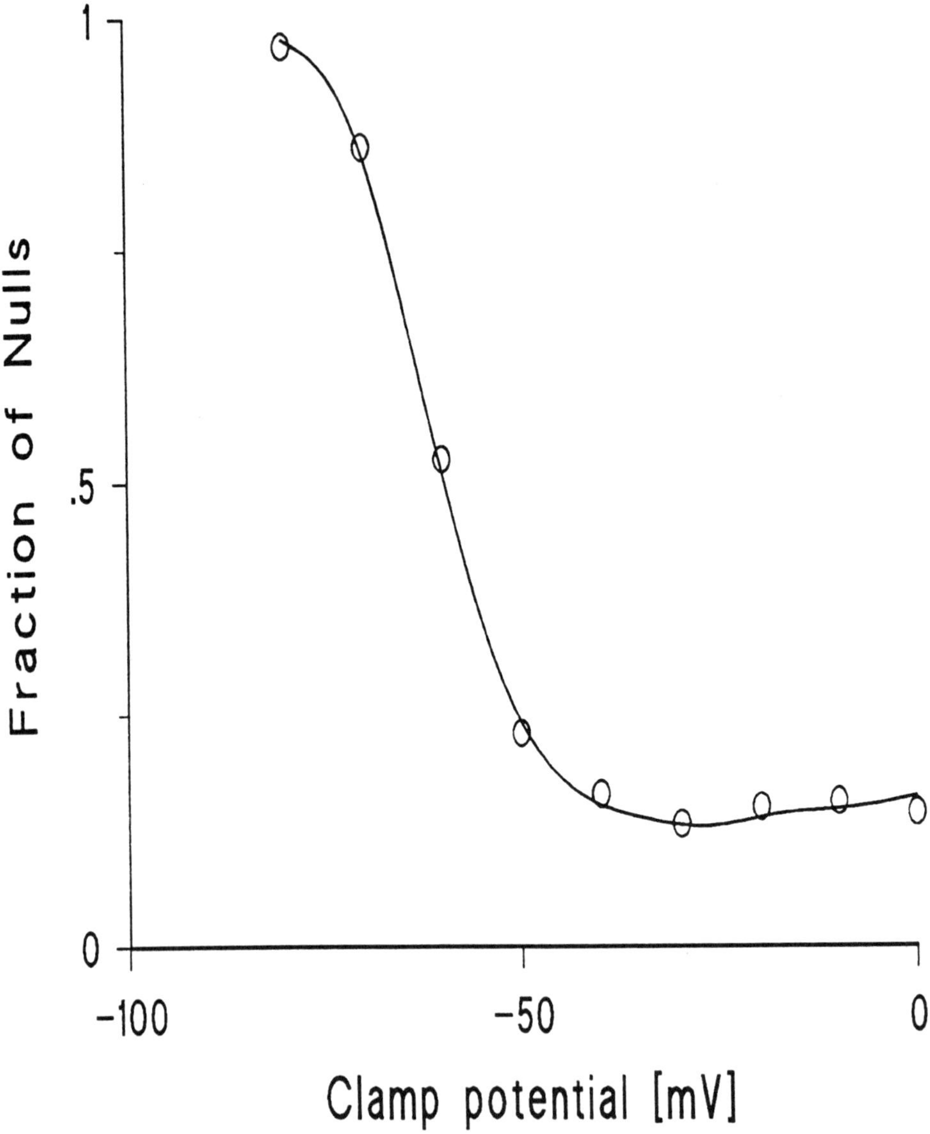

Figure 12. Blank sweeps.

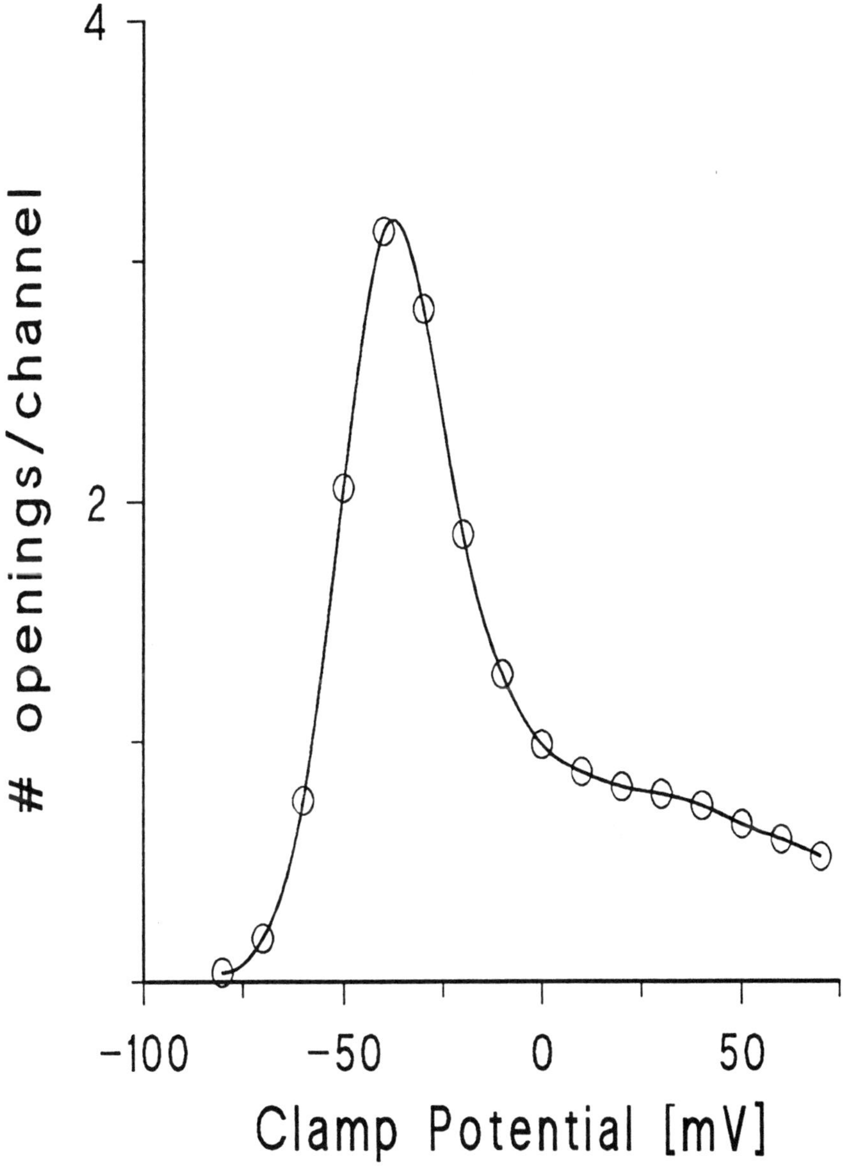

Figure 13. Number of openings.

11), but the number of reopenings decline (Fig. 13).
- Near −30 mV open times appear not very voltage-dependent although they are shorter at negative potentials (Fenwick et al., 1982) and longer at positive potentials (Grant and Starmer, 1987). However, upon further depolarization they shorten again (Fig. 14).
- Open times exhibit an exponential distribution, but careful analysis indicates a slight excess of long openings (Fig. 15; Aldrich and Stevens, 1983).
- Sodium channels exhibits at least 2 modes of openings; few openings and bursting mode. Bursting may span several consecutive sweeps indicating a duration of this mode of hundreds of milliseconds to seconds. Burst mode openings are longer than regular openings (Fig. 16; Grant et al., 1987).
- Inactivation may quickly follow channel opening and appears much slower from *rested* state. Moreover, rested state inactivation appears strongly voltage-dependent, whereas *open* state inactivation appears much less voltage-dependent.

3. *Accurate reproduction of drug effects*
   - Block of sodium channels by antiarrhythmic agents develops in a use-dependent fashion. Moreover, the block is more marked the faster the heart rate. Depolarization of the membrane potential also increases the block.
   - At the single channel level, not much data is available yet, but lidocaine induces use-dependent reduction of P_o and it shortens open time slightly (Bennett, unpublished observations). Mean open time is reduced without reducing single channel conductance. Bursting channels appear more sensitive to lidocaine (Fig. 17), as bursting can be virtually abolished when the early peak sodium current is virtually not reduced (Bennett, 1988).

The above list must be satisfied but is by no means comprehensive.

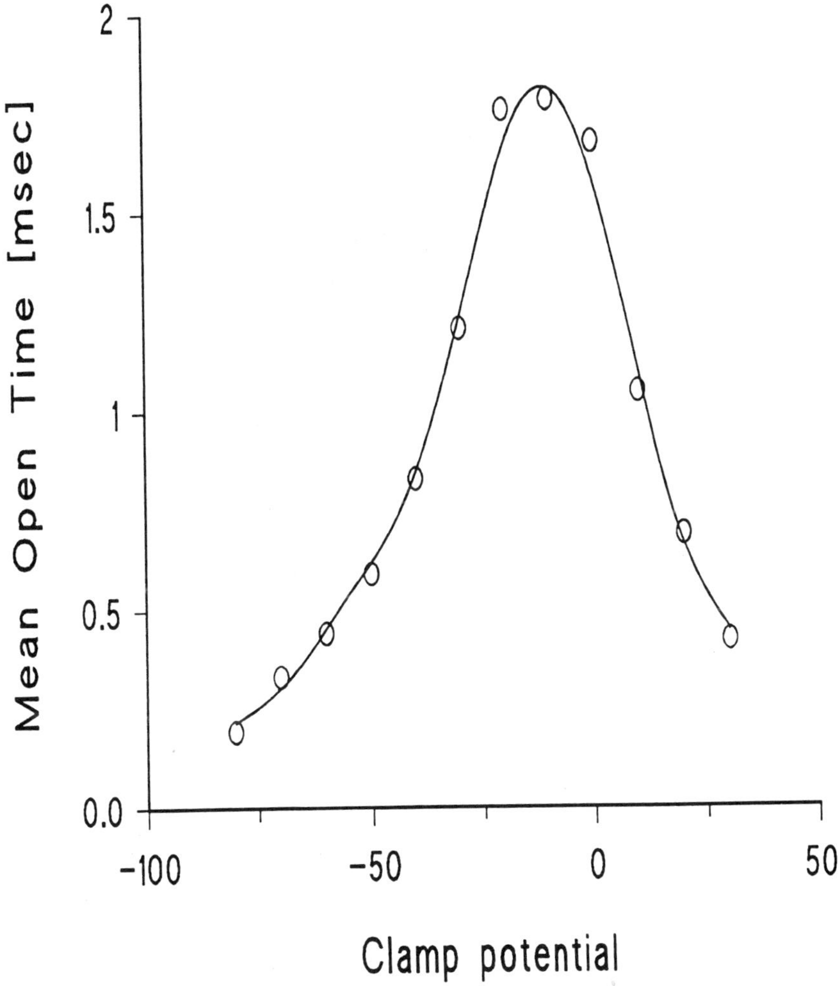

Figure 14. Mean open time.

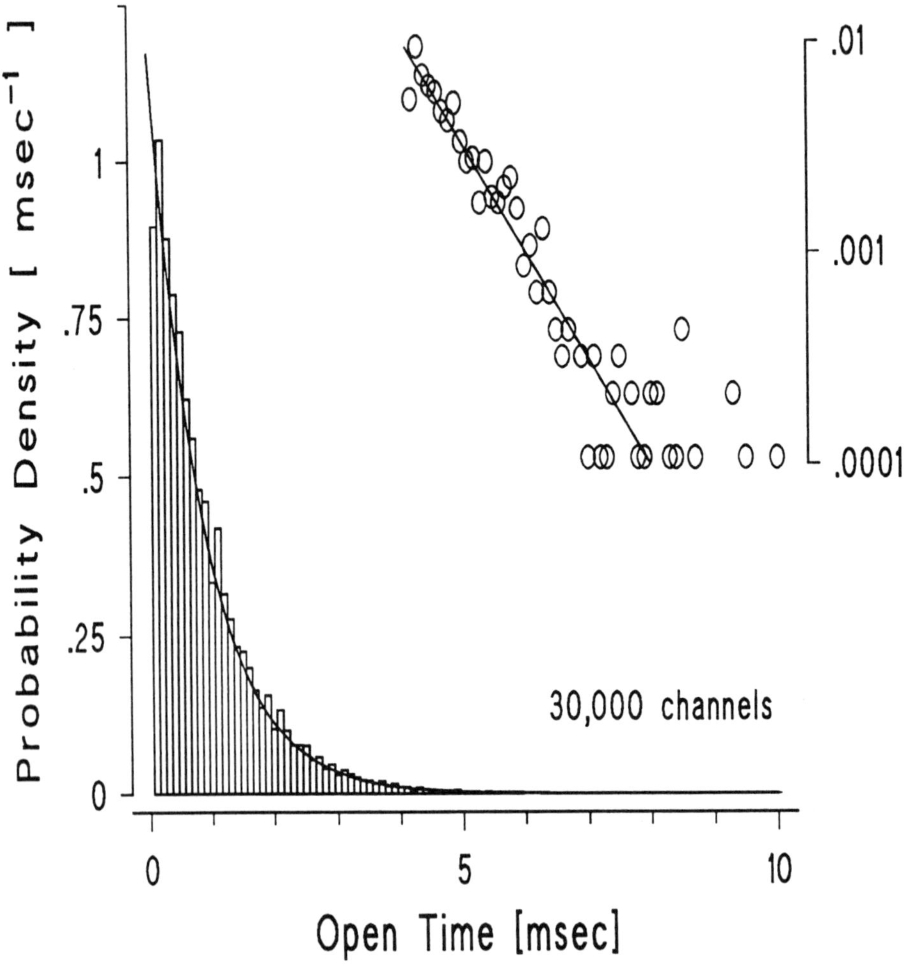

Figure 15. Open time histogram.

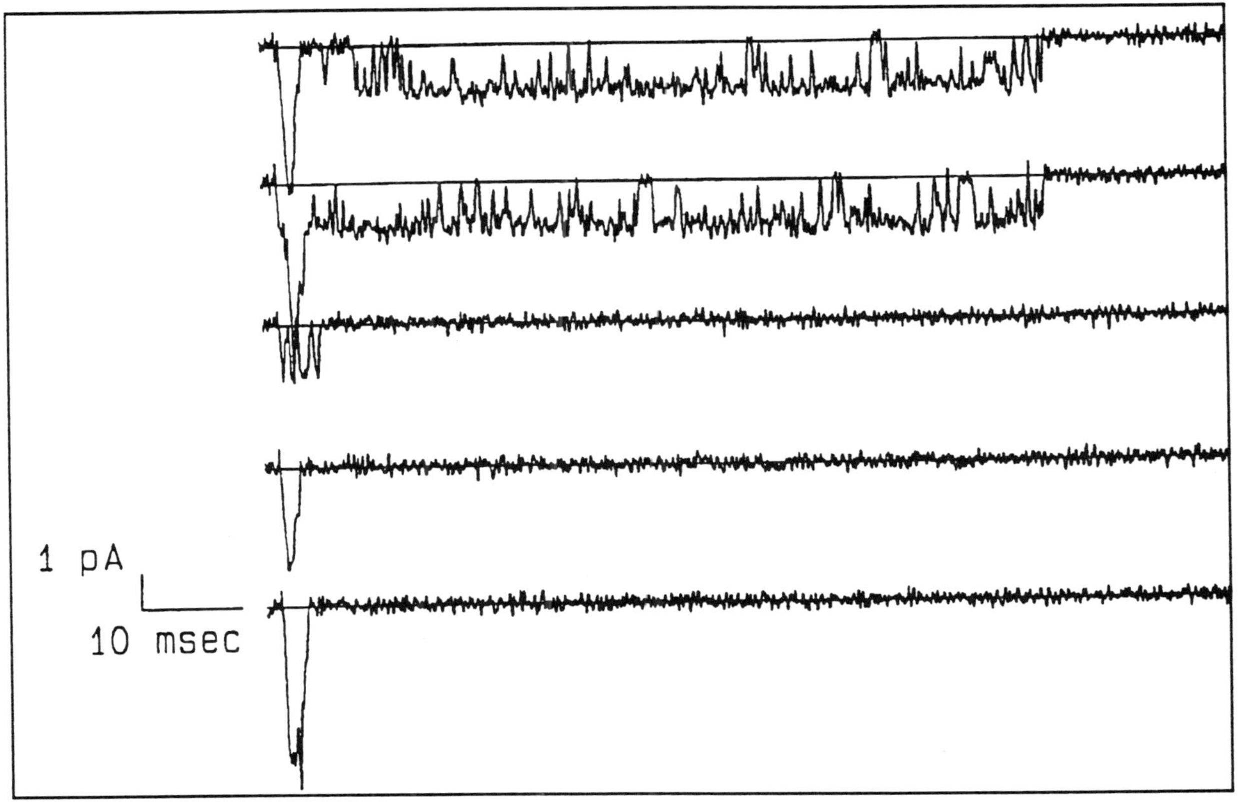

Figure 16. Flicker mode (mode 0) of cardiac sodium channel occurs in less than 1% of sweeps. Probability of observing 2 consecutive sweeps for random and independent events is 1 in 10,000 suggesting that the behavior shown represents the conversion of one channel into mode 0 for several seconds.

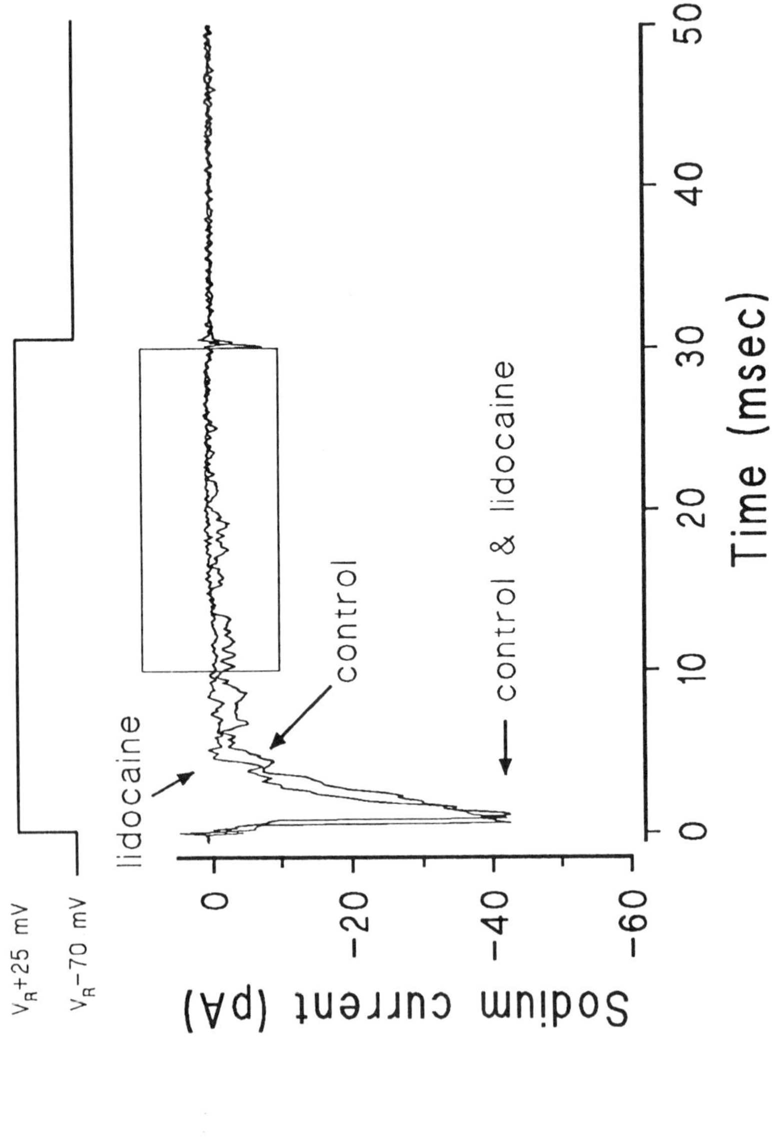

Figure 17. Lidocaine supresses late opening Na^+ channels with little or no effect upon the early peak I_{Na} after a rest period. A multichannel patch was used to optimize visualization of late channels. Lidocaine reduced opening probability of late opening, but single-channel amplitude was not changed.

BASIS FOR NEW SODIUM CHANNEL MODEL

Current models of single sodium channel behavior (Vandenberg and Horn, 1984; Kunze et al., 1985) are adequate to simulate their single channel data in the respective papers. However, as pointed out in both papers these models do not produce fully satisfactory macroscopic sodium currents over a broad range of voltages and times. We therefore found it necessary to construct an alternate model that could simulate both single channel data and macroscopic sodium currents.

Most groups working on the structure of the sodium channel (Noda et al., 1984; also see Guy, chapter 9) agree that the channel has four homologous domains, each containing a highly positively charged chain, proposed to be involved in activation. We therefore decided that our sodium channel model should have four activation units. For similar reasons, we assumed a single inactivation unit, which is most likely located on the cytoplasmic side of the membrane. Inactivation is functionally coupled to activation (Armstrong and Bezanilla, 1977; Nonner, 1980), in such a way that it develops quickly following activation. Since inactivation must be coupled to at least one activation process, we will assume that in its simplest form activation of only one specific activation unit leads to inactivation (also see Guy, chapter 9).

Activation is controlled by membrane potential, and until proven otherwise, we shall make the simplest assumption that all four activation units have a similar voltage-dependence and act independently—if experimental results indicate differently, it is rather straightforward to incorporate a cooperative index—inactivation then is triggered by activation of the 4th unit:

$$D_1 \underset{k_{DA}}{\overset{k_{AD}}{\Longleftrightarrow}} A_1$$

$$D_2 \underset{k_{DA}}{\overset{k_{AD}}{\Longleftrightarrow}} A_2$$

$$D_3 \underset{k_{DA}}{\overset{k_{AD}}{\Longleftrightarrow}} A_3$$

$$D_4 \underset{k_{DA}}{\overset{k_{AD}}{\Longleftrightarrow}} A_4 \underset{k_{AI}}{\overset{k_{IA}}{\Longleftrightarrow}} I$$

Thus, three of the activation processes move between their deactivated (D) and activated (A) conformation according to:

$$dA_i/dt = k_{AD}D_i - k_{DA}A_i \quad \text{where} \quad i = 1, 2, \text{or } 3 \qquad [1]$$

The fourth activation process and its associated inactivation move between deactivated, activated and inactivated (I) conformations according to:

$$dA_4/dt = k_{AD}D_4 + k_{AI}I - (k_{DA} + k_{IA})A_4 \qquad [2]$$

where the k's are a function of voltage (It is possible that interactions between the gating units also induce changes in the rate constants, in which case the rate constants would switch values, i.e., become state-dependent). Only when all four units are activated is the sodium channel open:

$$I_{Na} = N\gamma(E_m - E_{Na})A_1(t, v)A_2(t, v)A_3(t, v)A_4(t, v) \qquad [3]$$

where N is the number of sodium channels, γ the single channel conductance, E_m the membrane potential, E_{Na} the sodium equilibrium potential, A_1 through A_4 the voltage-dependent probabilities of occupying an activated conformation.

In order to account for burst behavior, the channel can have several modes for inactivation. At this time we have only implemented mode 0 (where the channel does not inactivate; Fig. 18) and mode 1 (normal inactivation). For longer pulses, especially at depolarized potentials, it also will become necessary to let the channels exhibit slow and ultra-show inactivation upon prolonged depolarization (Clarkson et al., 1984; Saikawa and Carmeliet, 1982).

NOTE: These slow inactivation processes are not purely controlled by membrane potential. They are also modified by metabolic conditions. For example, the action of certain antiarrhythmic agents can be markedly dependent upon these slow inactivated states (Coromilias et al., 1986; Hondeghem and Matsubara, 1988). Moreover, we have recently observed that block by flecainide during slow inactivation is both more marked and faster in the presence of isoproterenol (unpublished observation by Anno and Hondeghem). Such behavior could result from a metabolic modification of the channel (e.g., phosphorylation/dephosphorylation; Catterall et al., 1986).

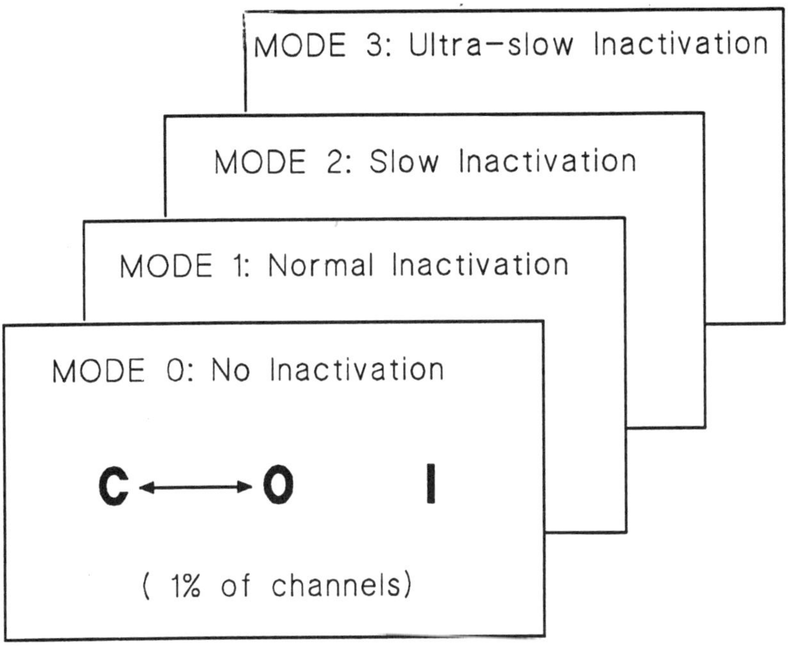

Figure 18. Modes of channel inactivation.

We have reproduced single channel behavior using Monte Carlo simulations of the model described above. However, in order to find suitable rate constants, in collaborations with Dr. Jeffrey Balser we are developing a global fitting procedure to search for the optimal rate constants. We have not yet incorporated mode 0 into the fitting procedure. As a result the rate constants used in the Monte Carlo simulations for Figures 7–10 are not fully optimized. We anticipate that once the flicker mode is incorporated into the fitting procedure, that rate constants will be further improved.

Interestingly, the simplex fitting algorithm converged to a set of rate constants that also reproduces known single channel behavior (Figs. 11–15). We do not know whether this is a coincidence or whether the information contained in the 56 different data sets used constrained the system to converge on a unique solution.

Since our model has a structural basis—has only 4 independent rate constants and reproduces the drug-free sodium currents rather faithfully—we used it to incorporate modulated receptor parameters.

INCORPORATION OF MODULATED RECEPTOR

Since it is postulated that there exists a specific single receptor for local anesthetic-like sodium channel blockers (Clarkson and Hondeghem, 1985), and since it has been known for a long time that block is intimately involved with both inactivation (Weidmann, 1955) and activation of the channels (Johnson and McKinnon, 1957), we assume that the modulated receptor is associated with this activation-inactivation pair (Fig. 19). Thus, when this pair is deactivated the sodium channel receptor has the **R** state affinity; when this pair is activated, the receptor is in the **A** state (**but not necessarily open,** since open requires that all four gates are activated: A^3A_4 in Figure 20), and when it is inactivated the receptor is in the **I** state. When the receptor is in the **R** state, but other units are **ACTIVATED** (A_1, A_2 or A_3), this may actually represent an early part of activation (left dashed box in Fig. 20). (Alternatively, the channel may be *open* when fewer gates are open. This would result in channels with more than one open state. We and others (Nagy, 1987; Scanley and Fozzard, 1987) have observed possible multiple open states, but this phenomena requires further study before incorporation into a quantitative model.) During this time drug interactions may have a mix of rested state affinity and activated state kinetics. Similarly, there could also be a late part of activation (right dashed box in Fig. 20). In this way, activation could be composed of at least four components: an early transient with **R** state affinity, a closed and open **A** state, and a late transient **I** state. Different pulse patterns may render the low or high affinity substates more or less important, so that activation may induce block or unblocking, depending in part on the pulse pattern and in part on the distribution between the states just prior to activation. Actually, it is possible to elicit activation-induced block without opening the channel (Wang and Strichartz, 1984; Chapter 15). Whether it is also possible to elicit activation-induced unblocking without opening the channel remains to be tested.

Drug-associated channels do not conduct and have a less steep voltage-dependence for inactivation, which is shifted to more negative potentials. When the channels are closed by activation gates, or by the inactivation gate, then drug interactions with the receptor proceed slowly and are primarily limited to the neutral form of the

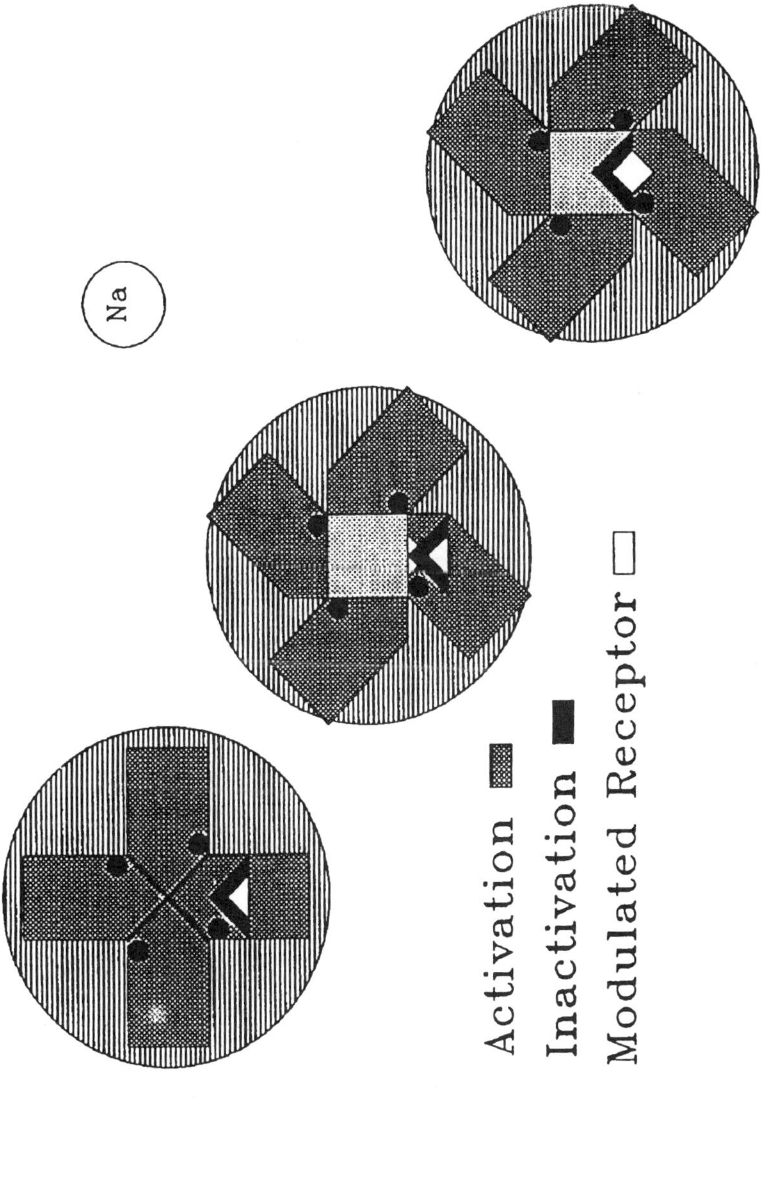

Figure 19. Diagrammatic representation of interaction of activation-inactivation unit and drug molecule: left RESTED, middle ACTIVATED, and right INACTIVATED.

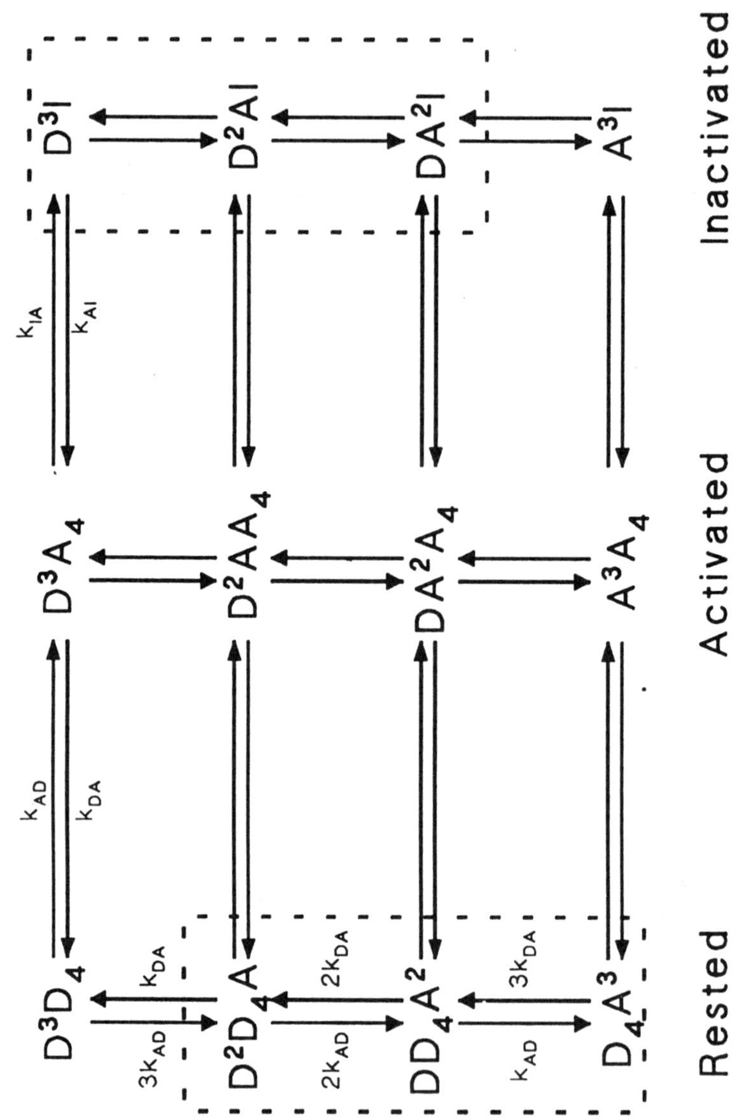

Figure 20. Single-channel modulated receptor (see text for explanation).

drug. The charged form of the drug can only interact with the receptor during activation. This interaction must have fast kinetics, as activation is too short lived to allow significant contributions by slow processes. If the membrane potential is not made very negative between pulses, the blocked channels will accumulate in **ID** and result in use-dependent block.

Attachment of binding (k_A) and unbinding (l_A) modulated rate constants provides an additional pathway to exit from open activated channels (A^3A_4; in Fig. 20) and consequently is predicted to shorten the observed open time. This prediction has been observed for lidocaine (Bennett, 1988; Nilius et al., 1987).

Channels in mode 0, spend more time in the high affinity activated state and therefore, may reach equilibrium block more quickly. As a result they are predicted to be more sensitive to block (see Fig. 17).

Drug-associated channels have their inactivation shifted to more negative potentials and will remain trapped in the **ID** pool, thus yielding more null sweeps in the presence of drug. However, for strong depolarizations, inactivation can be overcome and channel activity can be recovered (Nilius et al., 1987).

It should be noted that the activated state has 3 closed states from which inactivation can occur, but they can also become blocked. Thus, the activated state block during the first pulse in a train can be much larger than is apparent from the first pulse reduction. This explains how a fast activated state blocker like lidocaine can markedly reduce the second pulse in a train while not reducing much of the first pulse (much of the activated state block developed invisibly during the first pulse).

Reduction of open time will contribute to tonic block. There are two additional mechanisms for tonic block: **R** state blocking (usually negligible for therapeutic concentrations of antiarrhythmic agents), and **I** state blocking in combination with the voltage shift (see Hondeghem and Katzung, 1984).

Thus, at the single channel level, the main mechanisms for reduction of the sodium current are reduction of probability for opening: more blank sweeps and shorter open times. Mode 0 channels appear especially sensitive to block by antiarrhythmic agents. The latter may contribute to shortening of action potential duration.

CONCLUSION

The affinity of the receptor is modulated by membrane potential such that rested channels usually have a low affinity, while activated and/or inactivated channels have a high affinity. Upon binding, the drug alters the voltage-dependence of inactivation so that inactivation occurs at more negative potentials. The drug may also block the sodium channel. As a result sodium channels are less likely to open and may open for a shorter time. The sum of fewer and shorter single sodium currents yields reduced ensemble or macroscopic sodium currents. The reduced sodium currents lead to a reduced depolarization rate of the upstroke of the action potential, which in turn results in slowed conduction. The latter is responsible for the lengthening of the HV-internal and the widening of the QRS complex (Davis et al., 1986).

Acknowledgments: This work was supported by NIH Grant HL36020 and the Stahlman endowment. The authors thank Mrs. Betty Hondeghem for her editorial assistance.

BIBLIOGRAPHY

Aldrich RW, Stevens CF. Inactivation of open and closed sodium channels determined separately. Cold Spring Harbor Symposium. *Quant Biol* 48:147–153, 1983.

Armstrong CM, Bezanilla F. Inactivation of the sodium channel. II. Gating current experiments. *J Gen Physiol* 70:567–590, 1977.

Bennett PB. Kinetics and block of single sodium channels in voltage clamped cardiac cell membranes. *Biophys J* 53:227a, 1988.

Bennett PB. Mechanisms of antiarrhythmic drug action: block of sodium channels in voltage clamped cardiac cell membranes. *J Appl Cardiol* 2:463–488, 1987.

Bennett PB, Balser JR, Snyders DJ, Hondeghem LM. Modulated receptor: a review and update (unpublished data, 1989).

Catterall WA. Molecular properties of voltage-sensitive sodium channels. *Annu Rev Biochem* 55:953–985, 1986.

Chen CM, Gettes LS, Katzung BG. Effect of lidocaine and quinidine on steady state characteristics and recovery kinetics of (dV/dt)max in guinea pig ventricular myocardium. *Circ Res* 37:20–29, 1975.

Clarkson CW, Hondeghem LM. Evidence for a specific receptor site for lidocaine, quinidine, and bupivacaine associated with cardiac sodium channels in guinea pig ventricular myocardium. *Circ Res* 56:496–506, 1985.

Clarkson CW, Matsubara T, Hondeghem LM. Slow inactivation of V_{max} in guinea pig ventricular myocardium. *Am J Physiol* 247:645–654, 1984.

Coromilias J, Kidwell GA. Voltage dependence of inactivation block by quinidine and flecainide: relationship to slow inactivation of the sodium channel. *Circulation* 74:20, 1986.

Courtney KR. Mechanism of frequency dependent inhibition of sodium currents in frog myelinated nerve by the lidocaine derivative GEA 968. *J Pharmacol Exp Ther* 195:225–236, 1975.

Courtney KR. Quantifying antiarrhythmic drug blocking during action potentials in guinea-pig papillary muscle. *J Mol Cell Cardiol* 15:749–757, 1983.

Courtney KR. Review: quantitative structure/activity relationships based on use-dependent block and repriming kinetics in myocardium. *JMCC* 19:319–330, 1987.

Courtney KR, Kendig JJ, Cohen EN. The rates of interaction of local anesthetics with sodium channels in nerve. *JPET* 207:594–604, 1978.

Davis JD, Matsubara T, Scheinman MM, Katzung BG, Hondeghem LM. Use-dependent effects of lidocaine on conduction in canine myocardium: application of the modulated receptor hypothesis in vivo. *Circulation* 74:205–214, 1986.

de Senac JB. *Traite de la Structure du Coeur, de son Action, et de ses Maladies*. Paris: Vincent; 1749.

Duff HJ, Roden D, Primm RK, Oates JA, Woosley RL. Mexiletine in the treatment of resistant ventricular arrhythmias: enhancement of efficacy and reduction of dose-related side effects of combination with quinidine. *Circulation* 67:1124, 1983.

Fenwick EM, Marty A, Neher E. Sodium and Calcium channels in bovine chromaffin cells. *J Physiol* (*Lond*) 331:599–635, 1982.

Gintant GA, Hoffman BF. Use-dependent block of cardiac sodium channels by quaternary derivatives of lidocaine. *Pflugers Arch* 400:121–129, 1984.

Grant AO, Trantham JL, Brown KK and Strauss HC: pH-dependent effects of quinidine on the kinetics of dV/dt_{max} in guinea ventricular myocardium. Circ Res 50:210–217, 1982.

Grant AO, Starmer CF, Strauss HC. Unitary sodium channels in isolated cardiac myocytes of rabbit. *Circ Res* 53:823–829, 1983.

Grant AO, Starmer CF. Mechanisms of closure of cardiac sodium channels in rabbit ventricular myocytes: single channel analysis. *Circ Res* 60:897–913, 1987.

Hille B. Local anesthetics: hydrophilic and hydrophobic pathways for the drug-Receptor reaction. *J Gen Physiol* 69:497–515, 1977.

Hille B. The pH-dependent rate of action of local anesthetics on the node of Ranvier *J Gen Physiol* 69:475–496, 1977.

Hodgkin AL, Huxley AF. A quantitative description of membrane current and its application to conduction and excitation in nerve. *J Physiol (Lond)* 117:500–544, 1952.

Hondeghem LM. Antiarrhythmic agents: modulated receptor applications. *Circulation* 75:514–520, 1987.

Hondeghem LM, Katzung BG. Antiarrhythmic agents: the modulated receptor mechanism of action of sodium and calcium channel-blocking drugs. *Annu Rev Pharmacol Toxicol* 24:387–423, 1984.

Hondeghemn LM, Katzung BG. Test of a model of antiarrhythmic drug action: effect of quinidine and lidocaine on myocardial conduction. *Circulation* 61:1217, 1980.

Hondeghem LM, Katzung BG. Time and voltage dependent interaction of antiarrhythmic drugs with cardiac sodium channels. *Biochim Biophys Acta* 472:373–398, 1977.

Hondeghem LM, Matsubara T. Quinidine blocks cardiac sodium channels during opening and slow inactivation in guinea-pig papillary muscle. *Br J Pharmacol* 93:311–318, 1988.

Johns JA, Anno T, Bennett PB, Snyders DJ, Hondeghem LM. Temperature and voltage dependence of sodium channel blocking and unblocking by O-demethyl encainide in isolated guinea pigs myocytes. *J Cardiovasc Pharmacol* 13:826–835, 1989.

Johnson EA, McKinnon MG. The differential effect of quinidine and pyrilamine on the myocardial action potential at various rates of stimulation. *JPET* 120:460–468, 1957.

Kunze DL, Lacerda AE, Wilson DL, Brown AM. Cardiac Na currents and the inactivating, reopening, and waiting properties of single cardiac Na channels. *J Gen Physiol* 86:691–719, 1985.

Lewis T. *The Mechanism and Graphic Registration of the Heart Beat.* London, England: Shaw and Sons, 359, 1925.

Mason JW, Hondeghem LM, Katzung BG. Block of inactivated sodium channels and of depolarization-induced automaticity in guinea pig papillary muscle by amiodarone. *Circ Res* 55:277–285, 1984.

Matsubara T, Clarkson C, Hondeghem L. Lidocaine blocks open and inactivated cardiac sodium channels. *Naunyn-Schmiedeberg's Arch Pharmacol* 336:224–231, 1987.

Nagy K. Evidence for multiple open states of sodium channels in neuroblastoma cells. *J Membr Biol* 96:251–262, 1987.

Nilius B, Benndorf K, Markwardt F. Effects of lidocaine on single cardiac sodium channels. *JMCC* 19:865–874, 1987.

Noda M, Shimizu S, Tanabe T, et al. Primary structure of electrophorus electricus sodium channel deduced from cDNA sequence. *Nature* 312:121–127, 1984.

Nonner WJ. Relations between the inactivation of sodium channels and the immobilization of gating charge in frog myelinated nerve. *J Physiol (Lond)* 299:573–603, 1980.

Saikawa T, Carmeliet. Slow recovery of the maximal rate of rise ($\dot{V}_{max}$) of the action potential in sheep cardiac Purkinje fibers. *Pflugers Arch* 394:90–93, 1982.

Scanley BE, Fozzard HA. Low conductance sodium channels in canine cardiac Purkinje cell. *Biophys J* 52:489–495, 1987.

Snyders DJ, Hondeghem LM. Effects of quinidine on the sodium current of guinea-pig myocytes: evidence for drug-associated rested state with altered kinetics. *Circ Res* 1989. In press.

Snyders DJ, Hondeghem LM. Use-dependent unblocking of quinidine-blocked sodium channels: slowed activation and inactivation. *Circulation* 76:150, 1987.

Snyders DJ, Hondeghem LM. Voltage- and temperature-dependent recovery of quinidine- blocked cardiac sodium channels. *Biophys J* 51:260a, 1987.

Starmer CF, Grant AO, Strauss HC. A model of the interaction of local anesthetics with Na channels. *Biophys J* 41:145a, 1983.

Starmer CF, Grant AO, Strauss HC. Mechanisms of use-dependent block of sodium channels in excitable membranes by local anesthetics. *Biophys J* 46:15–27, 1984.

Strichartz GR. The inhibition of sodium currents in myelinated nerve by quaternary derivatives of lidocaine. *J Gen Physiol* 62:37–57, 1973.
Vandenberg C, Horn R. Inactivatio viewed through single sodium channels. *J Gen Physiol* 84:535–564, 1984.
Wang GR, Strichartz GR. Local anesthetics produce phasic block of sodium channels during activation. *Biophys J* 45:286a, 1984.
Weidmann S. Effects of calcium ions and local anaesthetics on electrical properties of Purkinje fibres. *J Physiol* 129:568–582, 1955.
Wenckebach KF. *Die unregelmassige Herztatigkeit und ihre klinische Bedeutung*. Leipzig, East Germany: Engelmann, 1914.

Chapter 12

Membrane Pathway for Drug Binding to Protein Receptors

David W. Chester
Leo G. Herbette

INTRODUCTION

The molecular mechanisms involved in 1,4-dihydropyridine (DHP) antagonist/agonist interaction with voltage-dependent calcium channels are relatively unknown. Further, there is uncertainty in the interplay between drug stereoselectivity (and opposing inotropic activity of DHP enantiomers), membrane potential, receptor state, and the membrane itself as modulators of channel function. We have been interested in ascertaining the time-averaged location of these drugs in the bilayer where drug-membrane (both lipid and receptor) interactions are maximized. We have reasoned that if the membrane bilayer location is an important parameter in facilitating receptor binding, the physical chemical characteristics of that locale could induce drug conformations that differ substantially from that observed in crystal structure determinations where drug-drug interactions are maximized. In fact, molecular modelling calculations for the antiarrhythmic drug, amiodarone, suggest that there are several minimum energy conformations as a function of solvent (including air/water interfacial) interaction (Chatelain et al., 1986). In addition, we have shown that the energy minimized

Hondeghem, Luc (ed): Molecular and Cellular Mechanisms of Antiarrhythmic Agents, Futura Publishing Company, Inc., Mount Kisco, NY, © 1989.

structure for amiodarone in an isotropic environment (low dielectric medium) similar to its membrane bilayer location differs significantly from the crystal structure (Figs. 1A and 1B); Trumbore et al., 1988). More recently, Holtje and Marrer (1987), using a quantum mechanical calculation approach, have suggested that the minimum energy conformations of dihydropyridines (DHP) and the resulting molecular electrostatic potentials may play a role in defining antagonist versus agonist action on calcium channel gating even in the case of enantiomeric pairs of DHP.

DHP calcium channel antagonists inhibit voltage-dependent calcium channel *opening* in cardiac sarcolemma and a variety of other membranes (Janis and Triggle, 1984; Hess et al., 1984; Janis and Scriabine, 1983). The specific binding of these drugs to the membrane receptor has been shown by Belleman and coworkers (1983) to be highly stereoselective, saturable, and reversible with k_d values ranging between 0.1 and 5 nM (Janis and Triggle, 1984) with intrinsic *on rates* of 10^7 $(Ms)^{-1}$ (Rhodes et al., 1985; Herbette et al., 1986). Moreover, Lee and Tsien (1983) have demonstrated that receptor state is an important parameter in DHP binding. It appears that these ligands may bind more preferentially and with greater affinity to the inactivated state of the receptor, which is modulated by membrane potential (Bean, 1984; Lee and Tsien, 1983) and, possibly, receptor phosphorylation (Flockerzi et al., 1986). Flockerzi et al., (1986) have shown that phosphorylation of the α_1 subunit (M_r 142,000) of the t-tubule DHP receptor effects an increased probability of receptor complex/calcium channel opening.

High binding affinity and receptor stereoselectivity affect both drug action and activity. Langs and Triggle (1985) have demonstrated that subtle changes in the pyridine ring puckering or torsion angles between the antiparallel pyridine and aryl rings have substantial effects on drug activity as modulators of calcium channels. Crystallographic studies on a series of nifedipine analogs reveals a limited correlation between increasing distortion from pyridine ring planarity and pharmacological activity (Langs and Triggle, 1985; Triggle et al., 1980). As well, the orientation of the carboxylate carbonyl substituent relative to the pyridine ring double bond appears to be related to antagonist activity (Langs and Triggle, 1985). In general, a *cis* orientation places the ester group forward, toward the aryl ring, with the potential for stabilizing the antiparallel ring orientation. Further, since no functional *trans, trans* DHP isomers

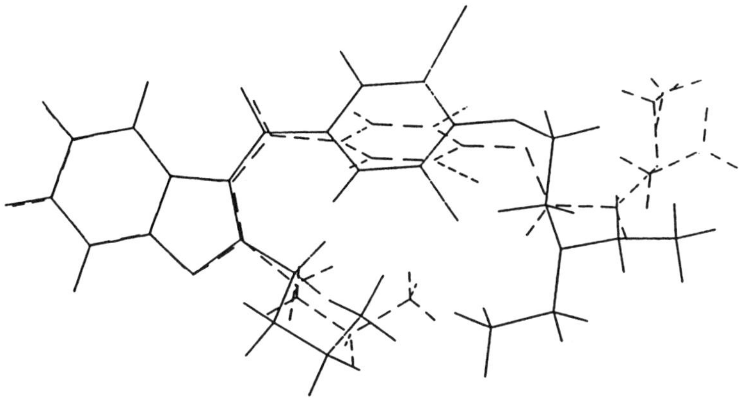

A

Figure 1A. The minimum energy structure of amiodarone (dashed bonds) calculated in a low dielectric constant medium with the program MMP2 superimposed on the crystal structure (solid bonds) of the drug.

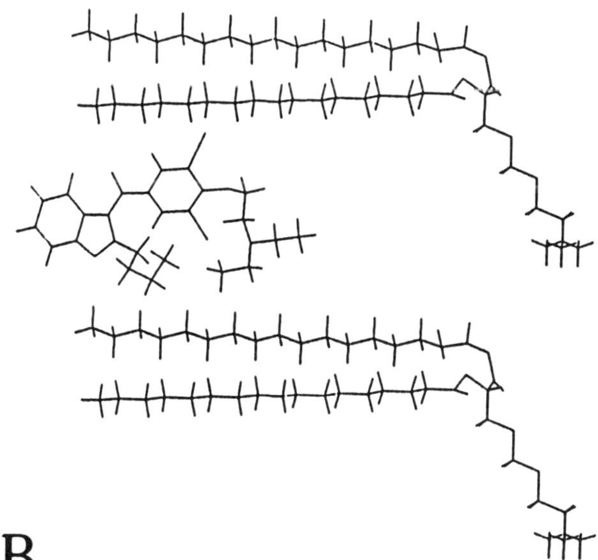

B

Figure 1B. Amiodarone incorporated into a membrane bilayer showing the position of the iodine atoms relative to the acly chains and the size of the molecule relative to the hydrocarbon core region.

have been identified, the *cis* orientation must convey some of the ligand activity (e.g., H bond potential, etc.).

Drug action is also markedly effected by ring substitution. The agonist BAY K 8644, containing a 3-nitro substituent to the pyridine ring, differs from a molecularly similar antagonist analog with a 3-carboxylate substitution (Langs and Triggle, 1985). Drug stereochemistry also impacts on activity since the enantiomeric pair of the DHP, Sandoz 202,791, exhibits both positive [S(+) isomer] and negative [R(-) isomer] inotropic activity (Hof et al., 1985; Kongsamut et al., 1985). Moreover, the S(+) agonist activity is converted to antagonist by membrane depolarization (Reuter et al., 1985). Thus, drug conformation and orientation are important criteria for consideration in the receptor ligand interaction as are the effects of membrane potential on the receptor site and functional activity.

A reasonable amount of progress has been made in the characterization, purification, and reconstitution of the voltage-dependent calcium channel from a variety of membrane sources. Initial work by Venter et al., (1983) and Curtis and Catterall (1984, 1986) yielded a DHP receptor of M_r 210–260,000 with an (M_r 135,000), (M_r 50,000), and (M_r 33,000) subunit structure. While there is disagreement in the literature regarding molecular weights and subunit composition, it appears that the receptor is comprised of a M_r 175,000 glycoprotein (α_2 or δ subunit), and nonglycosylated α_1, β and γ subunits of M_r 170, 50, and 33,000, respectively (Sharp et al., 1987; Takahashi and Caterall, 1987). The M_r 175,000 glycoprotein, as identified by wheatgerm peroxidase labeling, has been shown by a number of laboratories to migrate at ~M_r 150,000 under reducing conditions signifying that this subunit is coupled to a M_r 29–32,000 peptide via disulfide linkage(s). It is interesting to note, however, that there are differences between DHP receptor isolated from different sources. Horne et al., (1986) have isolated the DHP receptor from rat ventricular muscle with a variety of detergent regimes and determined an oligomeric complex molecular weight of M_r 370,000, which differs from that cited above. Rosenberg and coworkers (1986) have demonstrated through combined patch clamp and planar lipid bilayer electrophysiological studies that there are differences in the electrical characteristics of t-tubule and cardiac sarcolemmal voltage-dependent channels. Differences were identified in the gating properties between these two systems, namely, conductance, channel activity and channel activation, and open times. While there appears to be some functional (Rosenberg et al., 1986) and some antigenic (Takahashi and Catterall, 1987) differences between skeletal and cardiac DHP receptors, Takahashi and Catterall (1987) have shown that the two receptors share similar sedimentation coefficients with s values of 21 and 21.6 s for skeletal and cardiac channels, respectively. Recently, the complete amino acid sequence for the skeletal muscle DHP receptor was deduced from cDNA sequence analysis (Tanabe et al., 1987).

Several groups have prepared both mono- and polyvalent antibodies against these various components for the purpose of immunoprecipitation as well as to explore structural similarities between receptor sources. Antibodies (anti-140 and anti-32) prepared by Schmid et al., (1986) and Cooper and coworkers (1987) have demonstrated a clear relationship between the M_r 32,000 peptide and the M_r 175,000 DHP α_2 receptor glycoprotein. Moreover, they have used these antibodies to explore the structural similarities between receptor sources: skeletal muscle t-tubules, smooth muscle, and cardiac sarcolemma. It is interesting that antibodies generated against epitopes on the M_r 170,000 peptide (Leung et al., 1987) are capable of activating the calcium channel in planar lipid bilayer studies in the absence of added BAY K 8644. However, antibody binding does not appear to interfere with ligand binding, suggesting that the antibody does not have access to the BAY K 8644 binding site (Vilven et al., 1988). In yet another very interesting study, monoclonal antibodies derived against the skeletal muscle DHP receptor α_1) have been shown to specifically inhibit the slow inward DHP sensitive calcium current in BC3H1 myocytes in cell culture (Morton et al., 1988). Since they have demonstrated that their antibody does bind to a polypeptide in BC3H1 cells that is homologous to the DHP receptor in skeletal muscle, they postulate that this peptide is a functionally important component of the voltage-gated calcium channel rather than as a voltage sensor. One very exciting development is that Campbell et al., (1987) have been successful in preparing high affinity idiotypic antibodies against DHPs which could be used to probe the receptor binding domain. This antibody is very specific for DHP with K_d values in the femtomolar range and no observed binding for other calcium channel ligands.

Receptor activity may be modulated by phosphorylation, since Curtis and Catterall (1986) observed that the α_2 subunit is phosphorylated in intact t-tubule membranes, and both α and β subunits may be phosphorylated in vitro by the catalytic subunit of the cAMP dependent protein kinase. This observation has been disputed by

Imagawa et al., (1987) since they demonstrated, under their conditions, that the α_2 glycoprotein is not phosphorylated by the kinase. Moreover, they have identified an endogenous kinase, which is not regulated by either Ca^{+2}/calmodulin or cAMP, that phosphorylates the M_r 170,000 α_1 and M_r 52,000 β subunit proteins. Flockerzi et al., (1986) have suggested that cAMP dependent protein kinase phosphorylation of the α_1 subunit (M_r 142,000 in their system) is the functionally active site since the rate and extent of phosphorylation of this subunit is substantially greater than that observed for the β subunit. They have shown, in planar lipid bilayer reconstitution studies, that: (a) the isolated receptor is functional as a classical L-type calcium channel with single channel conductances of 20 pS; (b) these channels could be modulated by channel agonists (BAY K 8644) and antagonists (gallopamil); and (c) phosphorylation of the channel prolongs the channel open time and decreases the time interval between channel openings. These observations are consistent with the observations of Curtis and Catterall (1986) suggesting that the DHP receptor is the calcium channel itself since reconstituted receptor vesicles are active in facilitating DHP antagonist inhibitable calcium transport.

Rhodes and coworkers (1985) have proposed a two step model, the *membrane pathway* model, for DHP-receptor binding in which these drugs partition into and become oriented within the membrane bilayer before diffusing laterally on approach to the receptor binding site (Fig. 2). This pathway is in contrast to the *aqueous pathway* involving random diffusion through the bulk water phase outside the bilayer and subsequent binding to an exposed receptor site. Calculations of theoretical diffusion limited rates for anisotropic ligand-receptor binding indicates that the membrane pathway is 3 orders of magnitude faster than that of the aqueous pathway. The radioligand measured DHP binding rates of 10^7 $(Ms)^{-1}$ do not allow clear distinction between these two pathways since these values are within the range of the theoretical forward rate constants calculated for reasonably anisotropic ligands by an aqueous approach. From the preceeding discussion, it is clear that neither the ligand nor its binding is isotropic in nature and receptor binding is dependent upon several parameters in addition to diffusion. The calculated diffusion limited rates do not take into account these other binding constraints such as receptor state and, as a result only reflect the theoretical maximum diffusion limited rates for binding. It appears, therefore, that the receptor binding process is not dif-

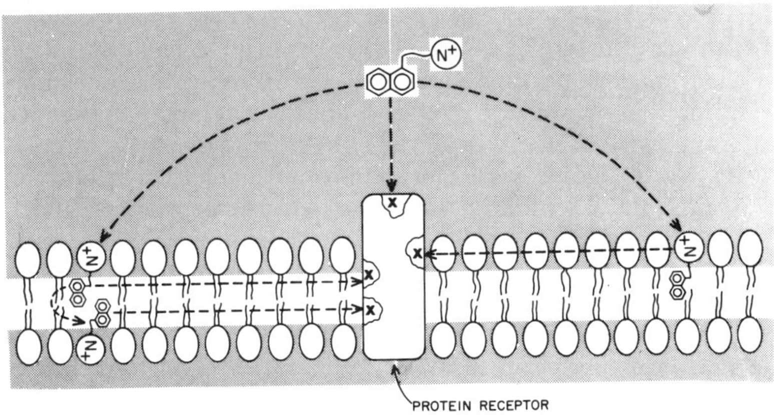

Figure 2. Drug receptor binding model illustrating a single step aqueous pathway to receptor binding (A) and a two step bilayer pathway (M). The components of the two step model are ligand partition into the membrane followed by lateral diffusion and subsequent interaction with a binding domain buried within the bilayer. An additional component is associated with flip-flop across the bilayer leaflet.

fusion limited such that the composite rates of the individual steps in the receptor binding process must be considered.

High membrane partition coefficients and an equilibrium position at the hydrocarbon core/water interface observed for these drugs (Herbette et al., 1986) support the notion that bulk lipid partitioning is a first step in the overall receptor binding mechanism. Moreover, the DHP nimodipine, has been shown by neutron diffraction studies to diffuse (*flip flop*) between the monolayers of the membrane bilayer (Herbette, 1986). This is consistent with recent studies conducted by Affolter and Coronado (1985, 1986) demonstrating that both DHPs (BAY K 8644) and phenylalkylamines (D-600) readily cross the bilayer to interact with asymmetrically reconstituted calcium channels in planar lipid bilayer systems.

Interaction and subsequent effects of drug on membrane structure and function has been a subject of interest and study for some time. Several biophysical techniques have been used to approach this problem (for comprehensive review, see Goldstein, 1984). The various techniques that have been applied involve (^{31}P, ^{2}H, ^{1}H, ^{13}C) nuclear magnetic resonance (NMR), electron spin resonance (ESR), differential scanning calorimetry, fluorescence spectroscopy, and x-ray and neutron diffraction. NMR [^{2H}] studies were used to determine the position of the local anesthetic, benzyl alcohol, in the mid-acyl chain region of the membrane bilayer. Another local anesthetic, dibucaine, was shown in ^{31}P NMR studies to interact with the membrane surface (Cullis and De Kruijff, 1979). Studies of phenothiazine (antipsychotic ligand: e.g., chlorpromazine)/ membrane interactions using differential scanning calorimetry, in concert with ^{13}C and ^{31}P NMR studies, have shown that the phenothiazine dialkylaminoalkyl chains are oriented near the phospholipid headgroups with the heterocyclic ring structure penetrating just beyond the glycerol backbone into the hydrocarbon region of the membrane (Frenzel et al., 1978). This bilayer position is similar to that observed by diffraction techniques for the β adrenergic receptor antagonist, propranolol (Herbette et al., 1983), which has similar structural characteristics. The location determined for the phenothiazine class of drug is consistent with a recent finding pertaining to its noncompetitive binding to the acetylcholine receptor (Giraudat et al., 1987). In these studies, it has been shown that chlorpromazine, as a noncompetitive channel blocker, was photoaffinity labelled to the hydrophobic spanning domain of the β subunit.

Traditional radioligand filtration assays have been used to measure receptor-ligand binding interactions. While these techniques are sufficient to study equilibrium conditions, the time-resolved capabilities are somewhat limited. The fluorescence spectroscopic approach has been used for both equilibrium (Bentley et al., 1985; Kolb et al., 1983) and time-resolved (for comprehensive review, see text edited by Shaafi and Fernandez, 1983) measurements of receptor-ligand interaction. The review by Bentley et al., (1985) highlights the use of fluorescence polarization as a means of examining steady state receptor binding parameters. The fluorescence redistribution after photobleaching (FRAP) technique has been successfully employed to ascertain the diffusional dynamics of various molecules (including a calcium channel antagonist (Chester et al., 1987) in a variety of membrane systems (Koppel, 1979; Shaafi and Fernandez, 1983). Moreover, this technique offers the potential of assessing, simultaneously, diffusion rates associated with fast and slow diffusing components of the membrane bilayer (Koppel and Sheetz, 1983).

In our studies, we have employed both diffraction and fluorescence spectroscopic techniques as an approach in addressing the question of ligand location and kinetics associated with drug-membrane bilayer and receptor interactions. The time-averaged drug location within the bilayer was determined by x-ray and neutron diffraction approaches. The use of isomorphous substitution techniques (identical drug structures with the exception that the analogs are deuterated at different specific locations within the molecule) in neutron diffraction studies has the potential to allow both orientational and possibly conformational assignments for these ligands in the membrane bilayer and at receptor sites, if the receptor site density in the membrane can be made sufficiently high. These time-averaged structures can then be compared to both calculated quantum mechanical minimum energy and crystal structures. The fluorescence studies examined the kinetics (time-resolved properties) of the microscopic events associated with the receptor binding pathway. It should be possible, with tandem use of these techniques, to distinguish between a one step aqueous route to receptor binding or a membrane bilayer pathway that involves bilayer partition, lateral diffusion, and receptor-ligand interaction for a variety of membrane protein receptors. Moreover, the fluorescence techniques offer the capacity to examine the relative effects of such things as membrane bilayer physical state on the receptor binding pathway.

While we feel the pathway to receptor binding is important, there are limits to evaluating relative receptor binding rates as a function of receptor site density. McClosky and Poo (1986) have suggested that only under the conditions of high ligand partition and low receptor site density would a substantial rate advantage be gained by a 2-step membrane bilayer pathway. In their analyses, they consider the receptor as a perfectly absorbing trap and ignore the potential for bilayer partitioning to facilitate equilibrium drug conformation/orientation. Interestingly, Colvin et al., (1985) and Herbette et al., (1985) have demonstrated that these prescribed conditions of high membrane partition coefficients for DHPs and low DHP receptor site density are met in cardiac sarcolemmal membranes.

METHODS OF APPROACH

Sample Preparation

Multilayer membrane samples for diffraction and fluorescence (FRAP) studies were prepared by the spin dry method as described in detail in a previous communication (Chester et al., 1987). Briefly, multilamellar vesicle preparations used in these studies were added to lucite sedimentation cells containing either a nonfluorescent "Aclar" (Dacron, Allied Chemical Co., NJ) or aluminum foil substrate used respectively for FRAP or diffraction measurements. The vesicles were sedimented onto the substrate after which the normal bucket caps were replaced with *spin dry caps* and the pelleted vesicles spin dried under centrifuge vacuum at 65,000 × g for 5 hours. On completion of the spin dry process, the samples were mounted and rehydrated over saturated salt solutions, which define specific relative humidities.

Diffraction

Small Angle X-ray and Neutron Diffraction

X-ray diffraction experiments with membrane lipid bilayers were carried out using a GX-18 rotating anode generator (Marconi Avionics, Borehamstead, England), equipped with a camera utilizing a single Franks' mirror as previously described in detail (Herbette et al., 1985). The diffraction patterns were collected on either film (Kodak NS-5T) or a Braun position sensitive proportional counting gas flow detector (Innovative Technology Inc., South Hamilton, Mass).

Diffraction samples were equilibrated to different relative humidities in sealed containers at 8°C. Diffraction peak intensities obtained from samples at various relative humidities were integrated and these appropriately phased (phasing of the structure factors by a swell analysis) structure factors were used to generate one dimensional electron density profile structures.

Neutron diffraction studies were carried out at the Brookhaven National Laboratory High Flux Beam Reactor (Upton, NY). For these studies, specifically deuterated drug analogs were used as isomorphous replacements for protonated drug to assign ligand location as a function of the deuterium location. The structure factors were phased either by a swell analysis, as in the x-ray case, or by plots of the structure factor against D_20/H_20 ratios to facilitate sample contrast variation.

Small Molecule Crystallographic Studies

Selected crystals of different drugs were mounted on a glass fiber. All diffraction was collected using a TEXRAY/Rigaku system equipped with a RU-200 generator, AFC-5 diffractometer, and TEXRAY control software. The entire system was obtained from Molecular Structure Corp. (College Station, Tex). Intensity data was collected by measuring counts at peak positions, and background corrected. Sample degradation was monitored by measuring the intensity of three standard reflections every 150 points. Crystal structures were solved by direct methods using the TEXSAN package of programs (Molecular Structures Corp., College Station, Tex.), including MITHRIL.

Fluorescence Studies

The fluorescence studies have involved both fluorescence redistribution after photobleaching (FRAP) and spectroscopy techniques as a means of addressing the time-resolved questions of ligand partition, lateral diffusion, and receptor binding. The FRAP studies used multilamellar stacks similar to those in the diffraction experiments. This allows us to work at very low probe to lipid concentrations while obtaining a very good signal to noise ratio. FRAP measurements of diffusion coefficients for $DiIC_{16}$ (phospholipid) and nisoldipine-lissamine rhodamine (Ns-R) were performed with an excitation wavelength of 5145 A on an Ortholux II fluorescence microscope (E. Leitz, Inc., Rockleigh, NJ) equipped with a vertical illuminator, water-cooled argon laser light source (Lexel), and a galvanometric scanning mirror. The basic design and geometry of the optical system has been previously described (Koppel, 1979). The diffusion coefficients were determined as a function of relative bilayer hydration as detailed by Chester et al., (1987). The initially uniform sample fluorescence was locally depleted (or bleached) by short (40 msec) exposure to a laser beam focused by a $10\times$ objective to a small, circularly symmetric spot. The fluorescence redistribution after photobleaching was followed with a series of 12-point scans with an attenuated monitoring beam. The percent recovery and recovery rate were determined with a 3 parameter non-linear least squares analysis of the time decay of the fluorescence depletion monitored coincident with the position of the bleaching pulse.

Molecular Modelling: Calculation of Drug Structures in the Membrane Bilayer

The molecular mechanics program MMP2, which assumes a homogeneous environment for the molecule, was used to estimate the minimum energy conformation of a ligand in the bilayer. Where necessary, due to the lack of needed parameters (e.g., iodine atom bond angles, bond energies, etc.) in the MMP2 parameter set, parameters used were based on published values. Initial starting coordinates for these analyses were obtained from crystallographic x-ray diffraction data. In order to determine the minimum energy conformation, energy minima were computed in a dielectric range from k = 2 to k = 80. At k = 2, the dihedral driver option of MMP2 was then used to generate several energy minimized sets of conformations related to the initial crystallographic conformation. These conformations were generated by torsion in 60° steps about bonds of interest. The total energies of the minimized structures derived from the crystal structures and the dihedral driver option were compared to determine whether a given structure was a local minimum. The conformation with the lowest total energy was deemed to be the global minimum for the study. The structure of lowest energy was then compared with the crystal structure using some common origin for the two structures and the relative differences noted. Some graphics and geometric calculations used CHEM-X, developed and distributed by Chemical Design Ltd., Oxford, England.

RESULTS AND DISCUSSION

As stated in the previous section, we have attempted to use the techniques of diffraction and fluorescence to assess both location and kinetics for a number of drugs in bilayers. The basic tenant behind these studies is summarized in Fig. 2, which represents a model for the pathways by which lipophilic ligands may bind to the membrane and interact with specific receptors. There is a reasonable amount of evidence from our laboratory and others (Kokubun and Reuter, 1984; Affolter and Coronado, 1985; Vilven et al., 1988) to suggest that partitioning of the ligand into membrane bilayers is an integral first step in the receptor binding pathway. With this pathway as our basic assumption, we embarked upon a series of studies to examine the location of several drugs in a variety of membrane preparations, and have begun to examine the kinetics of the steps involved in the overall receptor binding process: ligand partition, bilayer diffusion, and receptor interaction.

Figure 3 is a summary of the locations that have been identified for a β adrenergic antagonist (propranolol), uncharged DHP calcium

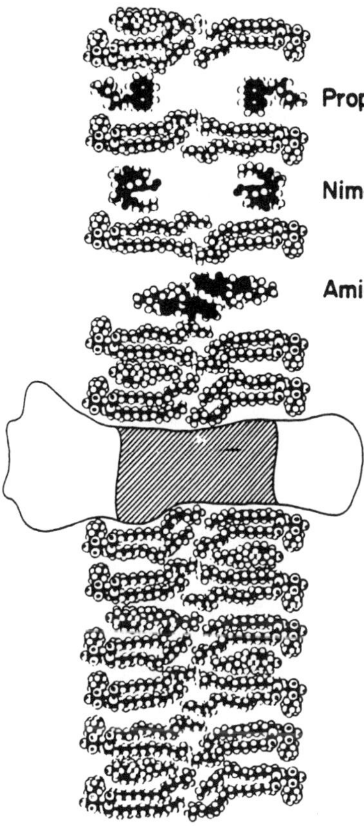

Figure 3. Illustration depicting the relative locations of propranolol, nimodipine and amiodarone in a membrane bilayer as determined by x-ray and neutron diffraction.

channel antagonist (nimodipine), and the antiarrhythmic agent amiodarone. We have been able to show that both DHP receptor agonists (BAY K 8644) and antagonists (nimodipine and BAY P 8857) share a similar position within the bilayer. This is interesting in light of the suggestion that agonists and antagonists compete for the same binding domain on the receptor (Janis et al., 1984; Hamilton et al., 1987). The charged DHP receptor antagonist, amlodipine, appears to be located in the same general location but is positioned slightly higher in the bilayer toward the phosphate headgroups. This location is reasonable since the quaternary amine moiety of this ligand would be expected to interact with the zwitterionic charge plane of the headgroup region of the membrane bilayer. This is consistent with the observations regarding the bilayer headgroup interactions with the charged moiety for propranolol. Drug partitioning to the bilayer hydrocarbon core/water interface would suggest that the physical chemical characteristics (charge character, abrupt change in dielectric about the interface, structured water phase, hydrogen bond potential, etc.) of this interfacial region would provide a minimum free energy environment for drug interaction. In our studies with amiodarone, we have determined that this drug is located below the bilayer interface. This location is consistent with its very high membrane partition coefficient of $\sim 10^6$. Moreover, the residence half-time for this drug in the membrane bilayer is very long and is comparable to the observed long clinical half-life (Herbette et al., 1988). This would suggest that amiodarone is relatively inaccessible to the bulk aqueous phase. From the structure studies, then, it appears that drugs that interact with the membrane have well defined time-averaged locations. These locations may be related to the position of the receptor binding domain along the bilayer normal. As such, the relative correlation between these two *sites* would have a dramatic effect on the effective ligand concentration at the binding site (see Fig. 7).

Ligand partition to the bilayer hydrocarbon core/water interface would, on a time-averaged basis, produce a steep concentration gradient of drug about this interface as illustrated in Figure 4. With regard to our proposed bilayer pathway model, either the membrane is functioning as an effective *sponge,* or drug partitioning into the bilayer is an integral first step in the receptor binding process. Since it appears from a number of studies (Affolter and Coronado, 1985, 1986; Kokubun and Reuter, 1984) with both DHP and phenylalkylamine calcium channel blockers that receptor binding site access must be gained via ligand partitioning into the bilayer, these data strongly support the latter contention for the nonspecific time-averaged drug location; that is, partition is the first step in the receptor binding mechanism. As such, drug partitioning to the bilayer hydrocarbon core/water interface would produce a plane of locally high drug concentration within which lateral diffusion would occur.

We have used the fluorescence redistribution after photobleaching (FRAP) technique with a fluorescent DHP, Nisoldipine-lissamine rhodamine (Ns-R, Fig. 5) to assess the diffusional dynamics of these ligands in pure cardiac sarcolemmal lipid bilayers. The drug

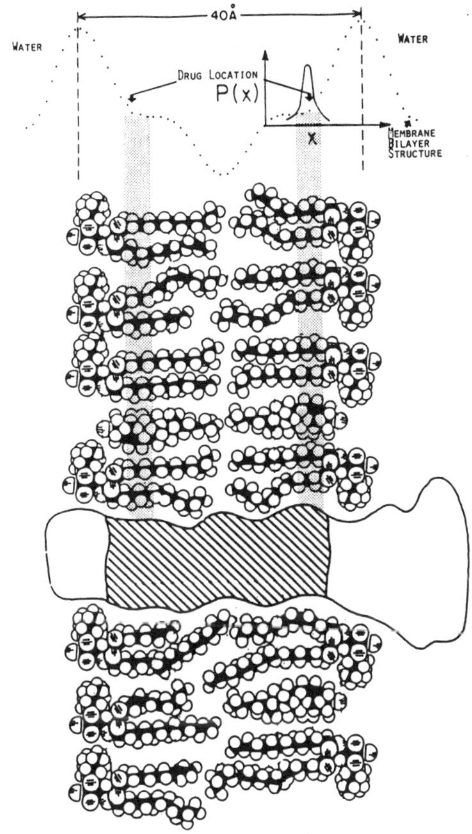

Figure 4. This figure illustrates a membrane with its x-ray diffraction profile structure and a drug concentration gradient centered about the hydrocarbon core/water interface. Ligand partitioning to this interface results in a plane of high drug concentration within which diffusion can occur.

diffusion data were compared with phospholipid diffusion using the probe $DiIC_{16}$ (Fig. 5). As a reference, a typical FRAP data set is shown in Figure 6A. Represented here are 3 basic data representations: (a) stacks of 12 point scans across the bleach point (indicated by the gaussian depletion); (b) the actual scan profile (fluorescence depletion followed by recovery back to the initial prebleached intensity); and (c) 3 parameter least squares fit of the data coincident with the bleach point. As the bilayers were maximally hydrated, the diffusion coefficients calculated for both the Ns-R and phospho-

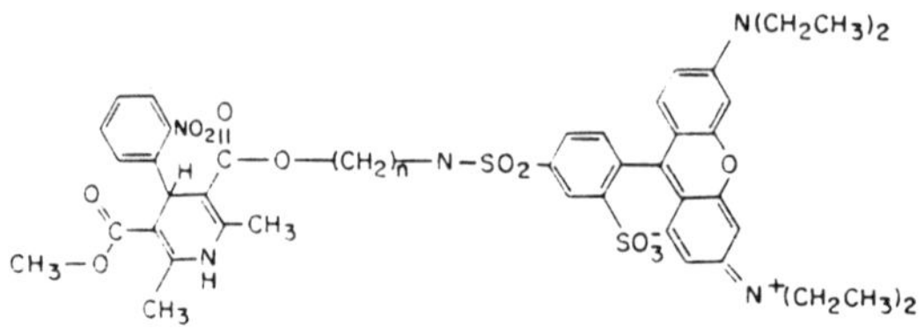

NISOLDIPINE-LISSAMINE RHODAMINE

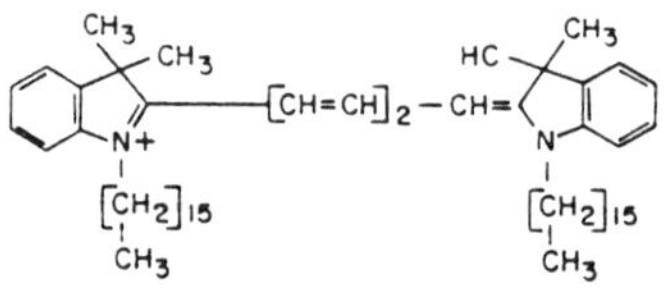

1,1'-DIHEXADECYL-3,3,3',3'-TETRAMETHYLINDOCARBOCYANINE
(DiI 16:0)

Figure 5. Structures for Nisoldipine-Lissamine Rhodamine (Ns-R) and $DiIC_{16}$ probes used in FRAP experiments for determination of drug diffusion coefficients.

lipid were essentially identical with a value of 4×10^{-8} cm^2/sec (Fig. 6B). Further studies with this and other probes have demonstrated that this value is a reasonable lower limit for drug diffusion in these membranes. We are currently in the process of determining the partition rates for these compounds into the membrane bilayer. Preliminary data indicate that drug partition is rapid with a half-time to completion of 5–6 seconds (unpublished observations, to appear in a separate communication). As such, we can begin to assess time constants for ligand partitioning into the bilayer and diffusion within the bulk lipid matrix en route to specific receptor binding.

It is clear that the physical chemical characteristics of the time-averaged bilayer location of a drug would have some potential ramifications on the orientation and conformation of the ligand in this environment. This conformation could be substantially different than that observed in crystal structure studies where drug-drug interactions are maximized. We have reasoned that the membrane conformation is the more relevant structure, and have suggested

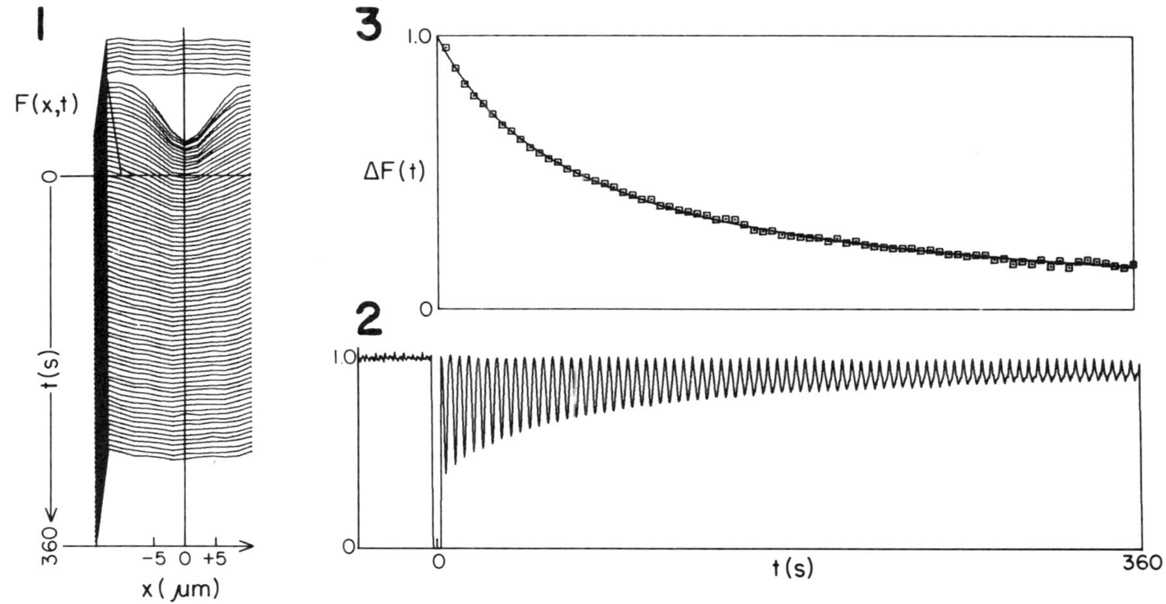

Figure 6A. Representation of a typical FRAP data set. (1) represents a stack of 84 individual 12 point scans through the bleached area (local fluorescence depletion); (2) represents the linear sequence of all scans during a series of fluorescence scans; and (3) represents a 3 parameter least squares fit of the data coincident with the bleach point.

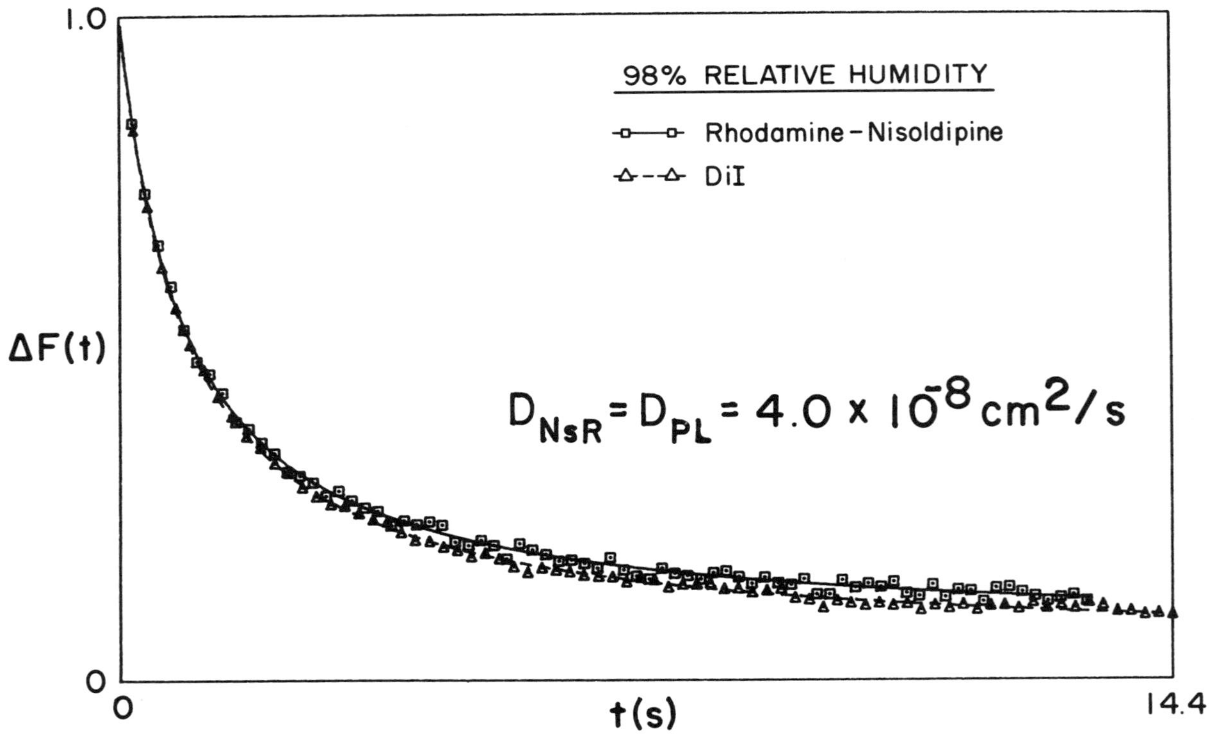

Figure 6B. Representation of 3 parameter least squares fit of data obtained for Ns-R and $DiIC_{16}$ at near maximum bilayer hydration (98% relative humidity), and demonstrates the similarity in diffusion coefficients for these two probes.

that an equilibrium conformation and orientation at a discrete location in the bilayer may facilitate receptor binding. This would be particularly true for highly anisotropic ligands where only specific conformations (and orientations) would result in successful receptor binding.

While we are attempting to determine directly the conformation and orientation of ligands in membranes using neutron diffraction techniques, it was of interest to examine quantum mechanically environmental effects on drug conformation. For these studies, minimum energy conformations for amiodarone were calculated for several different dielectric constant values using the MMP2 program, which assumes a homogeneous environment for the molecule. Crystal structure data were used for the initial starting coordinates. Since electronic interactions made only minor contributions to the total energy of the structure, increasing dielectric constant (k) from k = 2 to k = 80 had a negligible effect on the calculated conformation. While we realize the constraints to this assumption, our starting assumption is that the bilayer hydrocarbon core can be represented as an isotropic solution. Since, as discussed above, amiodarone assumes a time-averaged location deep within the bilayer, k = 2 was used to calculate the minimum energy structure of this drug in the bilayer. We anticipate that drug conformation changes would be even more pronounced when acyl chain interactions are taken into account.

Energy minimization of amiodarone under the aforesaid conditions produced significant changes in the membrane associated drug structure as compared with the crystallographic structure. The lowest energy structure showed an overall RMS shift of 1.36 A from the initial crystal structure. The largest change was a reorientation of the benzofuran ring with respect to the central 3,5-diiodophenyl ring. In the crystal structure, the torsion angle between these two rings was 81.84°. In the energy minimized bilayer structure, the benzofuran ring was more nearly parallel to the diiodophenyl ring with torsion angle of 40.85° as shown in Figure 1 (Trumbore et al., 1988). Shifts in the conformation of other regions of the molecule were not as pronounced but were significant. From these observations, we suggest that for membrane-active drugs, the structure of the drug in the bilayer is not necessarily the same as its crystal structure. Thus, drug design modalities for membrane-active drugs that rely on some structure-function activity information should be based on a structure data base that is derived from the relevant environment in which these drugs reside. To this end, our molecular modelling approaches must begin to evaluate the effects of bilayer anisotropy on ligand minimum energy comformations.

Figure 7 presents several model considerations that may have impact on drug pharmacokinetics as well as pharmacodynamics. Our initial hypothesis, highlighted in Figure 2, is that there are two basic pathways that can be considered with respect to drug receptor interaction: an aqueous pathway, and a membrane bilayer pathway. In the case of the acetylcholine receptor, the interaction of acetylcholine appears to occur via an aqueous route while the interaction of the noncompetitive inhibitor, chlorpromazine, occurs via the bilayer route (Giraudat et al., 1987). Our structure data and that of others clearly supports the concept that the membrane bilayer pathway may be operable for several amphipathic ligands and protein receptors in addition to the DHP receptor. With regard to the overall rates of receptor binding, however, there are a number of conditions that must be taken into account. McCloskey and Poo (1986) have shown that receptor site density is an important consideration when evaluating the advantage of one pathway over the other. These authors point out that at high receptor site density, binding rates via aqueous or membrane routes essentially would be inseparable. Conversely, at low receptor site density, there would be a substantial rate advantage gained by drug partitioning into the membrane bilayer. This is clearly the case with respect to DHP receptor interaction in cardiac sacrolemma where the density is approximately 1 receptor site per μ^2 (Colvin et al., 1985). Moreover, these membranes have a substantially increased lipid to protein ratio (approximately 2–3 mol lipid per mg protein) than that observed with other membrane sources (0.6–0.8 mol lipid per mg protein) (Colvin et al., 1985).

Our structure data has also revealed that different drugs do not always occupy the same general membrane locale. While it is clear that the hydrocarbon core/water interface does provide a highly anisotropic environment, which accommodates certain drug interactions, clearly other drugs such as amiodarone are not found at this position in the membrane profile structure. There is some recent preliminary evidence to suggest that phenylalkylamines, as well, interact at a position below the hydrocarbon core/water interface. Thus, for both amiodarone and phenylalkylamines, the bulk of the molecule is below the interfacial region. At this time, while we have tried to model these drugs in an environment that might *mimic* the

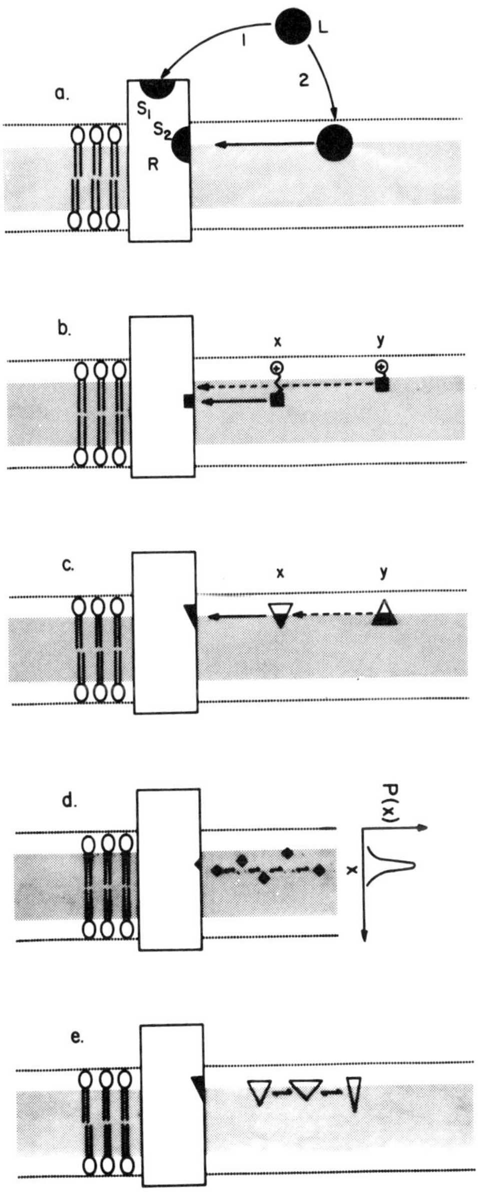

Figure 7. Molecular parameters that my define the basis for the design of membrane active drugs. (a) Drug L may reach a binding site on the surface of the membrane via an aqueous route (1) or by membrane bilayer pathway (2). (b) The highly ordered acyl chain pacing characteristics may restrict the depth of penetration of the ligand such as to change the local drug concentration at the level of the site. (c) Bilayer constraints on the orientation of the drug may affect binding ability. (d) Diffusion about an equilibrium position in the membrane as a function of the ligand concentration gradient centered about the interface. (e) Ligand conformational effects as a function of bilayer interaction.

hydrocarbon region of the bilayer, we can not ascribe definitive conformational and orientational characteristics to these drugs because the core region of the membrane cannot be adequately represented by an isotropic solution. Figure 7B illustrates the potential effects that bilayer structure may have on the level of ligand penetration. An interesting consideration for evaluation is the relative correlation between the location along the bilayer normal of the receptor binding domain and the time-averaged drug location. As shown, this could have impact on the absolute drug concentration at the level of the binding site as well as the absolute rate of specific receptor interaction. We also have observed recently that changes in bilayer physical state can have some impact on the observed location of drugs in the membrane.

Figures 7C and 7E illustrate the potential effects of bilayer location on drug orientation and conformation. A myriad of structure-activity studies have been performed demonstrating that, at least in the case of DHP, receptor binding is highly stereospecific. This stereospecificity mandates that the ligand, upon *presentation* to the receptor, would have to be in some reasonably well-defined conformation and orientation. That is to say, that with all degrees of freedom for drug rotation, translation, vibration, etc., an increased collision frequency would be required to obtain a *successful* interaction. Inherent in the drug molecule, there appears to be some molecular constraints that limit particular bond rotations and, hence, facilitate receptor binding (increased binding affinities). A case in point is the orientation of the DHP carbonyl groups relative to the pyridine ring. As pointed out previously, the *cis* configuration appears to place the ester substituents closer to the phenyl ring thereby stabilizing its antiparallel orientation relative to the pyridine ring plane (Langs and Triggle, 1985). On the other hand, the physical chemical characteristics of the drug interaction within the bilayer would tend to potentiate energy minimized drug conformations as a function of its environment. Phospholipid packing constraints, charge characteristics, hydrogen bond potential, counterion interactions, etc., would be anticipated to constrain *allowable* conformations and orientations of the drug in the membrane bilayer. We have reasoned that the equilibrium conformations and orientations would actually facilitate an increase in *successful* collisions with the receptor due partially to the reduced degrees of freedom allowed by drug partition to a discrete location in the bilayer. This discrete location and its relative impact on drug receptor interaction are highlighted in Figures 4 and 7D. Thus, the orientation and conformation of a drug in a membrane bilayer is highly coupled to the location that the drug assumes in this membrane.

While we have shown data and speculated on what we interpret to be the pathway for drug interaction with membrane receptors, it is interesting to speculate on the mechanism by which certain drugs exhibit differential effects on calcium channel activity as a function of membrane potential. In a number of cases opposing inotropic activity of drug enantiomers has been sighted (Hof et al., 1985; Kongsamut et al., 1985; Reuter et al., 1985). Moreover, in some cases (e.g., Sandoz 202,791 compound) changes in membrane potential can change agonist activity into antagonist activity (Reuter et al., 1985). Changes in membrane potential would not be expected to have their greatest effect on the physical chemical environment of the membrane and, hence, the drug's environment. Thus, the drug orientation and conformation would be expected to remain constant as constrained by its membrane environment. However, it's anticipated that the greatest effect would be on the receptor protein. This effect may occur as a function of a voltage sensor protein, which interacts with the DHP receptor, thereby changing the binding interaction, or via a direct effect on the receptor itself (binding domain configurational change) to facilitate the agonist to antagonist shift.

Recently, a quantum mechanical modelling paper showed that, as a function of minimum energy drug conformation, one could differentiate between agonists and antagonist in the electrostatic potential over the 5′ carboxylate of the DHP (Höltje and Marrer, 1987). They reasoned that the different electrostatic charge potentials for agonists and antagonists could effect the potential of the receptor protein. To examine this, they chose to model the interaction of tryptophan with the DHP, since this amino acid residue would tend to induce positive electrostatic potentials for a ligand in close proximity. Their conclusion is that the electrostatic charge potential of the tryptophan residue was influenced in direct proportion by the electrostatic potential of the DHP. One may postulate, then, that DHP interaction within the receptor binding domain may involve hydrophobic stacking interactions between ligand and aromatic amino acid residues in the binding pocket. As well, one may envision a myriad of hydrogen bond potentials between the ligand and charged amino acid residues in the binding pocket as well. Rebek (1987), in a very interesting publication, examined model building for molecular recognition. In his studies, a variety of parameters were assessed including binding forces, site selectivity, substrate character, microenvironment, etc., which would be expected to affect binding of substrate into the molecular recognition cleft. Some of these considerations may prove useful in evaluating the interaction of DHP with their receptors in the membrane, and in building new hypotheses regarding mechanisms for ligand inotropic activity as well as drug design.

CONCLUSIONS

An understanding of the molecular mechanism of drug binding to membrane proteins mandates that both the structure of the drug in different environments be determined and the kinetics of interaction with these different environments be known. In addition, a static and dynamic picture of how drugs interact with cell membranes can be used in the design of agents that exhibit an optimized pharmacokinetic and pharmacodynamic profile. With the advent of new biophysical approaches, these molecular parameters can now be determined. Thus, a rational approach to drug design and drug delivery may eventually be secured at a molecular level.

Acknowledgments: We would like to thank Drs. J. Moring and S.D. Wang for providing the crystallographic coordinates used in the molecular mechanics calculations, and Dr. A.M. Katz for continual discussions regarding drug-membrane interactions, which allowed us to relate these results to clinical questions. We also would like to thank Dr. D.G. Rhodes for his invaluable input into these studies, especially in the area of modelling. Graphics and geometric calculations in Figure 1 and accompanying discussion were provided by CHEM-X, developed and distributed by Chemical Design Ltd., Oxford, England. This work was supported by research grants HL-33026 and HL-07420 from the National Institutes of Health, by a grant from the Whitaker Foundation, and a gift from the Paterson Trust Foundation and RJR Nabisco, Inc. We also would like to thank our graduate students M. Trumbore and R.P. Mason who were supported by a Health Center Research Advisory Committee Graduate Student Fellowship. Dr. L. Herbette acknowledges his current affiliation as an Established Investigator of the American Heart Association. The work was carried out in the Biomolecular Structure Analysis Center at the University of Connecticut Health Center. We would also like to thank Ms. Tammy Wojtusik for preparing the final form of this manuscript for submission. The Structure Center acknowledges support from the State of Connecticut Department of Higher Education's High Technology Project and Grant Program.

BIBLIOGRAPHY

Affolter H, Coronado R. Agonists of Bay K 8644 and CGP 28392. Open calcium channels from skeletal muscle transverse tubules. *Biophys J* 48:341–347, 1985.

Affolter H, Coronado R. The sidedness of reconstituted calcium channels from muscle transverse tubules as determined by D-600 and D-890 blockade. *Biophys J* 49:197a, 1986.

Bean BP. Nitrendipine block of cardiac calcium channels: high-affinity binding to the inactivated state. *Proc Natl Acad Sci (USA)* 81:6388–6392, 1984.

Belleman P, Schade A, Towart R. Dihydropyridine receptor in rate brain labeled with (^{3}H)nimodipine. *Proc Natl Acad Sci (USA)* 80:2356–2360, 1983.

Bently KL, Thompson LK, Klebe RJ, Horowitz PM. Fluorescence polarization: a general method for measuring ligand binding and membrane microviscosity. *Biotechniques* 3:356–366, 1985.

Campbell KP, Sharp AH, Strom M, Kahl SD. High-affinity antibodies to the 1,4-dihydrophridine Ca^{2+}-channel blockers. *Proc Nat Acad Sci USA* 83(9):2792–2796, 1987.

Chatelain P, Ferreira J, Laurel R, Ruysschaert JM. Amiodarone induced modifications of the phospholipid physical state. A fluorescence polarization study. *Biochem Pharmacol* 35:3007–2013, 1986.

Chester DW, Herbette LG, Mason RP, Joslyn AF, Triggle DJ, Koppel DE. Diffusion of dihydropyridine calcium channel antagonists in cardiac sarcolemmal lipid multibilayers. *Biophys J* 52:1021–1030, 1987.

Colvin RA, Ashavaid TF, Herbette LG. Structure function studies of canine cardiac sarcolemmal membranes. I. Estimation of receptor site densities. *Biochim Biophys Acta* 812:601–608, 1985.

Cooper CL, Vandaele S, Barhanin J, Fosset M, Lazdunski M, Hosey MM. Purification and characterization of the dihydropyridine-sensitive voltage-dependent calcium channel from cardiac tissue. *J Biol Chem* 262:509–512, 1987.

Cullis PR, De Kruijff, B. Lipid polymorphism and the functional roles of lipids in biological membranes. *Biochim Biophys Acta* 559:399–402, 1979.

Curtis BM, Catterall WA. Purification of the calcium antagonist receptor of the voltage-sensitive calcium channel from skeletal muscle transverse tubules. *Biochem* 23:2113–2118, 1984.

Curtis BM, Catterall WA. Reconstitution of the voltage-sensitive calcium channel purified from skeletal muscle transverse tubules. *Biochem* 25:3077–3083, 1986.

Flockerzi V, Oeken HJ, Hofmann F, Pelzer D, Cavalie A, Twauntwein W. Purified dihydropyridine-binding site from skeletal muscle T-tubules is a functional calcium channel. *Nature* 323:66–68, 1986.

Frenzel J, Arnold K, Nuhn P. Calorimetric ^{13}C NMR and ^{31}P NMR studies on the interaction of some phenothiazine derivatives with dipalmitoyl phosphatidylcholine model membranes. *Biochim Biophys Acta* 507:185–197, 1978.

Giraudat J, Dennis M, Heidmann T, Haumont PY, Lederer F, Changeux JP. Structure of the high-affinity binding site for noncompetitive blockers of the acetylcholine receptor. [^{3}H]chlorpromazine labels homologous residues in the β and δ chains. *Biochem* 26:2410–2418, 1987.

Goldstein DB. The effects of drugs on membrane fluidity. *Annu Rev Pharmacol Toxicol* 24:43–64, 1984.

Hamilton SL, Yatani A, Brush K, Schwartz A, Brown AM. A comparison between the binding and electrophysiological effects of dihydropyridines on cardiac membranes. *Mol Pharmacol* 31:221–231, 1987.
Herbette LG, Chester DW, Rhodes DG. Structural analysis of drug molecules in biological membranes. *Biophys J* 49:91–93, 1986.
Herbette LG, Katz AM, Sturtevant JM. Comparison of the interaction of propranolol and timolol with model and biological membrane systems. *Mol Pharmacol* 24:259–269, 1983.
Herbette LG, MacAlister T, Ashavaid TF, Colvin RA. Structure-function studies of canine cardiac sarcolemmal membranes. II. Structural organization of the sacrolemmal membrane as determined by electron microscopy and lamellar x-ray diffraction. *Biochim Biophys Acta* 812:609, 1985.
Herbette LG, Trumbore M, Chester DW, Katz AM. Possible molecular basis for the pharmacokinetics and pharmacodynamics of three membrane-active drugs: propranolol, nimodipine, and amiodarone. *J Mol Cell Cardiol* 20:373–378, 1988.
Hess P, Lansman JB, Fox AP, Nowycky MC, Nilius B, McCleskey EW, et al. Calcium channels: mechanisms of modulation and ion permeation. *J Gen Physiol* 86:5a, 1985.
Hof RP, Reugg UT, Hof A, Vogel A. Stereoselectivity at the calcium channel: opposite action of the enantiomers of a 1,4-dihydropyridine. *J Cardiovasc Pharm* 7:689–693, 1985.
Höltje HD, Marrer S. A molecular graphics study on structure-action relationships of calcium-antagonistic and agonistic 1,4-dihydropyridines. *J Comput-Aided Mol Design* 1:23–30, 1987.
Horne WA, Weiland GA, Oswald RE. Solubilization and hydrodynamic characterization of the dihydropyridine receptor from rat ventricular muscle. *J Biol Chem* 261:3588–3594, 1986.
Imagawa P, Leung AT, Campbell KP. Phosphorylation of the 1,4-dihydropyridine receptor of the voltage dependent calcium channel by an intrinsic protein kinase in isolated triads from rabbit skeletal muscle. *J Biol Chem* 262:8333–8339, 1987.
Janis RA, Rampe D, Sarmiento JG, Triggle DJ. Specific binding of a calcium channel activator [^{3}]Bay K 8644 to membranes from cardiac muscle and brain. *Biochem Biophys Res Commun* 121:317–323, 1984.
Janis RA, Scriabine A. Sites of action of Ca^{2+} channel inhibitors. *Biochem Pharmacol* 32:3499–3507, 1983.
Janis RA, Triggle DJ. 14-Dihydropyridine Ca^{2+} channel antagonists and activators: a comparison of binding characteristics with pharmacology. *Drug Dev Res* 4:5425–5437, 1984.
Kokubun S, Reuter H. Dihydropyridine derivatives prolong the open state of Ca^{++} channels in cultured cardiac cells. *Proc Natl Acad Sci (USA)* 81:4824–4827, 1984.
Kolb VM, Koman A, Terenius L. Fluorescent probes for opioid receptors. *Life Sci* 33:423–426, 1983.
Kongsamut S, Kamp TJ, Miller RJ, Sanquinetti MC. Calcium channel agonist and antagonist effects of the sterioisomers of the dihydropyridine. *Biochem Biophys Res Commun* 130:141–148, 1985.

Koppel DE. Fluorescence redistribution after photobleaching. A new multipoint analysis of membrane translational dynamics. *Biophys J* 28:281–292, 1979.

Koppel DE, Sheetz MP. A localized pattern photobleaching method for the concurrent analysis of rapid and slow diffusion processes. *Biophys J* 43:175–181, 1983.

Langs DA, Triggle DJ. Conformational features of calcium channel agonist and antagonist analogs of nifedipine. *Mol Pharmacol* 27:544–548, 1985.

Lee LS, Tsien RW. Mechanism of calcium channel blockade by verapamil, D-600, diltiazem and nitrendipine in single dialysed heart cells. *Nature* 302:790–794, 1983.

Leung AT, Imagawa T, Campbell KP. Structural characterization of the 1,4-dihydropyridine receptor of the voltage-dependent Ca^{2+} channel from rabbit skeletal muscle. Evidence for two distinct high molecular weight subunits. *J Biol Chem* 262:7943–7946, 1987.

McClosky M, Poo MM. Rates of membrane associated reactions: reduction of dimensionality revisited. *J Cell Biol* 102:88–96, 1986.

Morton ME, Caffrey JM, Brown AM, Froehner SC. Monoclonal antibody to the α_1 subunit of the dihydropyridine-binding complex inhibits calcium currents in BC3H1 myocytes. *J Biol Chem* 263:613–616, 1988.

Rebek J Jr. Model studies in molecular recognition. *Science* 235:1478–1484, 1987.

Reuter H, Porzig H, Kokobun S, Prod'hom B. Voltage dependence of dihydrophyridine ligand binding and action in intact cardiac cells. *J Gen Physiol* 86:5a, 1985.

Rhodes DG, Sarmiento JG, Herbette LG. Kinetics of binding of membrane-active drugs to receptor sites. Diffusion limited rates for a membrane bilayer approach of 1,4-dihydropyridine calcium channel antagonists to their active site. *Mol Pharmacol* 27:612–623, 1985.

Rosenberg RL, Hess P, Reeves JP, Smilowitz H, Tsien RW. Calcium channels in planar lipid bilayers: insights into mechanisms of ion permeation and gatings. *Science* 231:1564–1566, 1986.

Shaafi RI, Fernandez SM. *Fast methods in physical biochemistry and cell biology*. Amsterdam: Elsevier Science Publishers, 1983.

Sharp AH, Imagawa T, Leung AT, Campbell KP. Identification and characterization of the dihydropyridine-binding subunit of the skeletal muscle dihydropyridine receptor. *J Biol Chem* 262:12309–12315, 1987.

Takahashi M, Catterall WA. Dihydropyridine-sensitive calcium channels in cardiac and skeletal muscle membranes: studies with antibodies against the subunits. *Biochemistry* 26:5518–5526, 1987.

Tanabe T, Takeshima H, Mikami A, Flookerzi V, Takahashi H, Kangawa K, et al. Primary structure of the receptor for calcium channel blockers from skeletal muscle. *Nature* 328:313–318, 1987.

Triggle AM, Shefter E, Triggle DJ. Crystal structures of calcium channel antagonists: 26-dimethyl-3,5-dicarbomethoxy-4- [2-nitro-3-cyano- 4-(dimethylamino)-, and 2,3,4,5,6-penta- fluorophenyl]-1,4-dihydropyridine. *J Med Chem* 23:442–445, 1980.

Trumbore MW, Chester DW, Moring J, Rhodes D, Herbette LG. Structure and location of amiodarone in a membrane bilayer as determined by molecular mechanics and quantitative x-ray diffraction. *Biophys J* 54:535–543, 1988.

Venter JC, Fraser CM, Schaber JS, Yung CY, Bolger G, Triggle DJ. Molecular properties of the slow inward calcium channel. I. Molecular weight determination by radiation inactivation and covalent affinity labeling. *J Biol Chem* 258:9344–9348, 1983.

Vilven J, Leung AT, Imagawa T, Sharp AH, Campbell KP, Coronado R. Interaction of calcium channels of skeletal muscle with monoclonal antibodies specific for its dihydropyridine receptor. *Biophys J* 53:556a, 1988.

Chapter 13

Structure-Function Correlations of 1,4-Dihydropyridine Calcium Channel Antagonists and Activators

David J. Triggle

INTRODUCTION

The Ca^{2+} antagonist drugs active at voltage-dependent Ca^{2+} channels constitute a major therapeutic group of agents that find significant use in cardiovascular disorders. These drugs, including the clinically available verapamil, nifedipine, and diltiazem, and the Ca^{2+} channels with which they interact are discrete molecular species, or groups of species, distinct from other ion channels and their modulating drugs. Nonetheless, there are many similarities between drug action at Ca^{2+} channels and other classes of ion channels. In all cases a chemically heterogeneous group of agents serves to block or to activate channels. The modulation thus achieved reflects drug interactions at different sites and by different mechanisms, but common principles of drug access and voltage-dependence of action are found. This similarity of behavior of drug action at cation channels likely reflects underlying homologies in structure and function (Tanabe et al., 1987; Tempel et al., 1987).

Hondeghem, Luc (ed): Molecular and Cellular Mechanisms of Antiarrhythmic Agents, Futura Publishing Company, Inc., Mount Kisco, NY, © 1989.

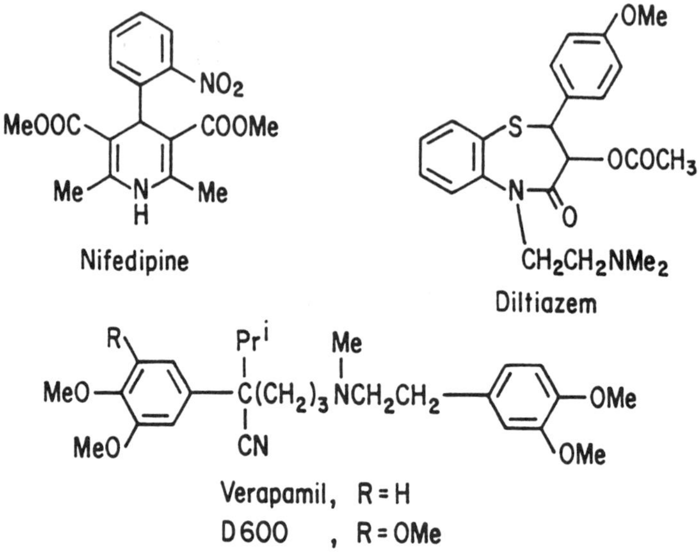

Figure 1. Chemical structures of representative Ca^{2+} channel antagonists of the 1,4-dihydropyridine, benzothiazepine and phenylalkylamine classes.

The Ca^{2+} Channel Antagonists

The Ca^{2+} channel antagonists, introduced into clinical medicine over the past fifteen years, constitute a chemically heterogeneous set of drugs representing the 1,4-dihydropyridine (nifedipine), phenylalkylamine (verapamil), and benzothiazepine (diltiazem) categories (Fig. 1). These agents are effective at one particular class of voltage-dependent Ca^{2+} channel, the L-channel. They are employed in cardiovascular medicine for a variety of disorders including angina in its several forms, supraventricular tachyarrhythmias, and hypertension, but their potential range of application is far wider, ranging from achalasia to vertigo (Janis et al., 1987; Triggle and Janis, 1987).

As might be anticipated from their chemical heterogeneity these agents show a corresponding lack of pharmacological and therapeutic homogeneity (Table I and II). Thus, while nifedipine, verapamil, and diltiazem are all effective, with minor quantitative differences, against angina, nifedipine is ineffective against cardiac arrhythmias, including supraventricular tachycardia and exerts

Table I
Therapeutic Uses of Calcium Channel Antagonists

Therapeutic Use	*Antagonist* Verapamil (I)	Nifedipine (II)	Diltiazem (III)
Angina:			
exertional	+ + +	+ + +	+ + +
spasm	+ + +	+ + +	+ + +
variant	+ + +	+ + +	+ + +
Arrhythmias:			
Supraventricular	+ + +	−	+ +
Atrial flutter	+ +	−	+ +
Hypertension	+ +	+ + +	+ +
Other:			
Hypertrophic cardiomyopathy	+ +	−	−
Raynaud's disease	+ +	+ +	+ +
Cardioplegia	+	+	+
Cerebral vasospasm	−	+	−

Classes I, II, and III as defined by the World Health Organization
Number of plus signs indicate extent of use

Table II
Hemodynamic Effects of Ca^{2+} Channel Antagonists

	Verapamil	Nifedipine	Diltiazem
Coronary blood flow	+ +	+ + +	+ +
Peripheral vasodilation	+ +	+ + +	+
Heart rate	+ −	0	0 −
Contractility	−	0 +	0 −
Preload	0	0 −	0
AV node conduction	− −	0	0
AV node erp	+ −	0	−
PR interval	+	0	+
AH interval	+	0	−

+ = increase; − = decrease; + − = variable effect; 0 = no effect.

relatively little cardiodepressant activity at vasodilating doses. Accordingly, in the cardiovascular system nifedipine and related 1,4-dihydropyridine antagonists are primarily vasodilatory, vascular smooth muscle selective agents, while verapamil and diltiazem enjoy both vasodilatory and cardiodepressant properties. These distinctions are embodied in the recent World Health Organization classification of verapamil, nifedipine, and diltiazem as representatives of group I, II, and III specific Ca^{2+} channel antagonists respectively.

The existence of these agents and the early pharmacological and electrophysiological evidence for their inhibitory actions at voltage-dependent Ca^{2+} channels (Fleckenstein, 1977; 1983) has raised a number of important questions:

1. Specific Actions?
   - selectivity
   - structure-activity relationships
   - stereoselectivity
   - specific binding sites (receptors)
2. Relationship to Ca^{2+}?
3. Specificity of action?
   - stimulus
   - tissue
4. Site(s) of action?
   - membrane
   - sidedness
   - intracellular
5. Sites and mechanisms of action?
   - single
   - multiple.

A considerable volume of work over the past decade has established that a primary site of action of the Ca^{2+} channel antagonists is at one type of voltage-dependent Ca^{2+} channel, the L-type high threshold, large conductance, slowly inactivating channel (Fox et al., 1987; Miller, 1987; Tsien et al., 1987), that plays a major role in supplying the Ca^{2+} demands of excitation-contraction coupling in smooth muscle, both vascular and nonvascular (Fig. 2). This work indicates very clearly that these actions are exerted through specific sites associated with the voltage-dependent Ca^{2+} channel and are

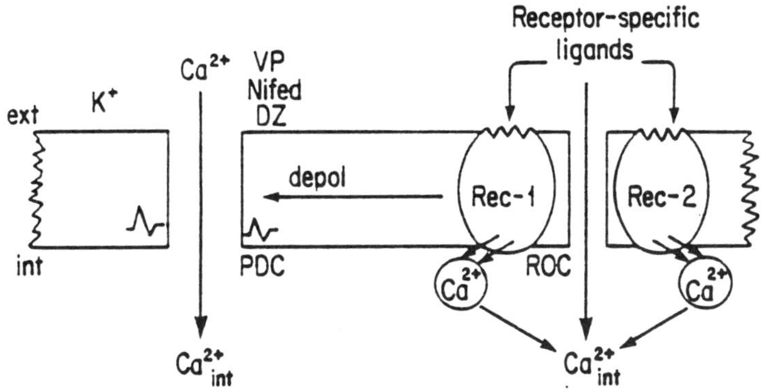

Figure 2. Representation of Ca^{2+} mobilization in an excitable cell. Depicted are three primary modes of activation including entry through potential-dependent channels (PDC), receptor-operated channels (ROC), and from receptor-linked intracellular Ca^{2+} pools (endoplasmic and sarcoplasmic reticulum).

not attributable to nonspecific membrane or cellular perturbation (Janis and Triggle, 1984; Triggle and Janis, 1987; Janis et al., 1987).

Accordingly, the specificity and selectivity of action of the Ca^{2+} channel antagonists derive from their blocking one of several pathways of Ca^{2+} mobilization and from the relative importance of this pathway according to stimulus demand and tissue type. The Ca^{2+} channels blocked are plasmalemmal entities, and thus to be distinguished from Ca^{2+} release channels in the endoplasmic and sarcoplasmic reticulum (Irvine et al., 1986; Lai et al., 1987).

Although all three major categories of Ca^{2+} channel antagonist drugs exert their principal actions at a single class of voltage-dependent Ca^{2+} channel, it is clear that they interact at discrete sites and that different routes of access to these sites likely exist according to the physicochemical properties of the drug and the channel equilibria between resting, open and inactivated states.

An additional subtlety to the analysis of ligand interactions at the Ca^{2+} channel has been the discovery of 1,4-dihydropyridines, including BAY K 8644 and 202 791 (Fig. 3), that function as activators of the channel with cardiotonic and vasoconstricting properties (Schramm et al., 1983; reviewed in Janis et al., 1987). The existence of both activator and antagonist ligands for the Ca^{2+} channel in the 1,4-dihydropyridine structure, and perhaps also for the

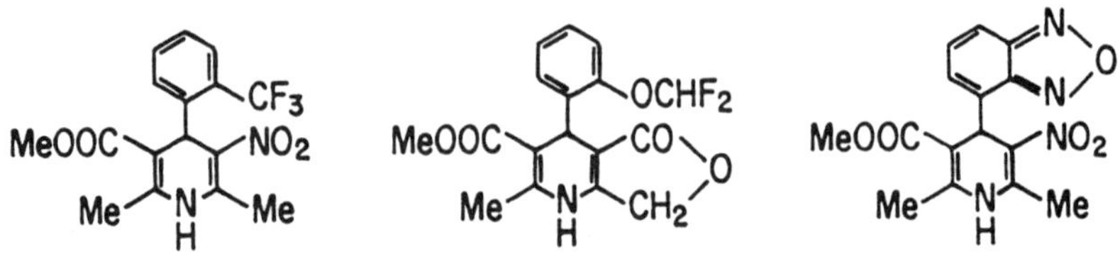

Figure 3. Chemical structures of 1,4-dihydropyridines with Ca^{2+} channel activating properties.

other ligand classes (Scott and Dolphin, 1987), raises several important questions. These include:

1. What are the structural demands for 1,4-dihydropyridine interaction at the Ca^{2+} channel?
2. What is the molecular basis for differentiation between activator and antagonist 1,4-dihydropyridines?
3. Do endogenous ligands exist that serve as physiological regulators of the Ca^{2+} channel and which are mimicked in structure and function by the 1,4-dihydropyridines?

1,4-Dihydropyridines: Structure-Function Relationships

Structure-function relationships for 1,4-dihydropyridine antagonists have been derived from both pharmacological (in vitro and in vivo) and biochemical (radioligand binding) studies. An early study by Loev and his colleagues (1974) demonstrated for in vivo antihypertensive effects that:

1. In a series of 2,6-dimethyl-3,5-dicarbomethoxy-4-substituted-1,4-dihydropyridines activity increases with increasing size of the 4-substituent, phenyl and substituted phenyl groups being optimum.
2. In the substituted 4-phenyl group small electron-withdrawing groups in the ortho- and meta-posi-

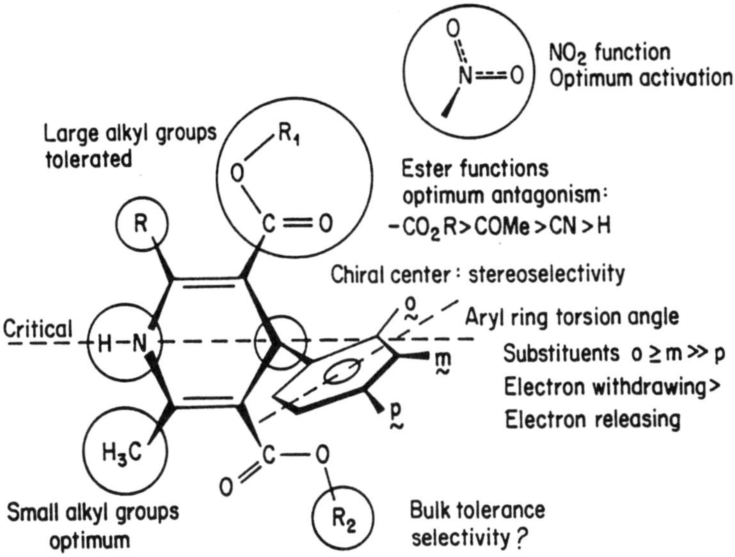

Figure 4. Structural features in 1,4-dihydropyridines important to the determination of activator and antagonist properties.

tions enhance activity, but any substituent in the para position reduces activity.

3. Oxidation of the 1,4-dihydropyridine ring to pyridine and substitution on N1 are both detrimental.
4. Ester groups at C-3 and C-5 of the 1,4-dihydropyridine ring confer optimum antagonist activity; other electron-withdrawing groups, including -CN and -COMe, reduce activity quite substantially.

These conclusions have been found to be generally valid in subsequent studies with isolated tissues and subcellular fractions (for review see Janis et al., 1987). These general features are represented in Fig. 4.

When the 1,4-dihydropyridine ring is asymmetrically substituted, C-4 becomes chiral and the anticipated stereoselectivity occurs (reviewed in Janis et al., 1987). Asymmetrically substituted diester derivatives are usually more active than their symmetric counterparts, suggesting an asymmetric character of the corresponding binding sites (Towart et al., 1981; Triggle and Swamy, 1984; Janis et al., 1987).

Although the substitution pattern at C-3, C-4 and C-5 of the 1,4-dihydropyridine ring has received the greatest attention, more recent efforts have focussed on the substituents at C-2 and C-6. Replacement of a C-2 methyl group by 2-aminoethoxymethyl yields the amlodipine series that is characterized by high potency, very high stereoselectivity and unusually slow onset of action and persistence of blockade (Burges et al., 1987). These characteristics suggest that a different binding orientation may be produced, relative to that adopted by nifedipine, because of the presence of the basic 2-substituent in the 1,4-dihydropyridine ring.

Most efforts to define quantitative structure-activity relationships in the 1,4-dihydropyridine series have been frustrated by small series of compounds covering a restricted range of activities (Mannhold et al., 1982; Janis et al., 1987). However, in an extensive series of nonchiral substituted 4-phenyl-2,6-dimethyl-3,5-dicarbomethoxy-1,4-dihydropyridines examined as antagonists of smooth muscle tension responses:

$$\log 1/IC_{50} = 14.23 + 1.96\sigma_m - 0.44L_m - 3.26B_{1p} - 1.51L_{m'} + 0.62\pi \qquad [1]$$

$$n = 46, \quad r = 0.90, \quad s = 0.67, \quad F = 33.93$$

where m and m′ represent orientations of the meta-substituents away from and over the plane of the 1,4-dihydropyridine ring respectively, σ_m is the electronic constant and π is the hydrophobic constant (Coburn et al., 1988). The size of the Verloop steric length constants indicates the relative importance of unfavorable steric interactions as a function of position and orientation. These interactions are least for the ortho positions and greatest for the para positions and are larger for substituents that are forced into a position over the 1,4-dihydropyridine ring.

The effects of phenyl ring and ester group substitution pattern are expressed independently. Thus, in the 3,5-dicarbomethoxy (nifedipine) and 3-carbomethoxy-5-carboxyisobutyl (nisoldipine) series the same rank order of phenyl ring substituent activity is expressed (Fig. 5); (Fossheim et al., 1988).

The precise conformation adopted by 1,4-dihydropyridines at their receptor site is not known. However, solid state structures and the synthesis of rigid analogs have been very useful in this regard. In the solid state the phenyl ring is in a pseudoaxial orientation

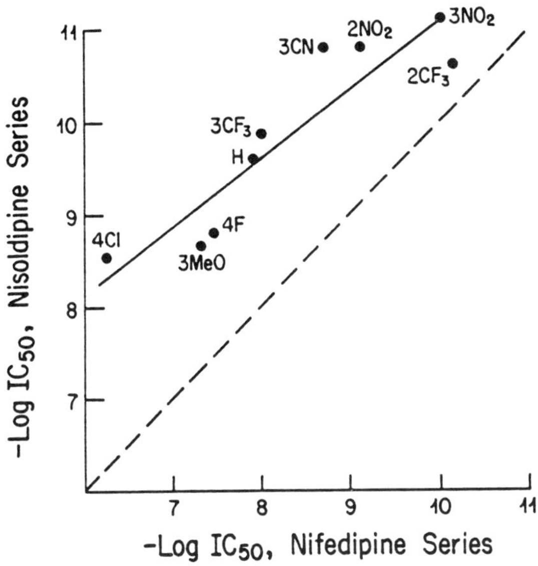

Figure 5. Correlation between the abilities of phenyl substituted nifedipine and nisoldipine derivatives to inhibit K+ depolarization-induced tension responses in intestinal smooth muscle (Data from Joslyn et al., 1988).

approximately bisecting a 1,4-dihydropyridine ring that is in a flattened boat conformation (Fig. 6); (Fossheim et al., 1982, 1988). The significance of this conformation is reinforced by the activities of a series of rigid analogs where activity increases with increasing bridge length and inter-ring angle (Fig. 7A); (Seidel et al., 1984) and by the activities of the rigid 1,3-benzothiazocines analogs (Fig. 7B) where the beta diastereomers are the more potent (Baldwin et al., 1987).

The role of the C-3 and C-5 ester groups in determining activity is receiving increased attention. It is clear that large variations in ester size can be tolerated without significant loss of activity and with the apparent demonstration of modest degrees of vascular bed selectivity (Fig. 8); (Freedman and Waters, 1987; Janis et al., 1987). An asymmetric disposition and character of the ester binding sites is likely.

Solid state structures reveal that a *cis, trans* ester group orientation placing an ester group *(cis)* close to the aryl ring is the most common geometry. Some *cis, cis* arrangements are known, but

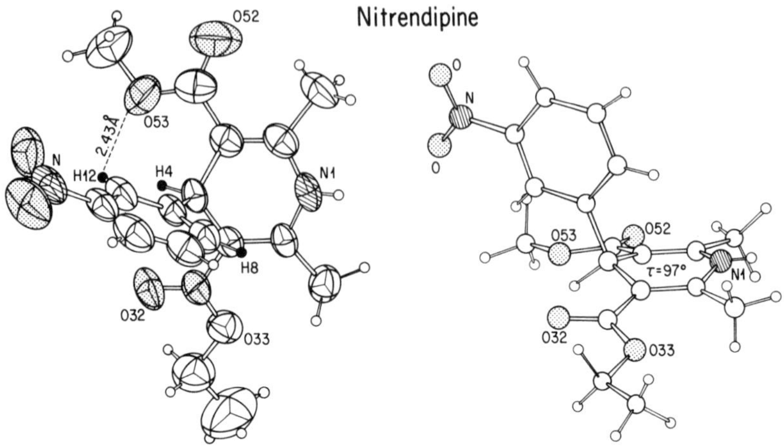

Figure 6. Two views of the solid state structure of nitrendipine. Structural features of particular importance are the flattened 1,4-dihydropyridine ring, and the pseudoaxial orientation of the phenyl ring bisecting the 1,4-dihydropyridine ring (Fossheim et al., 1982, 1988).

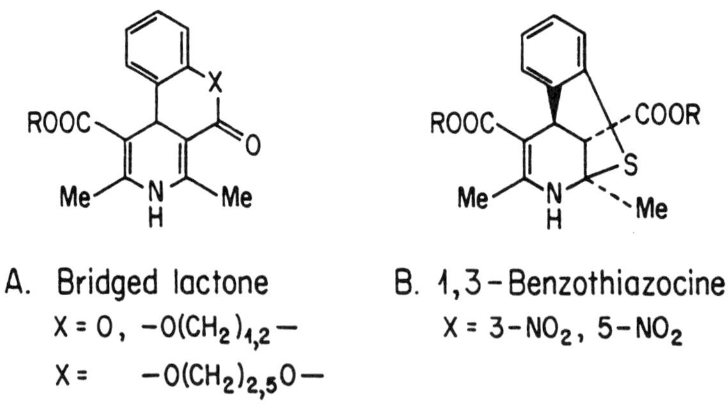

Figure 7. Conformationally rigid analogs of 1,4-dihydropyridines.

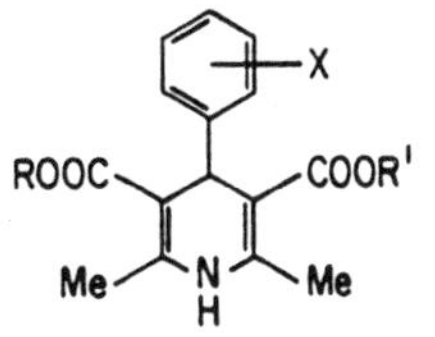

Nifedipine: X = 2-NO_2, R = R' = Me
Nitrendipine: X = 3-NO_2, R = Me, R' = Et
Nimodipine: X = 3-NO_2, R = Me_2CH, R' = $MeOCH_2CH_2$
Nisoldipine: X = 3-NO_2, R = Me, R' = Me_2CHCH_2
Nicardipine: X = 3-NO_2, R = Me, R' = $C_6H_5CH_2N(Me)CH_2CH_2$
Felodipine: X = 2,3 Cl_2, R = Me, R' = Et

Figure 8. Structural formulae of analogs of nifedipine that are in clinical use or clinical trial.

no *trans, trans* geometries have been reported (Fig. 9); (Langs and Triggle, 1985; Triggle et al., 1988).

However, steric factors are not the sole determinant of biological activity. Inactive molecules share identical or very similar conformations. Thus, the 2- and 4-nitrophenyl substituted 2,6-dimethyl-3,5-dicarbomethoxy-1,4-dihydropyridines differ by greater than 10^4-fold in activity but share very common solid state structures. Furthermore, very similar solid state structures are found in antagonist and activator structures (Langs and Triggle, 1985). Additionally, the remarkable enantiomeric discrimination revealed in several pairs of 5-nitro substituted 1,4-dihydropyridines whereby the [R] and [S] enantiomers have antagonist and activator properties respectively (Fig. 10); (Hof et al., 1985; Franckowiak et al., 1985) indicates that the interpretation of structure activity relationships in the 1,4-dihydropyridines demands analysis both in terms of ligand and binding site structures. This view is strengthened by the observation that many 1,4-dihydropyridines considered as solely an-

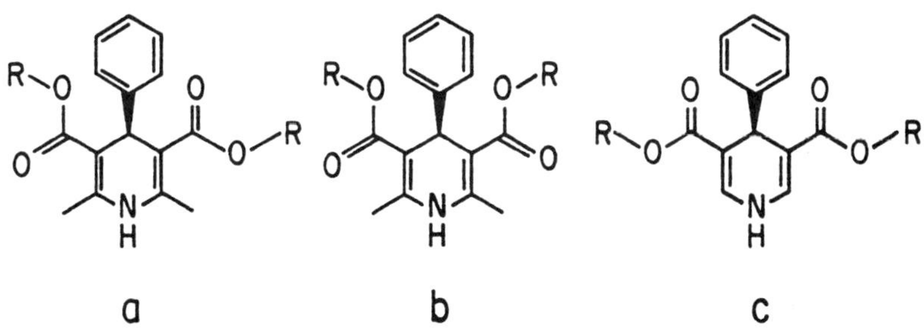

Figure 9. Conformations of C-3 and C-5 ester groups in 1,4-dihydropyridines. a. cis, trans; b, cis, cis; c. trans, trans.

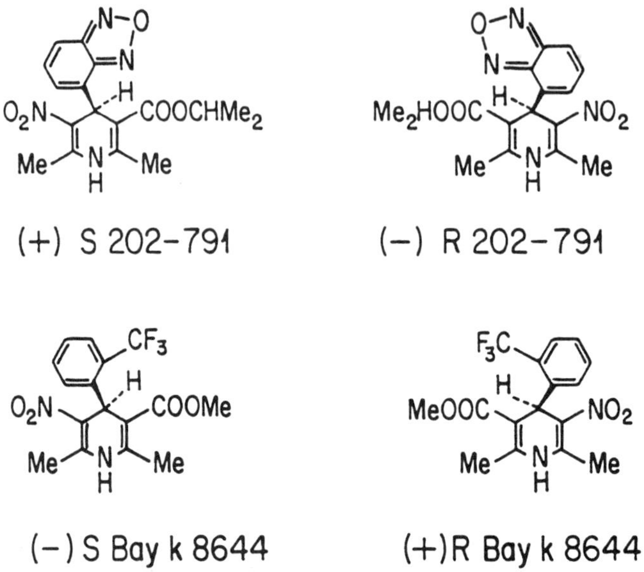

Figure 10. Enantiomeric 1,4-dihydropyridine pairs where the S and R configurations are activator and antagonist respectively.

tagonist or activator species, and including nifedipine and nitrendipine, may also have activator properties under certain conditions (Brown et al., 1984, 1986; Schwartz et al., 1984; Hess et al., 1984; Scott and Dolphin, 1987).

1,4-Dihydropyridines: Mechanisms of Action

The relationship of the receptor site for the 1,4-dihydropyridine antagonists and activators to the functional machinery of the Ca^{2+} channel remains to be established. However, it is clear from electrophysiological studies that interaction of the 1,4-dihydropyridines to the L-type of channel is strongly modulated by voltage and that the apparent affinity of the 1,4-dihydropyridine antagonists is significantly increased by membrane depolarization (Sanguinetti and Kass, 1984; Bean, 1984; Triggle and Janis, 1987). Accordingly, the interactions of 1,4-dihydropyridines (and other classes of Ca^{2+} channel antagonists) must be interpreted in terms of state-dependent binding (the *modulated receptor* hypothesis) processes, whereby ligand affinity is determined by selective interactions with and access to the resting, open or inactivated states of the Ca^{2+} channel (Hondeghem and Katzung, 1984).

State-dependent binding processes likely underlie the well-established observations that high affinity binding of [3H]1,4-dihydropyridines, K_D values of 10^{-9}–10^{-11}M, is very readily detectable in membrane fragments from excitable cells, but that the correlations between radioligand binding and pharmacological affinities vary considerably. This ratio varies from approximately 1:1 in K+ depolarized smooth muscle, to 1:100 in electrically paced cardiac muscle, and to the frequently observed pharmacological inactivity of the 1,4-dihydropyridines in neuronal systems. These differences are, of course, consistent with the therapeutic profile of the 1,4-dihydropyridines as primarily vasodilators with little cardiac depressant activity and, in common with other Ca^{2+} channel antagonists, normally negligible CNS activity (Triggle and Janis, 1984, 1987; Janis et al., 1987). Despite the major quantitative differences in observed biological activity exhibited by the 1,4-dihydropyridines, the same rank order expression of activities is found when the activities of a series is compared in different tissues, and the same high affinity binding is found in plasmalemmal membrane fragments regardless of the sensitivity of the cell response (Bolger et al., 1983; Janis et al., 1984, 1987).

These observations indicate that a common receptor is being expressed in different states according to the stimulus conditions. It is likely that the high affinity binding to (depolarized) membrane fragments corresponds to the high affinity interactions with the inactivated channel state that are detected electrophysiologically. Accordingly, the observed affinity and activator/antagonist character of the 1,4-dihydropyridines will depend upon their affinities to the several available states of the channel, upon access pathways to these states, and upon the allosteric constants governing state equilibria. Similar considerations apply to ligand interactions at other channel categories (Hondeghem and Katzung, 1984).

1,4-Dihydropyridines that interact with and stabilize the open channel state will be activators while those that interact with the inactivated state will be antagonists. Additionally, a third group of ligands should exist that interact with the resting state of the channel. These should also be antagonist species, but no completely characterized member of this class has yet been reported.

The preceding considerations demonstrate the importance of

state-dependent considerations to the elucidation of the significance of the structure-activity relationships for 1,4-dihydropyridines active at L-type Ca^{2+} channels. The excellent 1:1 correlations observed between pharmacological activities in depolarized smooth muscle and binding affinities in depolarized membranes are thus due to the dominance of the same inactivated state of the Ca^{2+} channel in both types of preparation. In contrast, the approximately 100-fold difference between binding and pharmacological activities in cardiac muscle may be attributed to the relative dominance of low affinity resting states of the channel in paced cardiac preparations. Similarly, the 10–100-fold lower sensitivity of the phasic (initial) relative to the tonic (later) component of contraction in many smooth muscles likely reflects the relative importance of ligand equilibration with resting and inactivated states of the channel respectively (Bolger et al., 1983; Yousif and Triggle, 1986). The elucidation and interpretation of the structure-activity relationships of 1,4-dihydropyridines must accommodate such state-dependent differences in interactions.

Radioligand binding studies of [3H]1,4-dihydropyridines in intact functional cells permit, in principle, the elucidation of structure-activity relationships according to channel state. Some reports of voltage-dependent binding of 1,4-dihydropyridines have appeared (Kokubun et al., 1986; Lee et al., 1987; Kamp and Miller, 1987). Binding of [3H]PN 200 110 to neonatal rat cardiac myocytes is strongly potential-dependent, affinity increasing approximately 100-fold from the resting to the depolarized state without change in the maximum number of binding sites. This change in affinity is due solely to a decrease in ligand dissociation rate in the depolarized state (Table III). Thus, the effect of depolarization is to enhance the interaction between the 1,4-dihydropyridine ligand and the binding site: the approximately 100-fold change in K_D corresponds to some 2.5 KCal interaction energy or one additional hydrogen bond in the drug-receptor interaction in the depolarized state.

The binding of activator-antagonist 1,4-dihydropyridine pairs to polarized and depolarized cells confirms that binding of the [R]-enantiomers (antagonists) is accompanied by a significant affinity shift, approximating that seen with PN 200 110, but that the affinity shift of the corresponding activator enantiomers is much smaller (Fig. 11). This has also been observed in other preparations (X. Y. Wei and D. J. Triggle, unpublished observations). This suggests that

Table III

Voltage Dependent Binding of [^{3}H]PN 200 110 Binding to Neonatal Rat Heart Cells (Wei et al., 1989b)

	[^{3}H]PN 200 110 Binding			
K^+, mM	k_1 min^{-1} M^{-1}	k_{-1} min^{-1}	K_D[a] M	B_{max}[a] fmole mg^{-1}
5.8 (polarized)	2.2×10^8	0.53	3.5×10^{-9}	47.2
50.0 (depolarized)	2.3×10^8	0.018	6.3×10^{-11}	50.1

[a] The corresponding values for neonatal rat heart cell membranes were $K_D = 5.5 \times 10^{-11}$ M, $B_{max} = 307$ fmoles mg^{-1}.

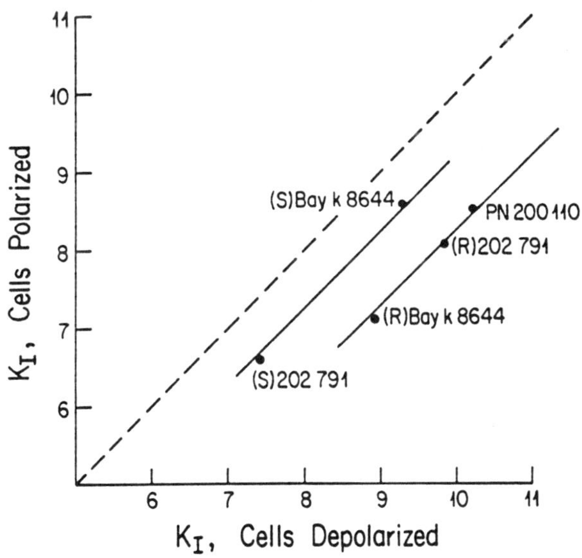

Figure 11. Correlation between the K_I values for competition with [3H]PN 200 110 binding to polarized (5 mM K^+) and depolarized (50 mM K+) cultured rat ventricular myocytes. The discrepancies between the two sets of K_I values are clearly larger for the antagonist than for the activator 1,4-dihydropyridines. (Data from Wei et al., 1989b).

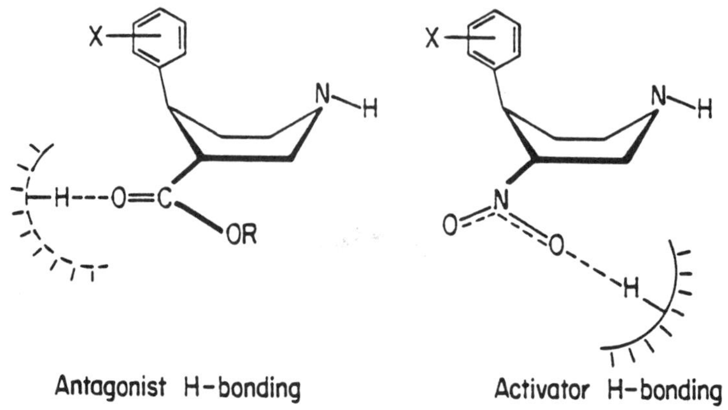

Figure 12. Representation of different modes of binding of 1,4-dihydropyridine activators and antagonists. A critical distinguishing role is attributed to the orientation of the H bond depicted. (After Mahmoudian and Richards, 1986).

state-dependent binding of these 1,4-dihydropyridine Ca^{2+} channel activators is less selective than for the antagonist species.

There are important implications to this proposal. First, consistent with previous suggestions and with ligand interactions in other receptor systems, it suggests that there will be a continuum of molecules whose properties are determined by their relative affinities for the open, resting, and inactivated states of this category of voltage-dependent Ca^{2+} channel. Second, it affords an explanation of why activator and antagonist properties exist within a single molecule (Williams et al., 1985; Kass, 1987; Wei et al., 1986), and indicates the possibility that 1,4-dihydropyridines exist with the appropriate balance of positive inotropic and vasodilatory properties—a therapeutically useful molecule (Janis et al., 1987). Thirdly, it suggests for the potent 3-carboalkoxy-5-nitro-substituted-1,4-dihydropyridines studied that the activator-antagonist selectivity arises from the relative inability of the antagonist enantiomers to interact with the open state, and not from the inability of the activator enantiomers to interact with the inactivated state (Fig. 12). Finally, this proposal accommodates the observation that, in contrast to the antagonist 1,4-dihydropyridines, there is little discrepancy in binding and pharmacological affinities for the activator enantiomers (Fig. 13).

The preceding conclusions are necessarily speculative. They are

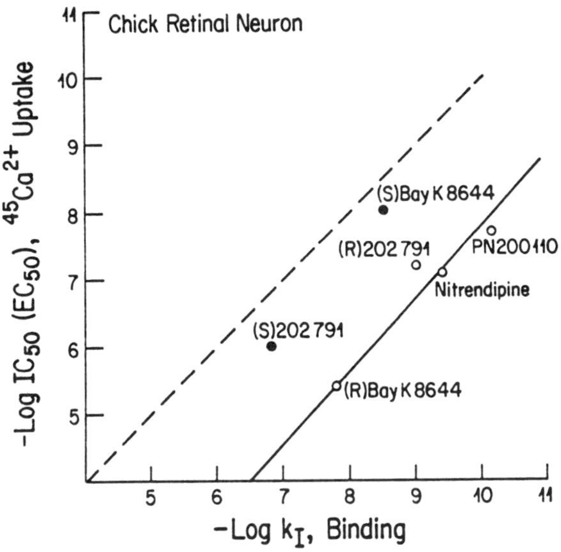

Figure 13. Correlation between binding and pharmacological affinities for a series of 1,4-dihydropyridine activators and antagonists in chick retinal neurons. The pharmacological activities are for the stimulation or inhibition of depolarization-sensitive 45 Ca^{2+} influx, and the binding affinities are for membrane fractions of chick retinal neurons. (Data from Wei et al., 1989a).

based on the behavior of a limited series of compounds acting in one cell type. It is probable that there exist subtypes of the L channels that may differ in several respects including their inactivation characteristics. The Ca^{2+} channels of pituitary cells appear to inactivate very slowly. Accordingly, [S] BAY K 8644 would not be expected to show antagonist properties and this is the case (McCarthy and Cohen, 1986). In chick retinal neurons the Ca^{2+} channels appear to inactivate very slowly and thus generate a discrepancy between the high affinity binding observed in membrane fragments and the low affinity pharmacology (Wei et al., 1989a). It is also certain that other variables exist that will also modulate the binding and pharmacological behavior of 1,4-dihydropyridines. Prominent among such possibilities are the G proteins, known to be associated with voltage-dependent Ca^{2+} channels, and whose activation promotes the stimulant effects of 1,4-dihydropyridines and other Ca^{2+} channel ligands in dorsal root ganglia (Scott and Dolphin, 1987).

The parameters defining 1,4-dihydropyridine—Ca^{2+} channel interactions are thus likely to be diffusely defined. The pharmacological and therapeutic behavior of these compounds will therefore be correspondingly flexible and will depend critically upon ligand structure, channel type, stimulus pattern, and metabolic state of the cell. 1, 4-Dihydropyridines may be considered as molecular chameleons of the Ca^{2+} channel, and the definition of their modes of action will have both basic and clinical benefits.

Clinical Implications

There are important clinical aspects to the definitions of the sites and mechanisms of action of the Ca^{2+} channel ligands. Although voltage-dependent Ca^{2+} channels are widely distributed in excitable tissues and can be readily detected by both electrophysiological and radioligand binding methods, the major therapeutic actions of the existing clinically available agents are exerted dominantly in the cardiovascular system. Factors determining the selectivity of action of these agents are, therefore, of particular importance.

In principle, several factors play roles in determining the observed selectivity of action of the Ca^{2+} channel antagonists. These factors include:

1. Pharmacokinetic factors: distribution and metabolism;
2. Source[s] of Ca^{2+} mobilized: relative extent of use of the several extracellular and intracellular pathways of Ca^{2+} mobilization;
3. Ca^{2+} channel class: different pharmacological profile of channel classes;
4. State-dependent interactions: affinity of drug depends upon channel state;
5. Pathological state: organ or tissue pathology may determine the relative importance of the above factors.

As previously discussed, state-dependent interactions are clearly of significance in determining apparent affinities of drugs for channel states and likely underlies the relative cardiac-vascular

Table IV
Properties of Plasmalemmal Ca^{2+} Channels[1]

	Channel Class		
	L	*T*	*N*
Activation range, mV	−60 to −10 mV	−70 mV	−30 mV
Inactivation range, mV	very slow	−100 to −60 mV	−120 to −30 mV
Inactivation rate	very slow	rapid	moderate
Conductance	35 ps	8 ps	13 ps
Kinetics	little activation	brief burst inactivation	long burst
Permeation	Ba2+ Ca2+	Ba2+ = Ca2+	Ba2+ Ca2+
Cd^{++} sensitivity	Sensitive	Insensitive	Sensitive
1,4-DHP sensitivity	Sensitive	Insensitive	Insensitive
w-Conotoxin sensitivity	Sensitive (neurons) Insensitive (muscle)	Insensitive	Sensitive

[1] Data computed from a variety of sources and are not intended to suggest that these properties are singularly characteristic of each channel class.

selectivity of the diltiazem, verapamil, and nifedipine categories. The relative importance of voltage- and frequency-dependence of interactions will be a major determinant (Hondeghem and Katzung, 1984). Additionally, the significant voltage-dependent interactions exhibited by the 1,4-dihydropyridines will also play a significant role in determining their relative selectivity for different vascular beds, affinity increasing with increasing vascular smooth muscle depolarization-induced tone. Kinetic factors also play an important role in determining the extent of interaction of drugs with Ca^{2+} channels. A transient opening of a channel may not permit equilibration of a ligand with a high affinity binding state.

A second major determinant of tissue selectivity is the existence of different channel classes and subclasses with different pharmacological characteristics. At the present time, three major channel classes are postulated, L, T, and N, which may be characterized by different voltage, kinetic, and permeation characteristics (Table IV. Additionally, these channel classes may be distinguished pharmacologically and it is the L channel class that dominates the functional pharmacology of the cardiovascular system that is sensitive to the existing clinically used groups of agents.

Finally, the expression and properties of these channels may be differentially modulated by pathological states including disease, chronic drug administration, and hormonal modulation. These aspects have been reviewed in detail elsewhere (Ferrante and Triggle, 1989) to document the changes that take place in alcohol dependence, myocardial ischemia, and thyroid hormone hyper- and hypofunction.

SUMMARY

The state-dependent interactions of 1,4-dihydropyridine Ca^{2+} channel antagonists and activators are important components of the definition of structure activity relationships and of the distinction between activator and antagonist structures. Improved understanding of these interactions will facilitate our definition of the quantitative and qualitative differences between ligand interactions at the several states of the Ca^{2+} channel. This is important to our further exploitation of the selectivity of action of these agents.

BIBLIOGRAPHY

Bean BP. Nitrendipine block of cardiac calcium channels: high affinity binding to the inactivated state. *Proc Nat Acad Sci USA* 81:6388–6392, 1984

Bolger GT, Gengo P, Klockowski R, Luchowski E, Siegel H, Janis RA, et al. Characterization of binding of the Ca^{2+} channel antagonist, [3H]nitrendipine, to guinea pig ileal smooth muscle. *J Pharmacol Exp Ther* 225:291–309, 1983.

Brown AM, Kunze DL, Yatani A. Dual effects of dihydropyridines on whole cell and unitary calcium currents in single ventricular cells of guinea pig. *J Physiol (Lond)* 379:495–514, 1986.

Brown AM, Kunze DL, Yatani A. The agonist effects of dihydropyridines on Ca channels. *Nature* 311:570–572, 1984.

Burges RA, Gardiner DG, Gwilt M, Higgins AJ, Blackburn KJ, Campbell SF, et al. Calcium channel blocking properties of amlodipine in vascular smooth muscle and cardiac muscle in vitro: evidence for voltage modulation of vascular dihydropyridine receptor. *J Cardiovasc Pharmacol* 9:110–118, 1987.

Coburn RA, Wierzba, Suto MJ, Solo AJ, Triggle AM, Triggle DJ. 1,4-Dihydropyridine antagonist activities at the calcium channel: a quantitative structure-activity relationship approach. *J Med Chem* 31:2103–2107, 1988.

Ferrante J, Triggle DJ. Drug-induced regulation of Ca^{2+} channels. *Pharmacol Rev* (Submitted for publication).

Fleckenstein A. *Calcium antagonism in heart and smooth muscle. Experimental facts and therapeutic propspects.* New York, NY: John Wiley & Sons, Inc., 1983.

Fleckenstein A. Specific pharmacology of calcium in myocardium, cardiac pacemakers and vascular smooth muscle. *Ann Rev Pharmacol Toxicol* 17:149–166, 1977.

Franckowiak G, Bechem M, Schramm M, Thomas G. The optical isomers of the 1,4-dihydropyridine Bay K 8644 show opposite effects on Ca channels. *Eur J Pharmacol* 114:223–226, 1985.

Fossheim R, Joslyn A, Solo AJ, Luchowski E, Rutledge A, Triggle DJ. Crystal structures and pharmacologic activities of 1,4-dihydropyridine calcium channel antagonists of the isobutyl methyl 2,6-dimethyl-4-(substituted phenyl)-1,4- dihydropyridine-3,5-dicarboxylate (nisoldipine) series. *J Med Chem* 31:300–305, 1988.

Fossheim R, Svarteng K, Mostad A, Romming C, Shefter E, Triggle DJ. Crystal structures and pharmacological activity of calcium channel antagonists: 2,6-dimethyl-3,5-dicarbomethoxy-4-(unsubstituted, 3-methyl, 4-methyl, 3-nitro, 4-nitro, and 2,4-dinitrophenyl)-1,4-dihydropyridine. *J Med Chem* 25:126–131, 1982.

Fox AP, Nowycky MC, Tsien RW. Kinetic and pharmacologic properties distinguishing three types of calcium currents in chick sensory neurones. *J Physiol (Lond)* 394:149–172, 1987.

Freedman DD, Waters DD. Second generation dihydropyridine calcium antagonists. Greater vasodilatory selectivity and some unique applications. *Drugs* 34:578–598, 1987.

Hess P, Lansman JB, Tsien RW. Different modes of Ca channel gating behaviour favored by dihydropyridine Ca agonists and antagonists. *Nature* 311:538–544, 1984.

Hof PR, Ruegg UT, Hof A, Vogel A. Stereoselectivity at the calcium channel: opposite action of the enantiomers of a 1,4-dihydropyridine. *J Cardiovasc Pharmacol* 7:689–693, 1985.

Hondeghem LM,Katzung BG. Antiarrhythmic agents: the modulated receptor mechanism of action of sodium and calcium channel-blocking drugs. *Ann Rev Pharmacol Toxicol* 24:387–423, 1984.

Irvine RF, Letcher AJ, Lander DJ, Berridge MJ. Specificity of inositol phosphate-stimulated Ca^{2+} mobilization from Swiss-mouse 3T3 cells. *Biochem J* 240:301–304, 1986.

Janis RA, Sarmiento JG, Maurer SC, Bolger GT, Triggle DJ. Characteriistics of the binding of [3H]nitrendipine to rabbit ventricular membranes: modifications by other Ca^{2+} channel antagonists and by the Ca^{2+} channel agonist Bay k 8644. *J Pharmacol Exp Ther* 231:8–15, 1984.

Janis RA, Silver P, Triggle DJ. Drug action and cellular calcium regulation. *Adv Drug Res* 16:311–591, 1987.

Janis RA, Triggle DJ. 1,4-Dihydropyridine Ca^{2+} channel antagonists and activators: a comparison of binding characteristics with pharmacology. *Drug Dev Res* 4:257–274, 1984.

Kamp TJ, Miller RJ. Voltage-dependent nitrendipine binding to cardiac sarcolemmal vesicles. *Mol Pharmacol* 32:278–285, 1987.

Kass RS. Voltage-dependent modification of cardiac calcium channel current by optical isomers of Bay K 8644: Implications for channel gating. *Circ Res* 61(Suppl I):1–5, 1987.

Kokubun S, Prod'hom B, Becker C, Porzig H, Reuter H. Studies on Ca channels in intact cardiac cells: voltage-dependent effects and cooperative interactions of dihydropyridine enantiomers. *Mol Pharmacol* 30:571–584, 1986.

Lai FA, Erickson HP, Rousseau E, Liu QY, Meissner G. Purification and reconstiution of the calcium release channel from skeletal muscle. *Nature* 331:315–319, 1988.

Langs DA, Triggle DJ. Conformational features of calcium channel agonist and antagonist analogs of nifedipine. *Mol Pharmacol* 27:544–548, 1985.

Lee RT, Smith TW, Marsh JD. Evidence for distinct calcium channel agonist and antagonist binding sites in intact cultured embryonic chick ventricular cells. *Circ Res* 60: 683–691, 1987.

Loev B, Goodman MM, Snador KM, Tedeschi R, Macko E. "Hantzsch-type" dihydropyridine hypotensive agents *J Med Chem* 17:956–965, 1974.

Mahmoudian M, Richards GW. A conformational distinction between dihydropyridine calcium agonists and antagonists. *J Chem Soc Chem Commun* 739–741, 1986.

Mannhold R, Rodenkirchen R, Bayer R. Quantitative and qualitative structure-activity relationships of specific Ca antagonists.*Prog Pharmacol* 5:25–52, 1982.

McCarthy RT, Cohen CJ. The enantiomers of Bay k 8644 have different effects on Ca channel gating in rat anterior pituitary cells. *Biophys J* 49:432abs, 1986.

Miller RJ. Multiple neuronal calcium channels. *Science* 235:46–52, 1987.

Sanguinetti MC, Kass RS. Voltage-dependent block of calcium channel current in calf cardiac Purkinje fibers by dihydropyridine calcium channel antagonists. *Circ Res* 55:336–348, 1984.

Schramm M, Thomas G, Franckowiak R. Novel dihydropyridines with positive inotropic action through activation of Ca^{2+} channels. *Nature* 303:535–538, 1983.

Schwartz A, Grupp I, Grupp G, Williams J, Vaghy P. Effects of dihydropyridine calcium channel modulators in the heart: pharmacological and radioligand binding correlations. *Biochem Biophys Res Commun* 125:387–394, 1984.

Scott RH, Dolphin AC. Activation of a G protein promotes agonist responses to calcium channel ligands. *Nature* 330:760–762, 1987.

Seidel W, Meyer H, Born L, Kazda S, Dompert W. Amer Chem Soc 187th National Meeting; St. Louis, MO, April 8–14, 1984. *Medicinal Chem* 14. Abstract.

Tanabe H, Takeshima H, Mikami A, Flockerzi V, Takahashi H, Kangawa K, et al. Primary structure of the receptor for calcium channel blockers from skeletal muscle. *Nature* 328:313–318, 1987.

Tempel B, Papazian DM, Schwarz TL, Jan YN, Jan LY. Sequence of a probable potassium channel component encoded at shaker locus of Drosophila. *Science* 237:720–775, 1987.

Towart R, Wehinger E, Meyer H. Effects of unsymmetrical ester substituted 1,4-dihydropyridine derivatives and their optical isomers on contractions of smooth muscle. *Naunyn Schmied Arch Pharmacol* 317:183–185, 1981.

Triggle DJ, Fossheim R, Hawthorn M, Joslyn A, Triggle AM, Wei X-Y. Calcium channels and calcium channel ligands: a dual perspective for structure-activity relationships. In: Melchiorre C, Gianella M, eds.*Proc 6th Int Camerino-Noordwijkerhout Symposium,* Camerino, Italy, 1987; Amsterdam: Elsevier;123–145, 1988.

Triggle DJ, Janis RA. Ca^{2+} channel antagonists. New perspectives from the radiuoligand binding assay. In: Back N, Spector S, eds. *Modern Methods in Pharmacology* Vol.2 New York, NY: Alan R. Liss Inc.;1–28, 1984.

Triggle DJ, Janis RA. Calcium channel ligands. *Ann Rev Pharmacol Toxicol* 27:347–369, 1987.

Triggle DJ, Swamy VC. Calcium antagonists: some chemical-pharmacological aspects. *Circ Res* 52(Suppl I):17–28, 1983.

Tsien RW, Hess P, McCleskey EW, Rosenberg RL. Calcium channels: mechanisms of selectivity, permeation and block. *Ann Rev Biophys Biophys Chem* 16:265–290, 1987.

Wei X-Y, Luchowski EM, Rutledge A, Su CM, Triggle DJ. Pharmacologic and radioligand binding analysis of the actions of 1,4-dihydropyridine activator-antagonist pairs in smooth muscle. *J Pharmacol Exp Ther* 239:144–152, 1986.

Wei X-Y, Rutledge A, Triggle DJ. Voltage-dependent binding of 1,4-dihydropyridine Ca^{2+} channel antagonists and activators in cultured neonatal rat ventricular myocytes. *Mol Pharmacol* 35:541–552, 1989b.

Wei X-Y, Rutledge A, Zhong Q, Triggle DJ. Ca^{2+} channels in chick neuronal retina cells characterized by 1,4-dihydropyridine antagonists and activators. *Can J Physiol* 67:506–514, 1989a.

Williams JS, Grupp IL, Grupp G, Vaghy PL, Dumont L, Schwartz A, et al. Profile of the oppositely acting enantiomers of the dihydropyridine 202–791 in cardiac preparations: receptor binding, electrophysiological and pharmacologic studies. *Biochem Biophy Res Commun* 131:13–21, 1985.

Yousif FB, Bolger GT, Ruzycky A, Triggle DJ. Ca^{2+} channel antagonist actions in bladder smooth muscle: comparative pharmacologic and [3H]nitrendipine binding studies. *Can J Physiol Pharmacol* 63:453–462, 1985.

Yousif FB, Triggle DJ. Inhibitory actions of a series of Ca^{2+} channel antagonists against agonist and K+ depolarization-induced responses in smooth muscle. An assessment of selectivity of action. *Can J Physiol Pharmacol* 64:273–283, 1986.

Chapter 14

Solid State Nuclear Magnetic Resonance Spectroscopy in the Study of Drug: *Membrane Interactions, Potential Applications with Antiarrhythmic Agents*

Alexandros Makriyannis
De-Ping Yang

INTRODUCTION

Although the molecular details for the mechanism of action of antiarrhythmic drugs are not well understood, it is generally believed that the effects of these molecules on the heart involve some type of interaction with cellular membranes. To study such effects one can turn to nuclear magnetic resonance (NMR) spectroscopy as a method of choice for obtaining structural and dynamical information on ligand:biopolymer interactions. During the past two decades numerous such studies have been carried out with soluble enzymes, other functional proteins, and nucleic acid preparations in solution using high resolution techniques. In such studies, information is obtained by observing the resonances due to the ligand molecule as a function of concentration, temperature, and other ex-

Hondeghem, Luc (ed): Molecular and Cellular Mechanisms of Antiarrhythmic Agents, Futura Publishing Company, Inc., Mount Kisco, NY, © 1989.

perimental conditions. Alternatively, spectral resonances due to the biopolymer can be used as the source of information. However, this is possible only with relatively small biopolymers (MW $< 25{,}000$) since large macromolecules tend to give broad and unresolved resonances.

High resolution NMR has also been used to study drug interactions with biological or model membranes. Such studies are much narrower in scope, principally because of the limitations inherent in the technique. Indeed, to obtain solution-type spectra using high resolution techniques it is necessary to have preparations in which the membrane is in the form of small vesicles (<250Å in diameter). Furthermore, interpretation of the data can be ambiguous because of the complexities involved in the analysis of spectral linewidths, the principal piece of information available from the spectra. The above difficulties can be circumvented with the use of solid-state NMR, a method which has been used successfully since the late 1970s to obtain information on the conformation and dynamics of proteins and lipid bilayers (Griffin, 1980; Seelig, 1977; Davis, 1983).

Over the past few years we have been successful in applying solid-state NMR techniques to study the interactions of membrane-active molecules with model phospholipid membranes. Using specifically ^{2}H and ^{13}C labeled phospholipids and cholesterol we have been able to obtain information on the drug-induced conformational and dynamical changes in the membrane bilayer. This allowed us to: (a) correlate drug structure and geometry with its ability to perturb the bilayer and thus provide a molecular basis for structure: function correlations; (b) use bilayer dynamical and conformational parameters to describe *membrane perturbation*. We have also used membrane preparations containing ^{2}H-labeled drug molecules to determine their orientation and study their dynamical behavior in the bilayer.

Our studies with cannabinoids and anesthetic steroids have provided us with evidence that the nature of the drug interaction with the membrane bilayer is highly dependent on drug geometry (Makriyannis et al., 1985; Makriyannis et al., 1986; Makriyannis et al., 1987). We also obtained evidence that the observed drug: membrane interactions are *amphipathic* where the polar and hydrophobic components of the drug molecule interact with the respective components of the membrane bilayer. This chapter will serve to illustrate how solid-state NMR can be used to study drug-membrane interactions and that similar studies can be used to probe the mechanism of action of antiarrhythmic drugs.

Model Membranes in the Study of Drug:Membrane Interactions

Model phospholipid membranes have been shown to share many of the conformational and dynamical properties of biological membranes and have been used extensively in studies aimed at obtaining information on the natural system (Rance, 1980; Davis, 1983). Additionally, model membranes have been used successfully to elucidate molecular mechanisms of drug action by providing information on drug: membrane interactions. The above studies employ a variety of biophysical methods including fluorescence, electron spin resonance, and high resolution NMR. However, the method that has provided the most detailed molecular information is solid-state NMR. The model membranes used for such studies are multilamellar bilayer semisolid phospholipid preparations in aqueous environments. In these experiments one or more nuclei in the membrane or the drug molecule serve as endogenous probes. This is an advantage over the frequently utilized fluorescence and ESR, which require the presence of bulky and potentially perturbing external probes.

Phosphatidylcholines as Model Membranes

The studies described in this chapter make use of L-α-dipalmitoylphosphatidylcholine (DPPC) as the lipid for the model membranes. Our choice was motivated by the consideration that phosphatidylcholines are major membrane components whose phase properties have been studied in detail. Calorimetric measurements with fully hydrated DPPC preparations show two endothermic transitions, namely, a broad low-enthalpy pretransition ($T_c' = 35.3°C$) and a main transition ($T_c = 41.3°C$). Below the pretransition, the phospholipid molecules are arranged in a lamellar gel phase ($L_{\beta'}$) in which the chains are tilted with respect to the plane of the bilayer and exist in an all *trans* conformation. Above the main transition the phospholipid bilayers exist in the liquid crystalline phase (L_α) with the chains perpendicular to the plane of the bilayer and their segments exist in two interconverting *gauche* and *trans* populations.

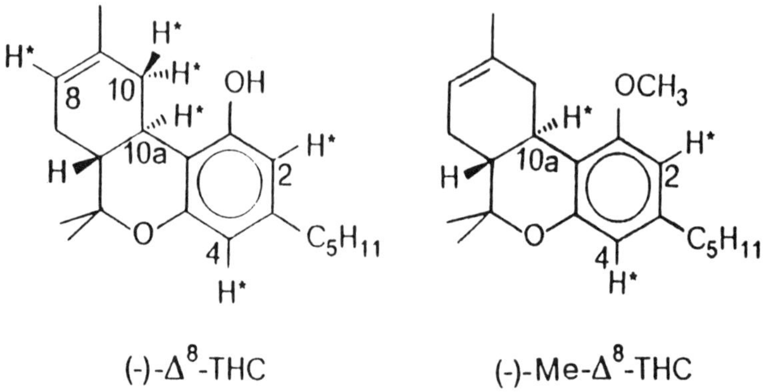

Figure 1. Structure of (-)-Δ^8-THC and (-)-Me-Δ^8-THC. Asterisks indicate the ^{2}H-labeled positions.

At temperatures between $T_c{}'$ and T_c, the preparation exists in the ripple phase ($P_{\beta'}$), which is believed to be composed of coexisting gel and liquid crystalline components.

MATERIALS AND METHODS

Materials

(-)-Δ^8-THC and (-)-O-methyl-Δ^8-THC (Fig. 1) were synthesized in our laboratory using known procedures. ^{2}H-labeled cannabinoids were synthesized according to procedures described elsewhere (Banijamali et al., 1987; Banijamali et al., 1988). L-α-dipalmitoylphosphatidylcholine (99 + %) was obtained from Sigma Chemical Company and purified chromatographically.

Samples for NMR experiments were prepared by dissolving the phospholipid and cannabinoid in 2 ml CH_2Cl_2. The solvent was then evaporated by passing a stream of nitrogen over the solution at 50°C and the residue was placed under vacuum (0.1 mmHg) for 12 hours. The cannabinoid/phospholipid mixtures were subsequently introduced in 7 mm glass tubes appropriately constricted and ^{2}H-depleted water (Sigma) was added to produce 50% w/w, lipid/water preparations. The samples were sealed under high vacuum and equilibrated at 50°C for 1 hour before recording the spectra. ^{2}H-NMR spectra were obtained on a home-built solid-state pulse spectrometer operating at 9.25 T (61.4 MHz) using a $90°_x$-τ-$90°_y$ quadrupole echo sequence (Davis et al., 1976). The ^{2}H 90° pulse width was 2.0–2.2 μs and τ = 30 μs while dwell times were 2 μs for gel-type spectra and 5 μs for L_α-type spectra. Recycle delays were 0.2 s and 8,000–16,000 echoes were accumulated for each spectrum.

^{2}H-Solid-State NMR in Membranes

In an oriented phase, the deuterium nucleus gives rise to a doublet due to the coupling of its quadrupole moment and the electric field gradient. This *quadrupole splitting* of the absorption line is equal to

$$\Delta \nu_Q = \frac{3}{4}\frac{e^2qQ}{h}\left(\frac{3\cos^2\theta - 1}{2}\right) \qquad [1]$$

where e^2qQ/h is the ^{2}H quadrupole coupling constant and θ is the angle between the magnetic field and the axis of molecular ordering. For rigid solids, all values of θ are possible and the spectrum has a *powder pattern* in which the two principal peaks correspond to θ = 90° with $\Delta\nu_Q = 3e^2qQ/4h$ and two shoulders for θ = 0° separated by $\Delta\nu_Q = 3e^2qQ/2h$.

The same powder pattern is observed in the spectra of ^{2}H-labeled multilamellar phospholipid bilayers in the liquid crystalline phase. However, in the latter case the ^{2}H-quadrupolar splitting is considerably narrowed because of rapid axial diffusion and/or *trans*:*gauche* isomerization in the chain (Fig. 2). In the gel phase, one observes a broad spectrum with no θ = 90° or θ = 0° edges. Therefore, the phase properties of the bilayer can be readily determined by examining the spectral lineshapes.

When specifically ^{2}H-labeled drug molecules are incorporated into the model membrane, their orientations in the bilayer can be determined by the following analysis. If, as expected, the drug molecule undergoes anisotropic motions in the bilayer, then each deuteron attached to the rigid tricyclic system will be expected to have an ^{2}H quadrupolar splitting described by the following equation:

$$\Delta \nu_Q = \frac{3}{4}\frac{e^2qQ}{h}\left(\frac{3\cos^2\alpha-1}{2}\right)\left\langle\frac{3\cos^2\theta-1}{2}\right\rangle \qquad [2]$$

where α is the angle between the C–^{2}H bond in question and the

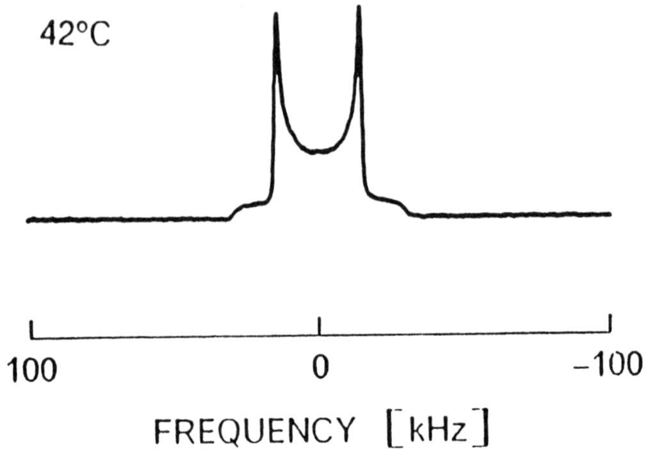

Figure 2. Solid-state ^{2}H NMR spectrum due to the 2[7′,7′-C^2H_2] segment of a DPPC aqueous dispersion at 42°C obtained using a $90°_x$-τ-$90°_y$ quadrupolar echo sequence (Davis et al., 1976) with a 90° pulse width of 2.1 μs; 8,000 echoes were signal-averaged.

rotational axis for the tricyclic component. The last term, which is known as the molecular order parameter (S_{mol}), describes the anisotropic motion of the ring system. Since S_{mol} should be identical for all ^{2}H atoms attached to the tricyclic molecular frame, the value of the observed quadrupolar splitting could be directly related to α. If the $\Delta \nu_Q$ values for a set of deuterons are available, one can then calculate both α and S_{mol} (Taylor et al., 1981), which give the geometric orientation and dynamic property of the molecule in the model membrane.

RESULTS AND DISCUSSION

Effect of (-)-Δ^8-tetrahydrocannabinol on the Phase Properties of DPPC Bilayers

Cannabinoids are believed to produce their biological properties, at least in part, by interacting with cellular membranes. In an attempt to understand their molecular mechanism of action, we have used ^{2}H-solid-state NMR to obtain information on their effects on membranes. The experiments described below make use of DPPC

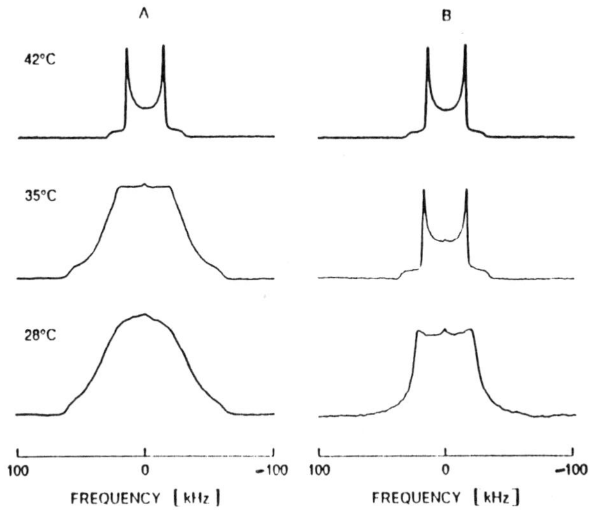

Figure 3. Temperature dependence of the ^{2}H-solid-state NMR spectra due to the 2[7′,7′-C^{2}H$_2$] segment of DPPC. (A) DPPC; (B) DPPC + (-)-Δ^8-THC (0.2M).

^{2}H-labeled at the 7-methylene segment of the *sn*-2 chain in aqueous dispersions into which the drug is incorporated.

The phase properties of hydrated DPPC preparations as described earlier are reflected in the respective ^{2}H-solid-state NMR spectra from 2[7′,7′-^{2}H$_2$] DPPC. Representative spectra obtained from the model membrane preparation in the absence and presence of (-)-Δ^8-tetrahydrocannabinol (Δ^8-THC), an active constituent of cannabis, are shown in Figure 3. The spectrum of DPPC in the L_α phase (Fig. 2) was described earlier (Makriyannis, et al., 1986). As the temperature is lowered below that of the main transition (T_c) the DPPC spectra broaden and do not display the sharp $\theta = 90°$ and $\theta = 0°$ edges that characterize the fast-limit spectra in the liquid crystalline phase. At temperatures just below the main transition and through the pretransition, the spectra acquire a flat top appearance with the $\theta = 90°$ and $\theta = 0°$ edges still discernible. This is a reflection of the coexistence of gel and liquid crystalline phases. Below the pretransition, all the *liquid crystalline* spectral features disappear. At 28°C the spectrum becomes rounded at the top. However, the spectral width is still less than one-half of that expected for the rigid lattice and is evidence that, even though in the gel phase, the DPPC chains continue to undergo diffusion along their long axes.

The most dramatic effects of Δ^8-THC on the ^2H lineshapes are produced during the transition between liquid crystalline to gel-type spectra. As is evidenced by the characteristic spectrum, at 35°C, the sample is present in the L_α phase. A general feature of the phase transition is that it is more gradual than with pure DPPC and that the spectra retain more liquid crystalline features. As the temperature is lowered below 35°C, the $\theta = 0°$ edges broaden while the center of the spectrum starts to fill. However, the $\theta = 90°$ edges maintain their sharp vertical features and the splitting is visible down to 28°C. Such spectra are characteristic of two components exchanging at an intermediate rate (Wittebort, 1982).

Our study, thus, shows that Δ^8-THC significantly decreases the phase transition temperature in model phospholipid membranes and increases the rate of acyl chain axial diffusion. In the liquid crystalline phase, the presence of Δ^8-THC results in no significant changes in the $\Delta\nu_Q$ values of 2[7′,7′-$^2H_2$] DPPC in contrast to the large changes produced by cholesterol in a similar preparation. For example at 42°C a 2[7′,7′-$^2H_2$] DPPC preparation containing cholesterol (0.15M) has a $\Delta\nu_Q$ value of 39 kHz compared to $\Delta\nu_Q = 28$ kHz for pure DPPC at the same temperature. This shows that unlike cholesterol, which produces a considerable increase in the *gauche*:*trans* conformer ratio of the methylene segments, Δ^8-THC does not affect this ratio when the measurements are carried out with the label in the 7-methylene segment close to the middle of the chain. We have shown elsewhere (Makriyannis et al., 1987) that in a 2[7′,7′-$^2H_2$] DPPC/cholesterol (0.85/0.15M) model membrane preparation, Δ^8-THC produces a significant decrease in the $\Delta\nu_Q$ values. This indicates that the drug increases the *gauche* conformer population in model phospholipid membranes containing cholesterol and, arguably, may produce similar effects on mammalian cellular membranes. Formation of larger numbers of *gauche* conformers in the phospholipid chains of membranes may be a molecular feature that can be associated with *membrane perturbation.*

Role of the Phenolic Hydroxyl Group in the (-)-Δ^8-THC:DPPC Interactions

To obtain more detailed molecular information on the Δ^8-THC:DPPC interactions, we have examined the effects of the drug

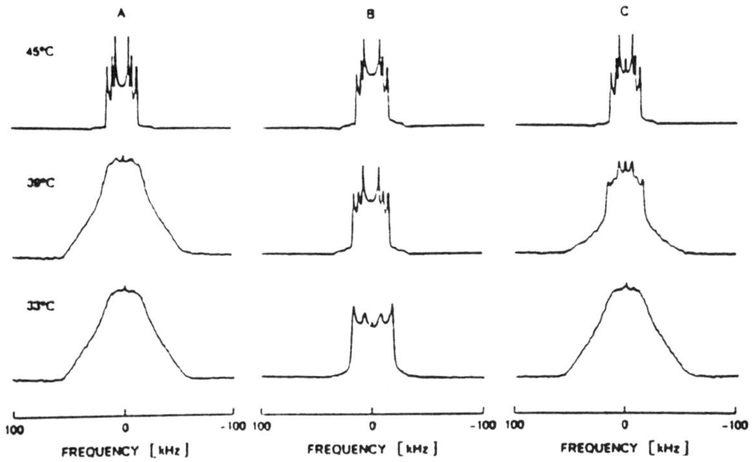

Figure 4. Temperature dependence of the ^{2}H-solid-state NMR spectra due to the 1,2[2′,2′-C^2H_2] segments of DPPC. (A) DPPC; (B) DPPC + Δ^8-THC (0.2M); (C) DPPC + Me-Δ^8-THC (0.2M).

on a second site in the DPPC bilayer, namely the first methylene segment for each of the two phospholipid chains. Furthermore, to obtain information on the role of the cannabinoid phenyl hydroxyl group during its interaction with the membrane, we have included in our studies (-)-O-methyl-Δ^8-tetrahydrocannabinol (Me-Δ^8-THC). This is a cannabinoid analog in which the phenolic hydroxyl, a polar hydrogen donor, has been substituted by the considerably less polar OCH_3 group.

Shown in Figure 4 are ^{2}H spectra of 1,2[2′,2′-$^2H_2$] DPPC aqueous dispersions (Fig. 4A) at different temperatures as well as the corresponding spectra from preparations containing Δ^8-THC (Fig. 4B) and Me-Δ^8-THC (Fig. 4C). As can be seen, when in the liquid crystalline phase, the ^{2}H spectrum of DPPC shows three components represented by three quadrupolar splittings. According to an earlier assignment (Seelig et al., 1975), the largest splitting corresponds to the two deuterons at the C-2′ position of the *sn*-1 chain and the other two splittings to the corresponding deuterons on the *sn*-2 chain. The inequivalence of the spectra due to the *sn*-1 and *sn*-2 α-C^2H_2 segments has been attributed to the different average conformations of the chains in the region of the glycerol backbone. The net result is that the beginning of the *sn*-1 chain is oriented per-

Table I
^2H Quadrupolar Splittings for 1,2[2′,2′-$^2H_2$] DPPC Preparations in the Absence and Presence of Drug Molecule (0.2M) at 45°C

	$\Delta\nu_Q$(*kHz*)		
Chain	*DPPC*	*DPPC + Δ⁸-THC*	*DPPC + Me-Δ⁸-THC*
sn-1	26.8	27.4	26.5
sn-2	17.8	19.3	17.7
	12.0	14.1	12.1

pendicular to the bilayer surface while the corresponding segments in the *sn*-2 chain are parallel to it. These interpretations are compatible with x-ray data for the crystalline phospholipid (Pearson et al., 1979).

It can be seen in Fig. 4 that Δ^8-THC produces significant changes in the spectra of 1,2[2′,2′-$^2H_2$] DPPC while its O-methyl ether analog has little effect. As with 2[7′,7′-$^2H_2$] DPPC spectra, Δ^8-THC (0.2M) decreases the main phase transition by 6°C while Me-Δ^8-THC (0.2M) produces a decrease of less than 2°C. At 39°C the spectrum from pure DPPC exhibits the flat top lineshape characteristic of the $P_{\beta'}$ phase, while that from the Δ^8-THC/DPPC preparation is a three component L_α type spectrum. Me-Δ^8-THC/DPPC gives a spectrum in which both the gel and the liquid crystalline phase are discernible. At 33°C the spectra from pure DPPC and Me-Δ^8-THC/DPPC are virtually identical with no sharp features in their lineshapes. On the other hand, the Δ^8-THC/DPPC spectra show the characteristic features described earlier with sharp $\theta = 90°$ edges but no $\theta = 0°$ edges. Only two of the three components observed in the L_α spectrum can be seen. The third, intermediate component is invisible probably due to broadening in the other two. Again, this type of spectrum is evidence for the presence of a mix of gel and liquid crystalline components undergoing intermolecular exchange at an intermediate rate.

Although the presence of Δ^8-THC produces no qualitative changes in the L_α bilayer lineshapes of DPPC, it does increase the quadrupolar splittings in all three spectral components (Table I). We notice that the increase is more significant with the two components representing the *sn*-2 chain. This effect may be interpreted to indicate a closer interaction of the drug molecule with the *sn*-2

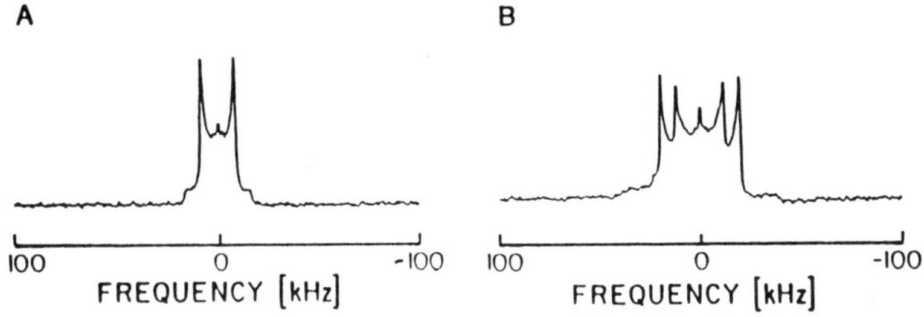

Figure 5. Representative ^{2}H-solid-state NMR spectra of ^{2}H-labeled (-)-Δ^8-THC (0.3M) in hydrated DPPC bilayers at 42°C. (A) 10a-d-(-)-Δ^8-THC; (B) 2,4-d_2-(-)-Δ^8-THC.

chain in the bilayer, and could be the result of a slight increase in the *gauche*:*trans* methylene conformer ratio. Alternatively, the increased $\Delta\nu_Q$ values may be associated with small drug-induced changes in the orientation of the α-C^2H_2 segment with respect to the bilayer surface. The methyl ether analog produces no significant changes in the quadrupolar splittings of the DPPC preparation.

The above data points to the significance of the phenolic hydroxyl group in cannabinoids during their interactions with membranes. These effects are almost entirely reversed when the hydroxyl hydrogen is substituted with the hydrophobic methyl group.

The Geometric Features of the Cannabinoid: DPPC Interaction

The conclusion regarding the essential role played by the phenolic OH during the cannabinoid:membrane interaction described in the previous section is further strengthened by our results from experiments aimed at determining the orientation of Δ^8-THC and Me-Δ^8-THC in DPPC multilamellar bilayers. The study required the introduction of ^{2}H labels in different positions of the three cannabinoid rings.

For our experiment, we synthesized Δ^8-THC with specific deuterium labels in the 2, 4, 8, 10α, 10β and 10a positions, and Me-Δ^8-THC in the 2, 4 and 10a positions. ^{2}H spectra were obtained for preparations containing one or more ^{2}H labels provided that these could be unambiguously assigned in the solid state spectra (Fig. 5). Our calculations, which will be described in detail elsewhere,

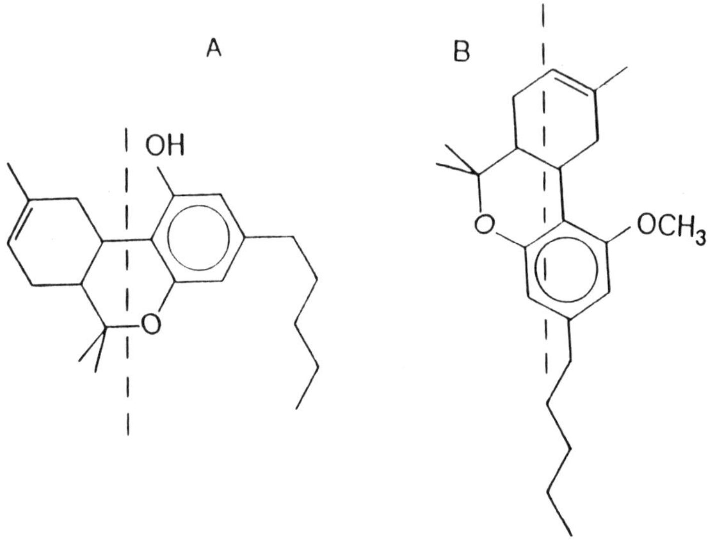

Figure 6. The orientations of (-)-Δ^8-THC and (-)-Me-Δ^8-THC in hydrated DPPC bilayers.

showed that Δ^8-THC orients with the long axis of its tricyclic structure perpendicular to the bilayer chains (Fig. 6A). Presumably, this *awkward* orientation occurs in order to optimize the interaction of the cannabinoid OH group with the polar membrane groups. On the other hand, our calculation showed that Me-Δ^8-THC assumes an orientation in which the long axis of the tricyclic structure is parallel to the lipid chains (Fig. 6B). From a geometrical and mechanical point of view, the fact that the rotation axis coincides with its natural long axis of the molecule points to the absence of hydrogen bonding between Me-Δ^8-THC and the lipid bilayer. This may explain the inability of this molecule to effectively perturb the membrane at the interface.

Based on the striking difference between the orientations of Δ^8-THC and its O-methyl ether analog in DPPC, it is tempting to speculate that the anchoring effect by the THC phenolic OH on the membrane is an essential requirement for cannabinoid activity. Therefore, the drug orientation in the amphipathic membrane may play an important role in determining the nature of the cannabinoid:membrane interaction and its ability to induce productive membrane perturbations.

The geometric requirement for drug: membrane interactions should be more stringent if the drug molecule has more than one hydroxyl group. In such a case, the preferred orientation of the drug at the active site would be one that allows all hydroxyl groups to be simultaneously oriented towards the polar side of the amphipathic bilayer. We have recently demonstrated this principle using two isomeric cannabinoids each containing two hydroxyl groups (Van der Schyf et al., 1988).

Experiments similar to those described in this chapter can be used to obtain unique information on the interactions of antiarrhythmic drugs with model and biological membranes. Such information may prove valuable for understanding the mechanism(s) of action of these drugs at the molecular level. At the same time, the molecular details of the drug: membrane interactions can provide the basis for rational design of novel antiarrhythmic agents.

Acknowledgments: This work was supported by grants from the National Institute on Drug Abuse (DA-3801) and the University of Connecticut Research Foundation (UCRF-35491). We would like to thank Professor R. G. Griffin for making the solid-state NMR spectrometer available for the deuterium NMR experiments.

BIBLIOGRAPHY

Banijamali AR, Abou Taleb N, Charalambous A, van der Schyf CJ, Makriyannis A. *J Labelled Compd Radiopharm* 25:73, 1988.
Banijamali AR, Charalambous A, van der Schyf CJ, Makriyannis A. *J Labelled Compd Radiopharm* 24:1479, 1987.
Davis JH. *Biochim Biophys Acta* 737:117, 1983.
Davis JH, Jeffrey KR, Bloom M, Valic MJ, Higgs TP. *Chem Phys Lett* 42:390, 1976.
Griffin R. *Methods in Enzymology* 79:108, 1980.
Makriyannis A, Banijamali AR, van der Schyf CJ. *Structure Activity Relationships of the Cannabinoids*. In: Rapaka R, Makriyannis A, eds. Rockville, MD: NIDA Research Monograph Series; Vol. 79, 1987.
Makriyannis A, Fesik SW. *Mol Pharmacol* 27:624, 1985.
Makriyannis A, Siminovitch DJ, Das Gupta SK, Griffin RG. *Biochim Biophys Acta* 859:49, 1986.
Pearson RH, Pascher I. *Nature (Lond)* 281:499, 1979.
Rance M, Jeffrey K, Tulloch A, Butler A, Smith ICP. *Biochim Biophys Acta* 600:245, 1980.
Seelig A, Seelig J. *Biochim Biophys Acta* 406:1, 1975.
Seelig J. *Q Rev Biophys* 10:353, 1977.
Taylor MG, Akiyama T, Smith ICP. *Chem Phys Lipids* 29:327, 1981.
Van der Schyf CJ, Mavromoustakos T, Makriyannis A. *Life Sci* 42:2231, 1988.
Wittebort RJ, Blume A, Huang TH, Das Gupta SK, Griffin RG. *Biochemistry* 21:3487, 1982.

Chapter 15

Binding Kinetics of Local Anesthetics to Closed and Open Sodium Channels During Phasic Inhibition: *Relevance to Antiarrhythmic Actions*

Daniel M. Chernoff
Gary R. Strichartz

INTRODUCTION

The blockade of impulses in excitable cells by local anesthetics results from the selective inhibition of voltage-gated sodium channels. Analysis of this inhibition to yield a mechanism at the molecular level is complicated by several factors. One is that sodium channels exist in a multiplicity of conformations. Channels take on different conformations or states in response to the membrane potential; transitions between some states are driven directly and strongly by potential, i.e., are *voltage-dependent,* whereas other transitions are only weakly voltage-dependent or are independent of potential. Many of these states are transitory in nature. At resting membrane potentials channels equilibrate between resting states (**R**) and inactivated states (**I**), and pass infrequently and transiently

Hondeghem, Luc (ed): Molecular and Cellular Mechanisms of Antiarrhythmic Agents, Futura Publishing Company, Inc., Mount Kisco, NY, © 1989.

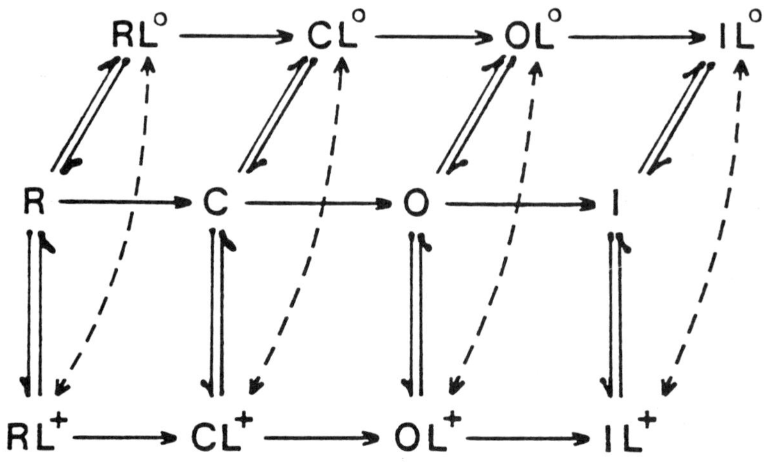

Figure 1. A general kinetic scheme for the binding of protonatable anesthetics to sodium channels. Sodium channels are depicted as existing in resting (*R*), preopen closed (*C*), open (*O*), and inactivated (*I*) states. Each state can bind anesthetic in either the neutral (1^0) or protonated (L^+) form, but both the rates of binding and equilibrium binding will in general depend on the channel conformation, the form of drug, and the concentrations in the compartments which have access to the binding site. Bound drug can gain or lose a proton by exchange with the extracellular compartment, but with rate constants and pK_a that may differ from those measured in bulk solution. Only *O* contributes to the macroscopic current.

to preopen (**C**) and open (**O**) states (Fig. 1). Rapid membrane depolarization, such as typically occurs during voltage-clamp experiments, alters all the voltage-dependent transition rates, and the channels relax through a sequence of **C, O,** and **I** states before reaching a new equilibrium, different from the one at rest.

The reactions of local anesthetics with the newly populated channel states differ from those for the states available at rest. The extent of local anesthetic (LA) binding is conventially measured by changes in the magnitude of peak Na^+ current (I_{Na}) elicited by a test depolarization. Binding is increased by preceding depolarizations indicating that certain voltage-gated states are more susceptible to inhibition by anesthetics. This phenomenon is called *use-dependent* or phasic inhibition. As schematized in Figure 1, the binding of local anesthetic (LA) to a channel state, shown by the transitions to *L complexed* forms, e.g. **R** to $\mathbf{RL^+}$ and $\mathbf{RL^\circ}$, is greater for *activated* states (**C** + **O**) and inactivated states (**I**) than for the resting state, **R.** Although earlier hypotheses emphasized the greater sensitivity of the inactivated states to anesthetic block, recent results show that for some LAs, binding to activated channels is sufficient to account for most use-dependent inhibition in axons (Strichartz and Wang, 1986; Wang et al., 1987). This follows from the briefness of the nerve impulse, when short depolarizations (~1 msec) strongly favor the more rapid binding reactions, which are typically to open or preopen *activated* states. (see Duration-dependence of Block, B_{ss}). Cardiac (ventricular) action potentials have plateau depolarizations lasting 100–200 times longer, during which many Na^+ channels reach an inactivated state that binds LAs tightly yet more slowly than the activated states. The inhibition of I_{Na} arising from this *late* binding is reversed slowly in the repolarized membrane and probably accounts for much of the antiarrhythmic and antifibrillatory actions of these drugs.

Ionization of LA also plays a critical role in the binding kinetics. Both cationic and base species of LA exist in the solutions bathing tissues at near neutral pH. It is possible that both species can bind to all states of the channel, as proposed by the binding reactions in the vertical and horizontal planes of Figure 1. Acid-base reactions involving bound drug may also occur (see Fig. 1: broken curves). It has been observed that when local anesthetics are applied at more alkaline pH, the decrease in I_{Na} is faster, and the final resting inhibition greater than for the same drug concentration applied at neutral pH (Hille, 1977b). *Use-dependent* inhibition, however, is less at alkaline than at neutral extracellular pH (Schwarz et al., 1977). The permeation of nerve membrane seems to be an important feature governing this local anesthetic action. The neutral (base) form of LA permeates more rapidly than the charged (acid) species, but once in the cytoplasm the drug will be protonated according to the pH of that phase. Studies with permanently charged quaternary local anesthetics imply that the cationic species is the more potent one for use-dependent block, if it can reach sites on the membrane or channel that are accessible from the cytoplasm (Frazier et al., 1970; Strichartz, 1973). Some permanently neutral local anesthetics, i.e., benzocaine, effect a resting block but produce negligible use-dependent inhibition (Hille, 1977a,b). Others produce both resting and use-dependent block (Chernoff and Strichartz, 1989), so the nature of the block cannot be identified with a single species of LA.

These separate observations have been integrated in a scheme where a single site for local anesthetics on a sodium channel is accessible by two pathways: a hydrophilic one, through the channel's pore from the cytoplasm; and a hydrophobic one, through the membrane (Hille, 1977a). The hydrophilic path is favored by charged drug molecules and kinetically restricted by the channel conformation, being only available in open channels; the hydrophobic path is always available to neutral drug molecules. In the original formulation, activated channels were envisioned as having a higher equilibrium affinity for local anesthetics than resting channels, aside from any kinetic limitations. But recent theories, evolving as a *guarded receptor hypothesis,* account for use-dependent inhibition by kinetic restrictions alone, postulating an anesthetic site of constant affinity but strongly state-dependent accessibility (Starmer et al., 1984). Regardless of the model being used, protonation of local anesthetics clearly is important for determining levels of resting and use-dependent inhibition.

The assays for inhibition of I_{Na} can confuse the analysis of local anesthetic mechanisms. Some reactions of drug molecules with channels may occur during the course of a test pulse, changing the size of the signal even as it is being measured. Protonation reactions of local anesthetics also may have relaxation times comparable to the lifetimes of channel states, particularly for bound drug molecules where the availability of proton donors and acceptors in the membrane or on the channel is probably different than in solution. Binding per se may alter a drug's pK_a, and in a reciprocal manner the degree of protonation will modify the binding.

All of these reactions are inferred from a distance, because the actual binding of local anesthetics to Na^+ channels has never been measured directly. All kinetic models of local anesthetic action assume that binding at an active site is sufficient to produce inhibition, and measured changes in I_{Na} are equated with fractional occupancy and used to calculate drug binding and dissociation. Although not explicitly addressed by our data, a microscopic mechanism of channel inhibition accompanies almost every kinetic model for local anesthetic action. We believe that the extensive evidence showing the drug-dependent immobilization of gating charge, and its exacerbation by repetitive depolarization indicates a major role for the inhibition of the activation process (Cahalan and Almers, 1979; Neumcke et al., 1981). On the other hand, data directly showing any blocking of normal open channels, i.e., a shortening of open channel lifetime, are lacking (Yeh et al., 1986). Local anesthetics appear to prevent at least some of the conformational changes underlying activation, but do not appear to *plug* open sodium channels.

Here, we have investigated the role of protonation in the kinetics of I_{Na} inhibition in myelinated nerve. By using a series of lidocaine homologues of different solution pK_a or hydrophobicity, we have observed different rates for the development and reversal of use-dependent inhibition. The pH-dependence of these rates provides a test for the relative contributions of hydrophobicity and protonation in local anesthetic binding reactions. Our results show that, while protonation of local anesthetic molecules can influence these reactions, both protonated and neutral forms do dissociate from closed channels. We have also examined the role of membrane potential in governing the onset and recovery kinetics of use-dependent block. Our results show several inconsistencies with any hypothesis that focuses exclusively on open or inactivated channels to account for use-dependent block and instead, suggest the involvement of preopen activated states in drug binding.

METHODS

Myelinated Nerve Fiber Voltage Clamp

Single myelinated nerve fibers from sciatic nerves of toad (*Bufo marinus,* Charles D. Sullivan Co., Nashville, TN) were isolated, mounted in a plexiglass chamber, and voltage clamped as described by Dodge and Frankenhaeuser (1958). All experiments were performed at 13 ± 1°C, the temperature maintained by a circulating temperature-controlled bath. Clamp settling time was <50 μsec in most experiments, and membrane potential reached 90% of the command potential within 20–30 μsec following a step potential change. Series resistance was partially compensated by using positive feedback around the voltage clamp amplifier (Sigworth, 1979). The volume of the pool bathing the node was about 0.1 ml, and the length of axon exposed to the test solutions was about 150 μm. Two ml of test solution were flushed through this pool in 15–30 sec to effect solution changes. Potassium currents were blocked by internal Cs^+ (120 mM). Linear membrane leakage and capacity currents were subtracted by an analog circuit with two adjustable time constants. The clamp was interfaced with an IBM-AT computer via a Labmaster A/D board (Scientific Solutions, Inc., Cleveland, OH) with

pCLAMP data acquisition software (Axon Instruments Inc, Burlingame CA). The current signal from the clamp amplifier was sampled at 25 kHz after passing through a 2-pole homemade low-pass Butterworth filter with 5 kHz corner frequency. The activation kinetics of sodium currents were too fast to be reliably recorded at this bandwidth, but the attenuation of peak currents by filtering was less than 5%. Membrane currents were estimated by scaling the clamp amplifier output by an assumed internodal resistance of 10 MΩ.

Solutions

External Ringer solutions contained (in mM): 110 NaCl, 2.5 KCl, 2.0 $CaCl_2$, 5 NaOH, and 10 H^+ buffer, where the buffer was either MES (pH 6.2), MOPS (pH 7.3), TAPS (pH 8.5), or CAPS (pH 10.4), titrated to final pH with NaOH. The internodes were cut in internal solution, containing (in mM): 120 CsCl, 5 NaOH, 10 MOPS, titrated to pH 7.2 with tetramethylammonium-OH. For some experiments in which the time course of use-dependent block at large depolarizations was studied, 30 mM internal CsCl was replaced with an equal amount of NaCl to produce larger (outward) currents.

Chemicals

Lidocaine·HCl and D-bupivacaine·HCl (the (+) optical isomer of bupivacaine) were the gift of Dr. Bertil Takman, Astra Pharmaceuticals, Westboro, MA. Glycylxylidide (compound III: GX) and PRG-030 (compound IV: 5-(diethylamino)pentano-2′,6′-xylidide) were generously provided as the HCl salts by Drs. Paul McMaster, College of the Holy Cross, and Eugene Byrnes, Assumption College, both in Worcester, MA. The chemical structures, pK_a, and octanol:buffer partition coefficients of these compounds are shown in Table I. Compounds I-III were prepared as 50 mM, 10 mM, and 100 mM stock solutions, respectively, in MOPS-Ringer. Compound IV was prepared as a 100 mM stock in ethanol. All stocks were stored at $-15°$ C in small aliquots. Individual aliquots were thawed and stored at 4° C for no more than seven days prior to use.

Modeling of Use-dependent Block

A three parameter model was developed to describe the decrease in peak I_{Na} produced by a train of pulses (use-dependent block). In

Table I

	Drug	M.W.	Structure	pKa[a]	p°	p+	IC50(μM)[d]
I	(lidocaine)	234	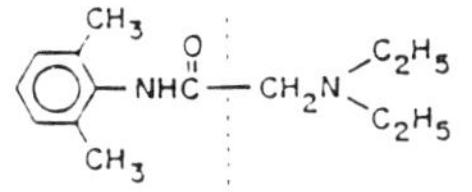	8.19	304[b]	0.06[b]	200
II	(bupivacaine)	288	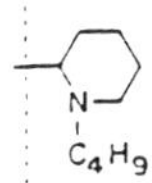	8.21	2565[b]	1.5[b]	25
III	(glycylxylidide)	178	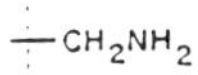	8.02	2.8[c]	?	800
IV	(PRG-030)	276	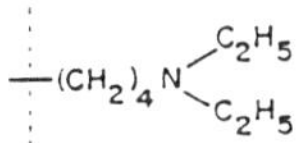	10.56	263[c]	?	1000

a. at 25°C in 0.17M NaCl-buffer
b. relative concentrations, between octanol and buffer, 25°C
c. relative concentrations, between octanol and H_2O, 37°C
d. concentration producing a 50% tonic decrease in P_{Na} at E_{hold} = -100mV, T=13°C

brief, the model separates the pulse train into two kinetically distinct intervals. During each depolarization, or *pulse,* channels enter states, s_i, which favor binding of drug. This increase in apparent affinity is produced by an increase in the forward binding rate (*guarded receptor*) and/or a decrease in the reverse binding rate (*modulated receptor*). In order to fully characterize the blocking kinetics, one needs to know, for each s_i, not only the forward and reverse binding rates, but also the mean dwell time of the channel in s_i as a function of pulse potential and duration. One approach to this problem is to assume that only a single state participates in binding (e.g., the open state: Starmer et al., 1986), with an access interval equal to the mean dwell time of Na channels in that state. As we shall show, this simplification is unlikely to be valid for all drugs, i.e., preopen and inactivated states appear to bind drug. We have chosen, therefore, to characterize binding during a depolarization by two dimensionless parameters: $B_d(\infty)$, representing an average of the equilibrium binding to each state, weighted by the dwell times; and k_d, describing the fractional increment in block per pulse. These empirically derived parameters assume only that binding is a first-order process, and both parameters will in general depend on

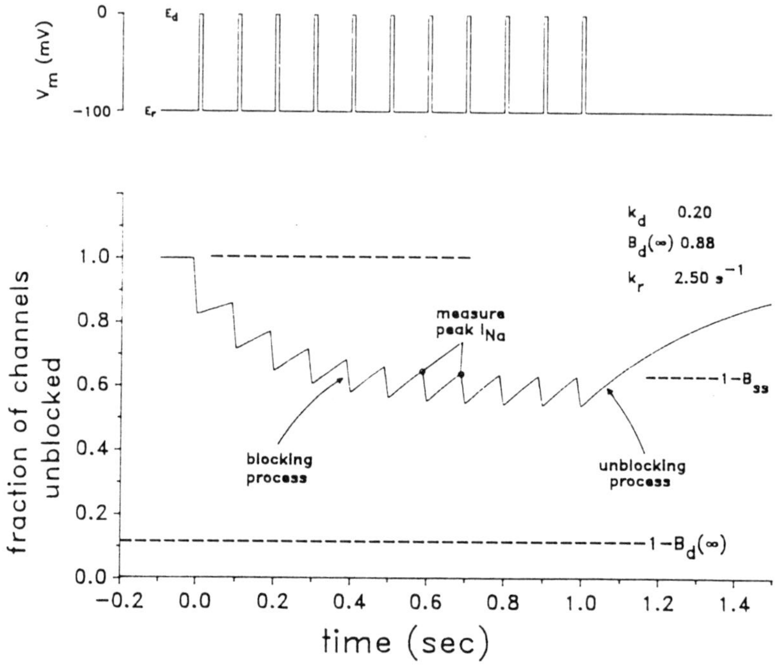

Figure 2. Simulation of use-dependent block in a voltage-clamp experiment. During each depolarization a fraction of the unblocked channels becomes blocked. During each repolarized interval, blocked channels continuously recover towards equilibrium (here assumed to be 0% block). Depending on the kinetics of binding during depolarization, peak I_{Na} may assay the fraction of channels unblocked at the start of depolarization (as drawn) or a smaller fraction if channels become blocked prior to peak I_{Na}. B_{ss} (equation 2) is 0.389 for the simulation shown (10 msec depolarization, 90 msec repolarization intervals).

pulse amplitude and duration. In the case of a single high affinity state, the characteristic time constant, tau, and the mean dwell time can replace k_d (Starmer and Courtney, 1986).

During each repolarized interval, recovery from the increased block is continuous and is described by an exponential rate parameter, k_r (units of sec^{-1}). A simulation based on this model depicts an increase in blocked channels during a 10 Hz pulse train (Fig. 2). A recursion relation for the fraction of channels blocked just prior to a given pulse in the train is

$$B_0 = 0 \quad [1a]$$

$$B_n = [B_{n-1}(1 - k_d) + k_d B_d(\infty)] \cdot \exp\{-k_r t_r\} \quad [1b]$$

where t_r is the interstimulus interval. The steady state block, B_{ss}, is

$$B_{ss} = \frac{k_d B_d(\infty) \cdot \exp\{-k_r t_r\}}{1 - (1 - k_d) \cdot \exp\{-k_r t_r\}} \qquad [2]$$

and a *pulse constant*, N, representing the number of pulses required to reach 1/e of steady state, is

$$N = [k_r t_r - \ln\{1 - k_d\}]^{-1} \qquad [3]$$

Curve Fitting

Fits of the model parameters described above, $B_d(\infty)$, k_r, and k_d, to use-dependent block data were performed using a nonlinear least-squares "Patternsearch" algorithm (Colquhoun, 1971). Peak currents from successive depolarizations at a given frequency were normalized to the size of the first peak in the pulse train. Data from runs at three or more repetition rates were weighted equally by the curve-fitting algorithm, which matched the observed change in peak current to the predicted change based on the recursion relation (equation 1) described above.

RESULTS

Analysis of Recovery Rates

The kinetics of recovery of sodium currents following use-dependent block by a wide variety of agents have been reported in the literature (reviewed by Courtney, 1987). When the time-course of recovery of peak I_{Na} is assessed by varying the interval between a train of conditioning pulses (to establish a steady-state level of inhibition) and a single test pulse, two exponential processes are usually observed—a fast component representing unblocked channels recovering from fast inactivation, and a slower component probably representing dissociation of drug from a binding site (Yeh and Tanguy, 1985). We refer to the rate constant of this slow component of recovery as k_r.

Dependence of k_r on Pulse Width and Potential

There is no *a priori* reason to believe that the rate of recovery from use-dependent block will be independent of the manner in

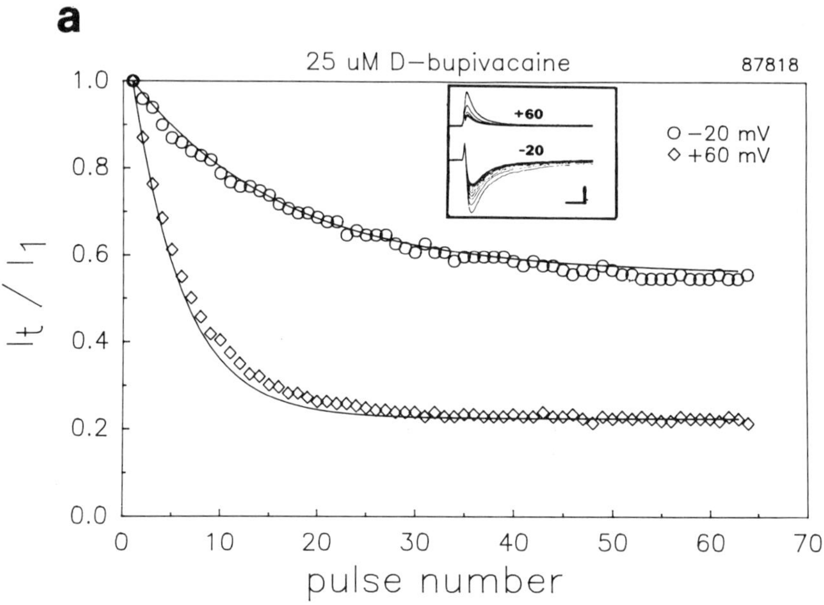

Figure 3A. The rate of recovery from use-dependent block is independent of pulse potential and duration. A. Following a period of rest at E_{hold} = −100 mV, use-dependent block is induced by a series of 16 msec pulses to −20 mV (circles) or +60 mV (diamonds) applied at 10 Hz. Raw current traces are also shown for the first and every fifth subsequent pulse (inset). The decreases in peak current were fit by the three parameter blocking model (continuous curves), with a common recovery rate k_r = 0.062 s^{-1}, and blocking parameters at −20 mV: k_d = 0.052, $B_d(\infty)$ = 0.508, or at +60 mV: k_d = 0.169, $B_d(\infty)$ = 0.809. Elevated internal Na^+ (35 mM) was used to produce larger outward currents. Parameter estimates were derived from the data shown together with separate trials at 4 and 1 Hz.

which the block was produced. For example, channels that are blocked while in the open conformation might recover at a different rate than channels that are blocked from the inactivated state. We tested this question experimentally by examining the dependence of k_r on the duration of the conditioning pulses and on the pulse potential (E_d).

The piecewise-linear kinetic model described in the METHODS section was used to fit a single exponential recovery rate to the use-dependent inhibition of peak I_{Na} data obtained at different rates of stimulation. In one such experiment with bupivacaine, changes in peak I_{Na} in response to pulses to +60 mV are compared to the same

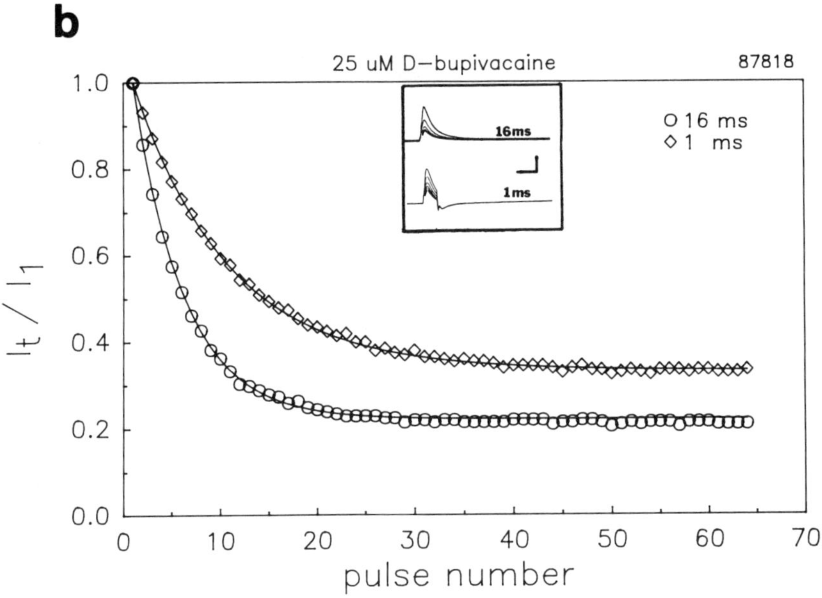

Figure 3B. Longer pulses potentiate block without affecting the recovery rate. A train of pulses to +60 mV with an interstimulus interval of 100 msec is shown for pulse durations of 16 msec (circles) or 1 msec (diamonds). Common recovery rate $k_r = 0.061\ s^{-1}$. Blocking parameters: $k_d = 0.169$, $B_d(\infty) = 0.809$ (16 msec pulses); $k_d = 0.091$, $B_d(\infty) = 0.715$ (1 msec pulses). 25 μM D-bupivacaine. Fiber 87818A. Scale bars 5 nA, 1 msec.

parameter kinetics obtained from pulses to −20 mV (Figs. 3A and 3B). We found that the kinetic model could fit both sets of observations with a common interpulse recovery rate of 0.061 s^{-1} (Fig. 3A, continuous lines). The greater block seen with large depolarizations can thus be entirely ascribed to more extensive LA binding during the conditioning pulses. Similarly, the potentiation of block with 16 msec pulses to +60 mV (producing complete inactivation) relative to that observed with pulses to the same potential but lasting only 1 msec (slightly longer than the time to peak I_{Na}) is consistent with a larger fraction of channels blocked with each pulse, not with a difference in the kinetics of recovery (Fig. 3B). Thus, blocked channels are not driven into slower recovering states by longer depolarizations. Experiments with the other anesthetics used in this study yielded similar results. We also point out that the number of pulses, N, required for peak I_{Na} to reach 1/e of steady-state is less for the conditions that produce greater steady-state block. If the potentiation of block were due to a slowing of recovery between pulses, an **increase** in N would be predicted (equation 3). We conclude that the rate of recovery from use-dependent block is independent of the size and duration of the conditioning pulses over the range tested (1–32 msec, −60 mV to +80 mV). If this result also holds for cardiac Na^+ channels, then antiarrhythmic potency will depend strongly on the duration of the plateau through the development of inhibition during depolarization, and reversal of inhibition during diastole will occur at a constant rate. We will return to consider this prediction further.

Dependence of k_r on E_{hold}

The rate of recovery from use-dependent block with a number of LAs has been reported to be modulated by the repolarization (holding) potential. For the quaternary lidocaine analog QX-314, the rate of recovery is increased by small depolarizing pulses consistent with a model wherein the drug can be trapped on its binding site when the Na channel is in the resting, closed conformation (Strichartz, 1973). In similar experiments in squid axon, where the rate of recovery was measured as a function of the holding potential alone, membrane hyperpolarization was shown to slow markedly the recovery from block with QX-314, with the homologous trimethyl derivative QX-222, and with 9-aminoacridine (a tertiary amine drug with a $pK_a > 10$, so that it exists almost completely in the charged form at physiological pH), (Yeh and Tanguy, 1985). In contrast, little voltage dependence of recovery was observed with lidocaine. These observations are consistent with the *m-gate* trapping model proposed as part of the guarded receptor hypothesis (Starmer et al., 1984), wherein the channel must gate to the open state to release a trapped anesthetic molecule; the same observations are difficult to reconcile with the modulated receptor hypothesis, in which hyperpolarization would be expected to *accelerate* drug dissociation from inactivated state(s) of the channel (Hondeghem and Katzung, 1977; Hille, 1977a). Under the guarded receptor hypothesis, the lack of voltage dependence observed with lidocaine is consistent with escape of the neutral species from the binding site of closed (or open) channels via a hydrophobic route, one which is energetically unfavorable for the charged molecule (Courtney and Starmer, 1986). The recovery

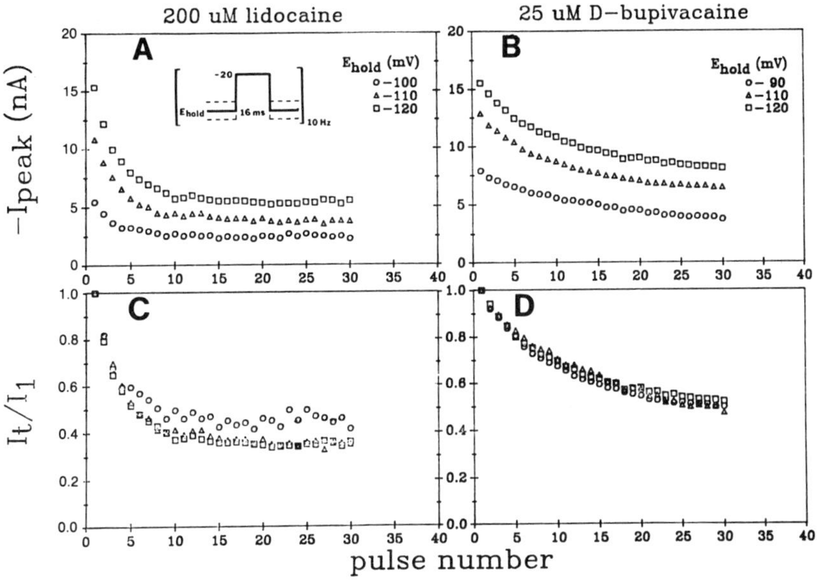

Figure 4. Effect of holding potential on use-dependent block with lidocaine and bupivacaine. Pulse protocol is shown in A (inset). A and B: Peak currents (unnormalized) are plotted in A (lidocaine) and B (bupivacaine), as a function of holding potential. C and D: The data from A and B are replotted after normalizing by the size of the first peak current in the pulse train. Little change in the time course of the use-dependent component of block is noted. Fibers 87N23 (lidocaine) and 87N22B (bupivacaine).

rate in this case will be limited by the rate of protonation/deprotonation and not by the frequency of channel gating.

We have examined the voltage dependence of k_r with lidocaine and bupivacaine for comparison with the results reported in other preparations. Varying the holding potential does not markedly affect the time course of use-dependent block with lidocaine or bupivacaine (Figs. 4A and 4B). Despite a large increase in tonic block and/or inactivation at more depolarized potentials (unnormalized peak currents, Figs. 4A and 4B), when the data are normalized to the amplitude of the tonically blocked current (Figs. 4C and 4D), the parameters of use-dependent block do not change significantly with E_{hold}. In particular, the recovery rate, k_r, estimated by applying the uptake model to these data and additional trials at 1 and 4 Hz, varied by less than 10% over the voltage range tested, −90 to −120 mV. This is noteworthy in that bupivacaine is a kinetically slow drug with a recovery rate at pH_o 7.3, comparable to that observed for QX-222 in squid by Yeh and Tanguy (1985), for which a strong voltage dependence was noted. It is possible that nodal Na channels from toad do not exhibit the same gating characteristics as those of squid axon, or that recovery from bupivacaine block, unlike QX-222, is not potentiated by the gating of channels towards the open state. These possibilities require further study.

pH_o Dependence of k_r

To what extent is the rate of recovery of sodium currents from use-dependent block governed by the charge of the anesthetic? The rate of approach to steady-state use-dependent block in frog skeletal muscle in the presence of lidocaine and procaine (but not the permanently charged QX-314 or neutral benzocaine) has been shown to depend on external pH (Schwarz et al., 1977). We have measured the kinetics of block with the four drugs used in this report over the pH range 6.2–10.4. Figure 5 shows examples with lidocaine (A) and bupivacaine (B). The pH-dependence of use-dependent block (measured at 2 or 3 stimulation rates) yields estimates of the model parameters k_d, $B_d(\infty)$, and k_r. There is a parallel increase in the values of all three parameters as pH_o is raised, although the mechanism responsible for the increase in k_r is likely to be different than that for the increase in the depolarization block parameters, as will be discussed later. Summary data for the four drugs tested is collected in Table II. Several features of these data are noteworthy: (1) k_r appears to increase monotonically with pH_o: Schwarz et al. (1977) have indicated that this pH dependence is a function of the degree of drug protonation and not a change in the binding site, since block by the quaternary QX-314 did not show significant pH dependence; (2) there is a flattening of the k_r-pH_o relationship at the extremes of pH, suggesting that distinct pH-dependent reactions may be rate-limiting at low and high pH; (3) a common recovery rate for all drugs at the extremes of pH is not observed, indicating that knowledge of the mean drug charge alone is insufficient to predict the recovery rate; (4) the drug with the highest pK_a (compound IV) displays the weakest k_r-pH_o relationship, consistent with the predominance of the protonated form of compound IV throughout the pH range explored.

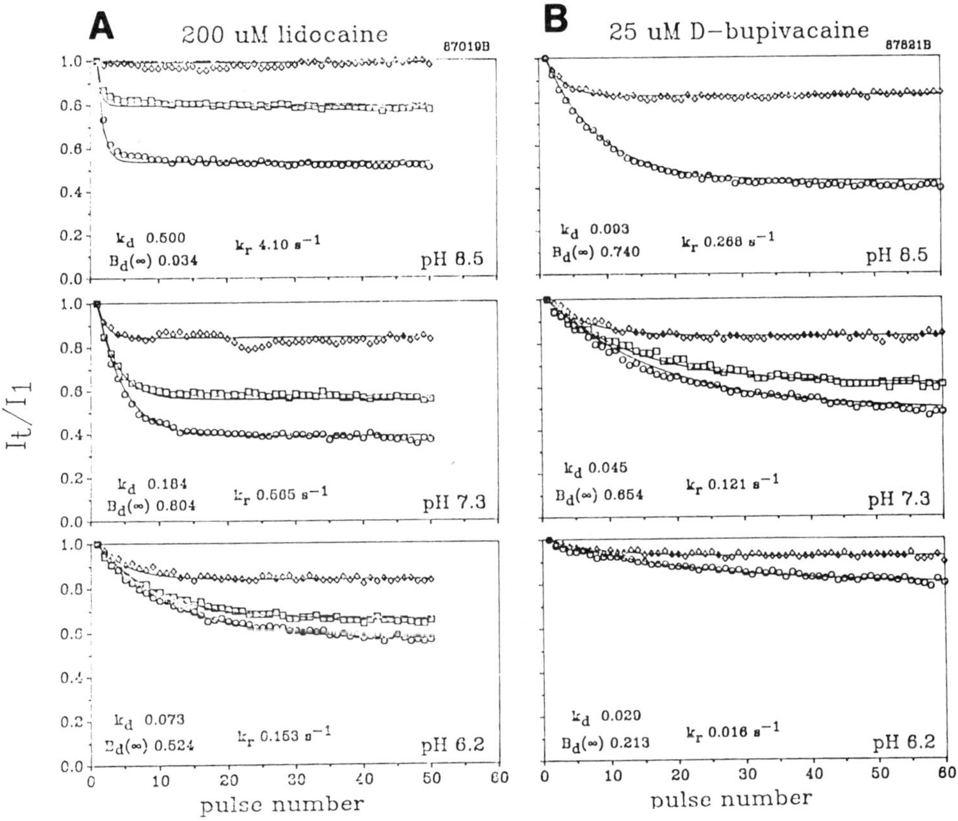

Figure 5. Effect of changes in pH_0 on use-dependent block with lidocaine (left panels) or bupivacaine (right panels). At a given pH_0, pulse trains (16 msec duration, 80 mV depolarization from E_{hold}) were applied at 10 Hz (circles), 4 Hz (squares) and 1 Hz (diamonds). Solution at a new pH was then washed in with the drug concentration held constant, and 5 minutes allowed for the system to re-equilibrate before pulse trains were applied. The calculated block parameters are shown below each data set and the fits of the model to the data are shown as the continuous curves. Fibers 87019B (lidocaine) and 87821B (bupivacaine).

Kinetics of Binding During Depolarization

Probing the kinetics of binding during depolarization presents a more challenging experimental problem than studying the kinetics of recovery. This is largely due to the transient nature of Na channel conformations during depolarization, each of which may

Table II
Kinetic Parameters of Use-Dependent Block

Compound		*External pH* 6.2	*n*	7.3	*n*	8.5	*n*	10.4	*n*
I	k_d	.071 ± .002		.156 ± .048		.360 ± .096		—	
	$B_d(\infty)$	.412 ± .112	3	.595 ± .143	9	.806 ± .164	5	—	
	$k_r(s^{-1})$	.182 ± .029		.651 ± .113		3.130 ± 1.42		—	
II	k_d	.041 ± .001		.074 ± .043		.108 ± .502		.111 ± .035	
	$B_d(\infty)$	.366 ± .125	2	.564 ± .144	10	.693 ± .204	7	.796 ± .130	3
	$k_r(s^{-1})$	.056 ± .026		.067 ± .031		.626 ± .361		1.68 ± .070	
III	k_d	.131 ± .012		.154 ± .058		.154 ± .046		—	
	$B_d(\infty)$	.278 ± .071	3	.451 ± .126	3	.644 ± .144	2	—	
	$k_r(s^{-1})$	.218 ± .069		.456 ± .153		1.59 ± .660		—	
IV	k_d	—		.031 ± .009		.080 ± .030		.181	
	$B_d(\infty)$	—		.511 ± .128	3	.754 ± .030	3	.833	1
	$k_r(s^{-1})$	—		.038 ± .005		.026 ± .008		.085	

determined from the development of block during trains of 1, 4 and 10 Hz pulses of 16 msec duration to −20 mV. T = 13°C.

bind drug at different rates. The problem is compounded when analyzing the binding of tertiary amine drugs, for which the charged and neutral conformers may exhibit different potency, rates of action, and routes of access to the binding site.

The estimation of rate and equilibrium binding constants during depolarization depends strongly on the model assumed. For example, in the original application of the guarded receptor model to lidocaine block of cardiac Na channels (Starmer et al., 1984), the calculated equilibrium binding constant, K_d, was three orders of magnitude smaller than that estimated using a modulated receptor model (Bean et al., 1983). In a more recent application of the guarded receptor hypothesis to ion channel block by tertiary amine drugs (Starmer and Courtney, 1986), it was postulated that the charged form interacts with the open conformation only (guard and trap functions proportional to m^3h) where m and h are Hodgkin-Huxley parameters, while the neutral form can bind to the inactivated channel as well but is not trapped (guard function = m^3, trap function = 1). Having established that the rate of recovery between pulses is independent of pulse magnitude and duration (see above), we have qualitatively tested the robustness of these guard and trap functions for charged and neutral forms of drug by examining the dependence of steady-state use-dependent block on the magnitude and duration of the conditioning pulses.

Duration- and Voltage-Dependence of B_{ss}

In Fig. 6, the dependence of B_{ss} on the size of the depolarization is plotted for each of the four drugs tested (at a stimulation rate of 10 Hz, duration of 16 msec, and with drug concentrations producing 50% tonic block). Superimposed on the plot is a dashed curve representing the integral of sodium permeability during a single 16 msec test pulse, as a function of the test pulse potential. There is a maximum in this integral due to an increasing rate of inactivation at more positive potentials coupled with a saturation in peak P_{Na} (Bean, 1981; Sutro, 1986).

Several features are noteworthy: (1) the local maximum in B_{ss} around −40mV, seen best for compounds III and IV, correlates with the maximum in the integral of P_{Na}; (2) B_{ss} continues to increase for potentials well beyond the saturation potential for P_{Na}; and (3) a significant use-dependent block is seen at potentials smaller than

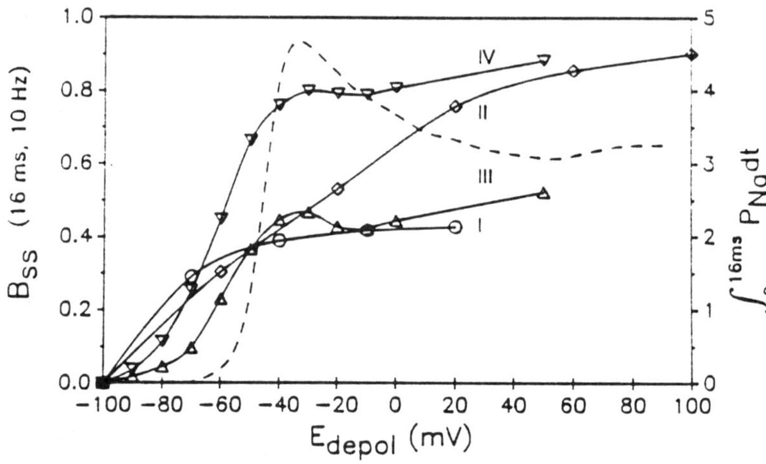

Figure 6. Voltage dependence of B_{ss}. Pulse trains (16 msec depolarizations @ 10 Hz) were applied in sufficient number to reach steady-state block. This steady-state block was then assayed by a standard pulse to −20 mV applied 100 msec following the last pulse in the train. For comparison with availability of the open channel state, the integral of P_{Na} is plotted as a function of the test pulse potential in arbitrary units (dashed curve), using the Goldman-Hodgkin-Katz equation to convert Na currents to permeabilities. Data for each drug at concentrations producing 50% tonic block are shown: 0.2 mM compound I (lidocaine), fiber 87708; 0.025 mM compound II (bupivacaine), fiber 87730; 0.8 mM compound III, fiber 88201; 1.0 mM compound IV, fiber 88309B. The smooth curves connecting the data points have no theoretical significance.

those required to produce measurable macroscopic currents. The first feature is consistent with the guarded receptor hypothesis, in which access is limited to open channels. The second feature is consistent with a binding site located within the membrane electric field. This location would produce voltage-dependent rates of binding of the charged species (Strichartz, 1973, but see also Wang et al., 1987). Alternatively, slower channel blocking reactions involving inactivated states may account for the continued increase in B_{ss} at large depolarizations, as channels appear to inactivate more rapidly and to a greater extent at more positive potentials. The third feature, however, seems quantitatively at odds with the open channels requirement of the guarded receptor hypothesis.

The dependence of B_{ss} on pulse duration is shown in Fig. 7, for a fixed depolarizing step of 80 mV from rest; the integrated sodium

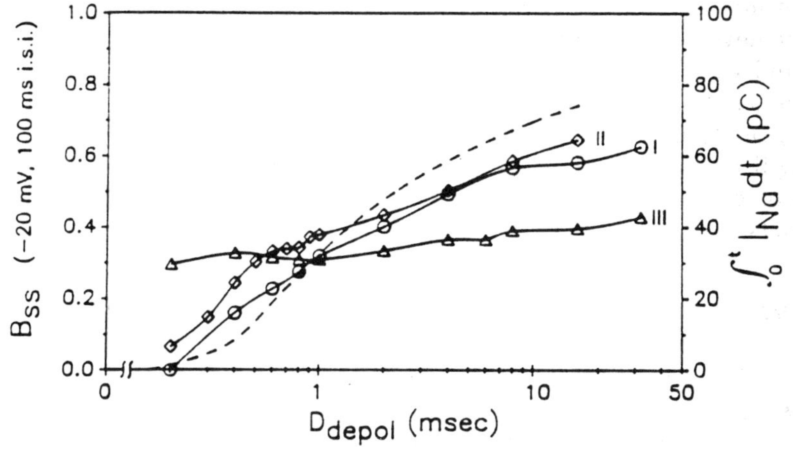

Figure 7. Duration dependence of B_{ss}. B_{ss} is plotted for compounds I–III as a function of the test pulse duration, maintaining the inter-stimulus interval (isi) constant at 100 msec and the pulse potential at −20 mV. The steady-state block is compared with the integral of sodium current for a single depolarization to −20 mV (dashed curve). A logarithmic abscissa is used to emphasize the block observed with short duration pulses. Compound 1, fiber 87N23; compound 2, fiber 87019A; compound 3, fiber 88201.

current, a measure of the total open time of the channels, is overlaid (dashed curve). All the drugs reduce I_{Na} proportionately more for short pulses than predicted by an open channel restriction. It is notable that the steady-state block with compound III is near-maximal for pulses of 0.2 msec duration, which is considerably shorter than the time to peak I_{Na}, ca. 0.5 msec. This behavior, which has also been observed with the lidocaine homologue GEA-968 (Strichartz and Wang, 1986), suggests that preopen states are the predominant substrates for rapid binding of some drugs.

The dependence of elicited inhibition on potential amplitude and duration should have important ramifications for antiarrhythmic actions. Subthreshold depolarizations are able to induce significant LA binding, even after only 16 msec, and thus the pattern of potential during diastole will have direct effects on the fraction of available Na^+ channels. During the plateau phase of depolarization the binding of LA also increases—in a manner strongly dependent on the particular drug. Some agents may bind slowly but persistently in this period, e.g., bupivacaine, providing a net inhibition that depends strongly on the duration of systole; others may achieve their full effect for the shortest systolic plateau (<100 msec) and will not be potentiated by longer depolarizations. The dependence on duration at negative potentials is also an important *therapeutic* parameter. Obviously, threshold for cardiac action potentials will be increased in a time-dependent mode by drugs that bind to preopen channels during diastole and to open and inactivated channels during systole.

pH_o Dependence of k_d

The kinetics of block during depolarizations are observed to vary with pH_o in a systematic fashion (see Fig. 5 and Table II). As pH_o is raised, the fractional block per pulse, k_d, and the theoretical equilibrium block, $B_d(\infty)$, both increase. These offsetting trends result in a steady-state block that can either increase or decrease with changes in pH_o, depending on the frequency of stimulation. In contrast, the characteristic pulse constant, N, always decreased under more alkaline conditions. These results are consistent with the interpretation of Schwarz et al. (1977), that raising external pH increases the rate of departure of drugs during the recovery interval by decreasing the degree of protonation; simultaneously, the rate of binding during the test pulse is increased by raising the concentration of drug in the membrane and cytoplasm through the higher membrane partitioning of the neutral species. Hydrophobic partitioning within the membrane thus brings LA molecules to a favored locus of reaction with the Na^+ channel's binding site, whereas the charge on the molecule (governed by extracellular pH) acts to retain drug molecules at the site.

DISCUSSION

The Association Kinetics of Use-dependent Block

These studies demonstrate that the inhibitory reactions of local anesthetics with neuronal sodium channels have association rates that vary with conditioning pulse potential, duration, and extracellular pH, the specifics depending on the particular anesthetic. It has not been attempted here to correlate all of the physico-chemical parameters of the drugs with the blocking kinetics, but several features deserve comment. Compound III, which has a pK_a near those of lidocaine and bupivacaine, but a far smaller octanol:buffer partition coefficient, is remarkable for the independence of steady-state block on pulse durations >0.2 msec that it exhibits (Fig. 7). Expected to be the least hydrophobic drug, and, therefore, to have the greatest selectivity towards open channel (hydrophilic) pathways, its variation of block with pulse potential parallels that of IV, a homologue with about 100-fold greater hydrophobicity, but accompanied by about 200-fold greater ionization at pH 7.3 (Fig. 6). By comparison, the block per pulse, k_d, of III at pH 7.3 is close to that of lidocaine (I), and they have the same solution pK_a yet about a 10-fold difference in hydrophobicity.

The parameter k_d is factored by the rates of binding to and dissociation from all the reactive states that contribute to phasic inhibition during a given test potential. Resolution of this complex parameter into the fundamental constituents will require more extensive experiments varying pulse duration at a variety of potentials, and vice-versa. A knowledge of the detailed dependence of these rate constants on channel state and on LA properties should provide insights on the fundamental association between drug and channel.

One general conclusion that can be drawn by examining Figures 6 and 7 is that potency ratios among drugs, even at the same pH, are not constant but will be highly dependent on the waveform of membrane potential. This emphasizes the undesirability of using action potentials, with their drug- and use-dependent shapes, for deriving fundamental kinetic parameters. As a particular conclusion, we note that both glycine xylidide (III) and GEA-968 (Strichartz and Wang, 1986), drugs of low hydrophobicity, produce almost full use-dependence with very short pulses, indicating a fast binding reaction with activated channels. The relatively high concentrations of these drugs required to produce block may account in part for the fast association, if one considers the aqueous and not the membrane phase as the source of free drug. However, if the drugs bind to the channel from within the membrane, then their local *free* concentrations are comparable to those of the more hydrophobic drugs. The more rapid equilibrium may then be due to their weaker hydrophobicity and correspondingly lower activation energy, both for passing from the membrane to the activated channel site and for dissociating from a somewhat hydrophobic activated site.

Two Kinetic Models for Recovery from Use-dependent Block

As Hille (1977a) has pointed out, there appear to be both hydrophilic and hydrophobic escape routes from the anesthetic binding site. It has generally been assumed that egress of ionized drug from the binding site is restricted to the hydrophilic pathway because of limited solubility in lipid, although one study (Broughton et al., 1984) postulates the direct dissociation of the charged form of tertiary amine drugs from the closed channel.

In the experiments reported here, the unblocking rates (k_r) were calculated for the interpulse periods when the membrane was repolarized. A given local anesthetic appears to dissociate from the blocked channel with the same rate regardless of whether block was effected by pulses that were large or small (Fig. 3A), short or long (Fig. 3B). Removal of channel inactivation by nonproteolytic chemical oxidants also has no effect on recovery from use-dependent block

a

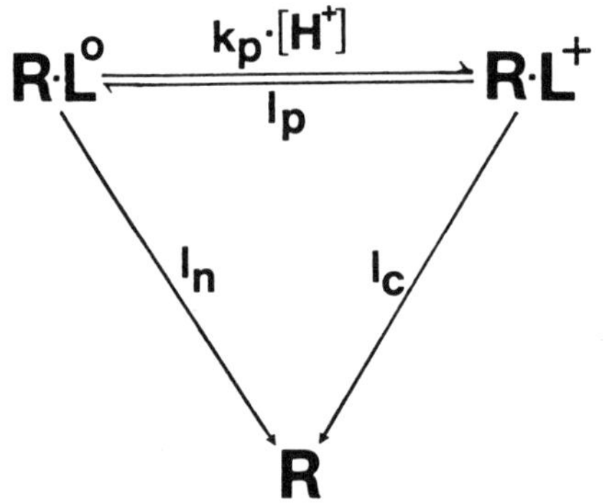

$$\tau_{slow} = \frac{l_c + l_n + l_p[1 + 10^{pK-pH}]}{l_p l_n + l_c[l_n + l_p 10^{pK-pH}]}$$

Figure 8A. Simplified models for recovery from use-dependent block. A. Recovery from block between pulses is shown as occurring from a single state, *R*, which may be the resting state (see text and compare with figure 1). Both the charged and uncharged form of drug can unbind from the channel, with characteristic rate constants l_c and l_n, respectively. Protonation rate constants (k_p and l_p) and hydrogen ion activity may differ from those extant in the external medium. This model is identical with that proposed by Broughton et al. (1984).

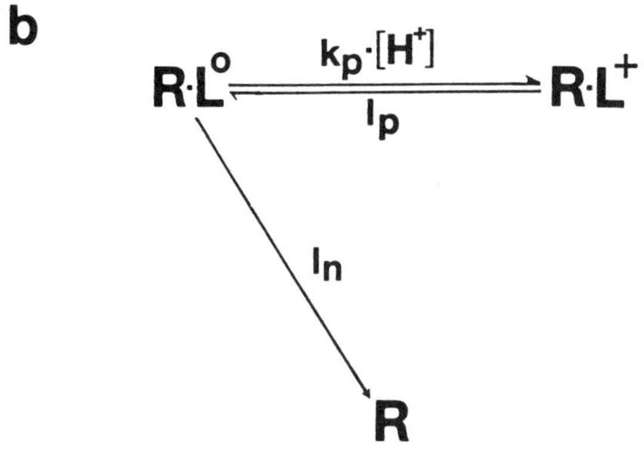

$$\tau_{slow} = l_p^{-1} + l_n^{-1}\,[1 + 10^{pK-pH}]$$

Figure 8B. More restrictive model (Starmer and Courtney, 1986). Protonated drug is trapped on the receptor, limiting dissociation to the l_n pathway. An approximate expression for the time constant, $\tau(= k_r^{-1})$, dominating recovery is shown beside each kinetic model.

in squid axon (Wang et al., 1987). For the analysis presented below, therefore, we treat all blocked channels as a single species, **RL**; **R** may, but need not, be equivalent to the closed resting form of the channel.

We consider two simple models to explain the pH dependence of recovery observed in the present study. In the first (Fig. 8A), dissociation of both forms of drug from the closed channel is permitted. In the second (Fig. 8B), only the neutral form is able to escape. In both models, the forward protonation rate for bound anesthetic (and thus the equilibrium fraction in the protonated form) is proportional to the extracellular hydrogen ion activity.

There are two time constants associated with a return to equilibrium of these systems following a perturbation. The slower of these time constants (shown beside each model) is generally dominant. We fit the free parameters of the models to match the observed recovery kinetics with lidocaine and bupivacaine (Fig. 9). At high pH_o, both models of Figure 8 predict an asymptotic rate of dissociation equal to the sum of the rates of deprotonation (l_p) and dissociation of neutral drug (l_n). However, only the less restrictive model (Fig. 8A) can account for the flattening of the k_r-pH_o relationship at low pH_o, where the nearly continuous protonation of drug reveals

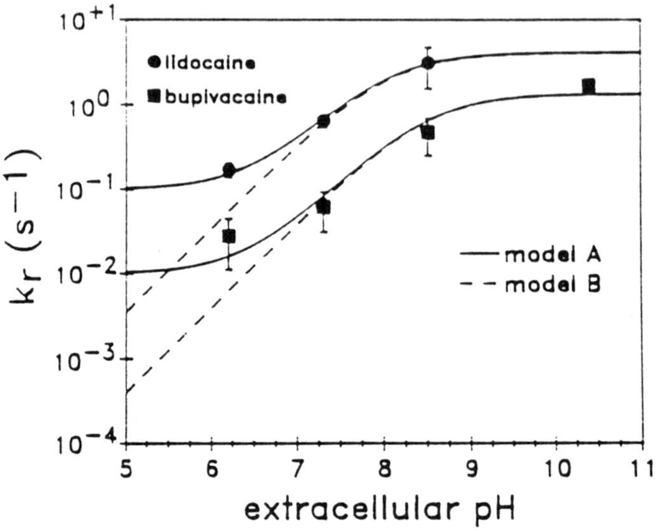

	k_p ($M^{-1}s^{-1}$)	l_p (s^{-1})	l_n (s^{-1})	l_c (s^{-1})	pH (binding site)	pK_a (binding site)
Model A						
lidocaine	$2 \cdot 10^9$	10	7	0.1	pH_0	8.3
bupivacaine	$2 \cdot 10^9$	4	2	0.01	"	8.7
Model B						
lidocaine	$2 \cdot 10^9$	10	7	-0-	"	8.3
bupivacaine	$2 \cdot 10^9$	4	2	-0-	"	8.7

Figure 9. Fit of the recovery models (figure 8) to the pH_0 dependence of recovery observed with two drugs (I and II), with k_r values from Table II. Solid lines: model A (two recovery pathways); dashed lines: model B (single recovery pathway). Model parameter values are shown beneath the graph.

the relatively slow pathway for dissociation of charged drug (rate constant l_c). This pathway by which a charged drug departs a closed channel may be hydrophobic (via the membrane), which would be consistent with the small yet measurable partitioning of the cationic species from water into relatively nonpolar octanol (Table 1).

Partitioning into biological membranes may be even greater. Recent studies show that the partition coefficient of the protonated species of tetracaine into vesicular phospholipid bilayers is 10^3-fold greater than the partition coefficient into octanol (although the partition coefficients of the neutral species are within an order of magnitude), (Sanchez et al., 1988). Studies on frog nerve show that a quaternary lidocaine derivative, QX572, can block Na channels upon external application, due apparently to slow permeation into or through the plasma membrane (Hille, 1977b). Likewise, the highly hydrophobic local anesthetic dibucaine, and its N-methyl quaternary derivative, pass into lipid vesicles at rates dependent on the membrane potential, implying a significant permeation by the charged species (Mayer et al., 1985; Mayer and Cullis, 1988). We also emphasize that the protonation rate constant and apparent pK_a of the bound drug are not directly observable—the values chosen for these parameters are simply empirical fits to the observed recovery rates. An alternative explanation for the asymptotic rate of recovery at low pH_o, i.e., that the drug escapes via random opening of Na channels at the resting potential, is unlikely. The shift of sodium activation to more positive potentials at low pH_o (Hille, 1968; Courtney, 1979) should make random openings at the holding potential less frequent, slowing recovery further still; such a continuous slowing at decreasing pH_o was not observed.

The relationship between tonic and use-dependent block by local anesthetics remains obscure. The kinetic models shown in Figure 8 do not allow for rebinding at the holding potential, and, therefore, implicitly require separate receptors for tonic and use-dependent effects. Although this model fits the data, we find a dual receptor premise less attractive both because it lacks parsimony and because it ignores the strong correlation between tonic and use-dependent potencies of most drugs. For example, the drugs listed in Table I produce 50% tonic block at concentrations that vary over two orders of magnitude, yet the calculated equilibrium use-dependent block, $B_d(\infty)$, produced at the same concentrations varies by less than a factor of 2 (Table II). Although a unified binding site is not required to explain the pH_o-dependence of recovery, we await more definitive experiments to resolve the question of independent tonic and use-dependent binding sites.

Duration- and Voltage-dependence of Use-dependent Block

Although the guarded receptor hypothesis has been successful in accounting for most aspects of use-dependent block, the use of Hodgkin-Huxley gating parameters as guard and trap functions, and the associated image of separate **m** and **h** gates forming a physical barrier to drug ingress/egress seem to us unduly restrictive and at odds with the more recent views of sodium channel gating derived from studies of gating current and single channels. It is apparent that *inactivation* is a measure of the availability of channels for activation, and not a physically separate gate or blocking mechanism (Armstrong and Bezanilla, 1977; Nonner, 1980). We prefer a simpler concept of channel function, wherein only one *gating* structure directly governs ion permeation. Furthermore, this gate need not be separate from the narrow regions of the pore that provide ion discrimination, the so-called *selectivity filter*. The molecular mechanisms of local anesthetics should be reconsidered with regard to all findings and not bound by notions introduced 10–15 years ago. An ecumenical vision of local anesthetic action permits block of activated channels without *plugging* the pore and requires only that the anesthetic molecules effectively hinder conformational changes that subserve sodium channel activation.

Relevance to Antiarrhythmic Actions

Although the experiments reported here were done exclusively on nerve, we believe that they may be extrapolated to cardiac Na^+ channels, with certain qualifications. Signal among these qualifications are the different conditions; both the higher temperature and the presence of physiological buffers (i.e., CO_2:bicarbonate, see Courtney, 1981) will alter the rates and equilibria of drug binding reactions as well as the transitions among channel states. A second concern is the difference in the channels themselves between different tissues. Mammalian ventricular myocardium contains Na^+ channels that differ from their neuronal counterparts in pharmacological (e.g., tetrodotoxin sensitivity; Cohen et al., 1981) and physiological properties (e.g., inactivation kinetics; Gettes and Reuter, 1974). Although the response to LA has common features in both tissues, the detailed kinetics are clearly different (Bean et al., 1983; Hondeghem and Katzung, 1984) even in tissues under very similar environmental circumstances.

Yet another issue for antiarrhythmic actions addresses the measurable inhibitions of cardiac K^+ and Ca^{2+} currents by LA agents. Both lidocaine (Josephson, 1988) and tetracaine (Carmeliet et al., 1986) inhibit these other currents at *therapeutic doses,* and thereby may alter the shape of the action potential and the level of threshold, thus modulating any ectopic pacemaker. Through the actions on these other currents a drug may prolong or shorten the plateau depolarization and modify the diastolic potential. These respective actions on the plateau will have positively or negatively synergistic effects on the same agent's ability to bind to Na^+ channels, which will itself alter the frequency and duration of impulses. Even in a single, isolated ventricular cell the reciprocal interactions between multiple inward and outward ionic currents and the ultimately determined action potential can be shaped in profound ways by subtle changes in voltage-dependent drug binding reactions. A *complete* model for antiarrhythmic agents (i.e., class I, and possibly class III) should begin with the complex relationships at the single cell level, one which includes the separate binding rates to the different states of all the proteins that contribute to the cardiac membrane potential.

BIBLIOGRAPHY

Armstrong CM, Bezanilla F. Inactivation of the sodium channel. II. Gating current experiments. *J Gen Physiol* 70:567–590, 1977.

Bean BP. Sodium channel inactivation in the crayfish giant axon. Must channels open before inactivating? *Biophys J* 35:595–614, 1981.

Bean BP, Cohen CJ, Tsien RW. Lidocaine block of cardiac sodium channels. *J Gen Physiol* 81:613–642, 1983.

Broughton A, Grant AO, Starmer CF, Klinger JK, Stambler BS, Strauss HC. Lipid solubility modulates pH potentiation of local anesthetic block of V_{max} reactivation in guinea pig myocardium. *Circ Res* 55:513–525, 1984.

Cahalan MD, Almers W. Block of sodium conductance and gating current in squid giant axon poisoned with quaternary strychnine. *Biophys J* 27:57–74, 1979.

Carmeliet E, Morad M, Van der Heyden G, Vereecke J. Electrophysiological effects of tetracaine in single guinea-pig ventricular myocytes. *J Physiol (Lond)* 376:143–161, 1986.

Chernoff DM, Strichartz GR. Tonic and phasic block of neuronal sodium currents by 5-hydroxyhexano-2′,6′-xylide, a neutral lidocaine homologue. *J Gen Physiol* 93:1075–1090, 1989.

Clarkson CW, Hondeghem LM. Mechanisms for bupivacaine depression of cardiac conduction: fast block of sodium channels during the action potential with slow recovery from block during diastole. *Anesthesiology* 62:396–405, 1985.

Cohen CJ, Bean BP, Colatsky TJ, Tsien RW. Tetrodotoxin block of sodium channels in rabbit Purkinje fibers. *J Gen Physiol* 78:383–411, 1981.

Colquhoun DC. *Lecture in Biostatistics.* Clarendon Press, Oxford, 1971.

Courtney KR. Extracellular pH selectively modulates recovery from sodium inactivation in frog myelinated nerve. *Biopsy J* 28:363–368, 1979.

Courtney KR. Review: quantitative structure/activity relations based on use-dependent block and repriming kinetics in myocardium. *J Mol Cell Cardiol* 19:1–12, 1987.

Courtney KR. Significance of bicarbonate for antiarrhythmic drug action. *J Mol Cell Cardiol* 13:1031–1034, 1981.

Dodge FA, Frankenhaeuser B. Membrane currents in isolated frog nerve fibre under voltage clamp conditions. *J Physiol* 143:76–90, 1958.

Frazier DT, Narahashi T, Yamada M. The site of action and active form of local anesthetics. II. Experiments with quaternary compounds. *J Pharmacol Exp Ther* 171:45–51, 1970.

Gettes LS, Reuter H. Slow recovery from inactivation of inward currents in mammalian myocardial fibres. *J Physiol (Lond)* 240:703–724, 1974.

Hille B. Charges and potentials at the nerve surface. Divalent ions and pH. *J Gen Physiol* 55:221–236, 1968.

Hille B. Local anesthetics: hydrophilic and hydrophobic pathways for the drug-receptor reaction. *J Gen Physiol* 69:497–515, 1977a.

Hille B. The pH-dependent rate of action of local anesthetics on the node of Ranvier. *J Gen Physiol* 69:475–496, 1977b.

Hondeghem LM, Katzung BG. Antiarrhythmic agents: The modulated receptor mechanism of action of sodium and calcium channel-blocking drugs. *Ann Rev Pharmacol Toxicol* 24:387–423, 1984.

Hondeghem LM, Katzung BG. Time- and voltage-dependent interactions if antiarrhythmic drugs with cardiac sodium channels. *Biochim Biophys Acta* 472:373–98, 1977.

Josephson IR. Lidocaine blocks Na, Ca and K currents of chick ventricular myocytes. *J Mol Cell Cardiol* 20:593–604, 1988.

Mayer LD, Bally MD, Hope MJ, Cullis PR. Uptake of dibucaine into large unilamellar vesicles in response to a membrane potential. *J Biol Chem* 260:802–808, 1985.

Mayer LD, Cullis PR. Uptake of N-methyldibucaine into large unilamellar vesicles in response to a membrane potential. *Biochemistry* (in press) 1988.

Neumcke B, Schwarz W, Stampfli R. Block of Na channels in the membrane of myelinated nerve by benzocaine. *Pflugers Arch* 390:230–236, 1981.

Nonner W. Relations between the inactivation of sodium channels and the immobilization of gating charge in frog myelinated nerve. *J Physiol (Lond)* 299:573–603, 1980.

Sanchez V, Ferrante FM, Cibotti N, Strichartz GR. Partitioning of tetracaine base and cation into phospholipid membranes: Relevance to anesthetic potency. *Regional Anesth* 13(suppl.):81, 1988.

Schwarz W, Palade PT, Hille B. Local anesthetics: Effect of pH on use-dependent block of sodium channels in frog muscle. *Biophys J* 20:343–367, 1977.

Sigworth FJ. Analysis of non-stationary sodium current fluctuations in frog myelinated nerve. Thesis, Yale University, 1979.

Starmer CF, Courtney KR. Modeling ion channel blockade at guarded binding sites: application to tertiary drugs. *Am Physiol Soc* H848–856, 1986.

Starmer CF, Grant AO, Strauss HC. Mechanisms of use-dependent block of sodium channels in excitable membranes by local anesthetics. *Biophys J* 46:15–27, 1984.

Starmer CF, Yeh JZ, Tanguy J. A quantitative description of QX222 blockade of sodium channels in squid axons. *Biophys J* 49:913–920, 1986.

Strichartz GR. The inhibition of sodium currents in myelinated by quaternary derivatives of lidocaine. *J Gen Physiol* 62:37–57, 1973.

Strichartz GR, Wang GK. The kinetic basis for phasic local anesthetic blockade of neuronal sodium channels. in *Molecular and Cellular Mechanisms of Anesthesia* (S.H. Roth and K.W. Miller, eds.). Plenum Press, New York, 1986, pp. 217–226.

Sutro JB. Kinetics of veratridine action on Na channels of skeletal muscle. *J Gen Physiol* 87:1–24, 1986.

Wang GK, Brodwick MS, Eaton DC, Strichartz GR. Inhibition of sodium currents by local anesthetics in chloramine-T treated squid axons: the role of Na channel activation. *J Gen Physiol* 89:645–667, 1987.

Yeh JZ, McCarthy WA, Quandt FN, Yamamoto D. Single channel analysis of the action of Na channel blockers 9-aminoacridine and QX-314 in neuroblastoma cells. in *Molecular Mechanisms of Anesthetics* (S.H. Roth and K.W. Miller, eds.). Plenum Press, New York, 1986.

Yeh JZ, Tanguy J. Na channel activation gate modulates slow recovery from use-dependent block by local anesthetics in squid giant axons. *Biophys J* 47:685–694, 1985.

Index